D1712502

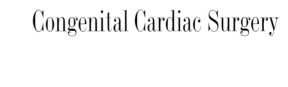

Congenital Cardiac Surgery

Congenital Cardiac Surgery

EDITED BY

BRUCE A. REITZ, MD

Professor & Chairman, Department of Cardiothoracic Surgery
Stanford University Medical Center, Stanford, California

DAVID D. YUH, MD

Assistant Professor, Division of Cardiac Surgery
The Johns Hopkins Hospital, Baltimore, Maryland

McGraw-Hill, Inc.
MEDICAL PUBLISHING DIVISION
New York Chicago San Francisco Lisbon London Madrid Mexico City
Milan New Delhi San Juan Seoul Singapore Sydney Toronto

McGraw-Hill

A Division of The McGraw·Hill Companies

CONGENITAL CARDIAC SURGERY

Copyright © 2002 by The **McGraw-Hill Companies**, Inc. All rights reserved. Printed in the United States of America. Except as permitted under the United States Copyright Act of 1976, no part of this publication may be reproduced or distributed in any form or by any means, or stored in a data base or retrieval system, without the prior written permission of the publisher.

234567890KGPKGP098765432

ISBN 0-8385-1542-8

This book was set in 10/12 Times Roman by TechBooks, Inc.
The editors were Martin J. Wonsewicz and Regina Y. Brown.
The production supervisor was Richard Ruzycka.
The cover designer was Mary McKeon.
The text designer was Robert Freese.
The illustrations were created by J·B Woolsey Associates.
The illustration manager was Charissa Baker.
The index was prepared by Jerry Ralya.
Quebecor World Kingsport was the printer and binder.

This book is printed on acid-free paper.

Library of Congress Cataloging-in-Publication Data

Congenital cardiac surgery / Bruce A. Reitz, David D. Yuh.
     p. ; cm.
    Includes bibliographical references and index.
    ISBN 0-8385-1542-8
    1. Congenital heart disease—Surgery.   2. Congenital heart disease in childern—Surgery.
3. Pediatric cardiology.   4. Heart—Surgery.   I. Reitz, Bruce A.   II. Yuh, David D. (David Daiho)
[DNLM: 1. Heart Defects, Congenital—Surgery—Infant, Newborn.   2. Cardiac Surgical
Procedures—Infant, Newborn. WS 290 C7477 2001]
RD598 .C626   2001
617.4′12—dc21

                                      2001030272

Contents

Contributors

M. GAIL BOLTZ, MD
Assistant Professor of Anesthesia
Stanford University Medical Center
Stanford, California

CLIFFORD CHIN, MD
Assistant Professor of Pediatrics
Division of Pediatric Cardiology
Lucile Salter Packard Children's Hospital
Stanford, California

ANNE M. DUBIN, MD
Assistant Professor of Pediatrics
Division of Pediatric Cardiology
Lucile Salter Packard Children's Hospital
Stanford, California

DANIEL FALCO, MD
Fellow, Pediatric Critical Care
Lucile Salter Packard Children's Hospital
Stanford, California

JEFFREY A. FEINSTEIN, MD, MPH
Assistant Professor of Pediatrics
Director, Pediatric Cardiac Catheterization Laboratory
Lucile Salter Packard Children's Hospital
Stanford, California

FERNANDO GUTIERREZ, MD
Director, Cardiac Radiology
Mallinckrodt Institute of Radiology
Washington University Medical Center
St. Louis, Missouri

LAUREEN L. HILL, MD
Assistant Professor of Anesthesia
Washington University Medical Center
St. Louis, Missouri

CATHY R. LAMMERS, MD
Assistant Professor
Department of Anesthesiology
UC Davis School of Medicine
Davis, California

PHILLIP MOORE, MD
Assistant Professor of Pediatrics
Director, Pediatric Cardiac Catheterization Program
University of California, San Francisco Medical Center
San Francisco, California

NANCY PIKE, RN
Clinical Nurse Specialist
Department of Cardiothoracic Surgery
Stanford University Medical Center
Stanford, California

BRUCE A. REITZ, MD
Professor & Chairman
Department of Cardiothoracic Surgery
Stanford University Medical Center
Stanford, California

DAVID N. ROSENTHAL, MD
Assistant Professor of Pediatrics
Division of Pediatric Cardiology
Lucile Salter Packard Children's Hospital
Stanford, California

FREDERICK TIBAYAN, MD
Resident in General Surgery
Department of Surgery
Stanford University Medical Center
Stanford, California

GEORGE VAN HARE, MD
Associate Professor of Pediatrics
Division of Pediatric Cardiology
Lucile Salter Packard Children's Hospital
Stanford, California

DAVID D. YUH, MD
Assistant Professor
Division of Cardiac Surgery
The Johns Hopkins Hospital
Baltimore, Maryland

Preface

The domain of pediatric cardiac surgery is a cloistered one, due largely to its anatomic, physiologic, and technical complexities. The clinical and emotional stakes are indeed high in this field, requiring deftness of judgement, operative skill, and a caring approach to the patients and their parents. There are several outstanding textbooks on the subject of pediatric cardiac surgery. Their comprehensive detail, however, makes them somewhat daunting for neophytes to the field and may fairly quickly become dated. Unlike these established references, this textbook is directed towards those newly entering this challenging field, the young cardiac surgeons, pediatric intensivists, pediatric cardiologists, and anesthesiologists, who, early in their course of training, must rapidly assimilate the basic principles of diagnosis and treatment.

This book is divided into three main sections. The first section is dedicated to the preoperative evaluation of pediatric patients with congenital cardiac defects. The second and largest portion of this text outlines the medical and operative management of these defects, in addition to giving a thumbnail sketch of the pathologic processes involved. Each defect is outlined with 1) a schematic diagram to display the major anatomic anomalies and abnormal blood flow patterns, 2) a summary box listing pertinent features, 3) a more descriptive narrative of these features, and 4) atlas-style illustrations of key aspects of the palliative or corrective operations. The third and final section of this book deals with the relevant issues encountered in the early postoperative care of patients undergoing these operations.

We hope that this first edition will gently introduce many young surgeons and physicians to this exciting field and serve as a stimulus for further intellectual and technical development. In addition, we hope that it will contribute in some small way to further progress.

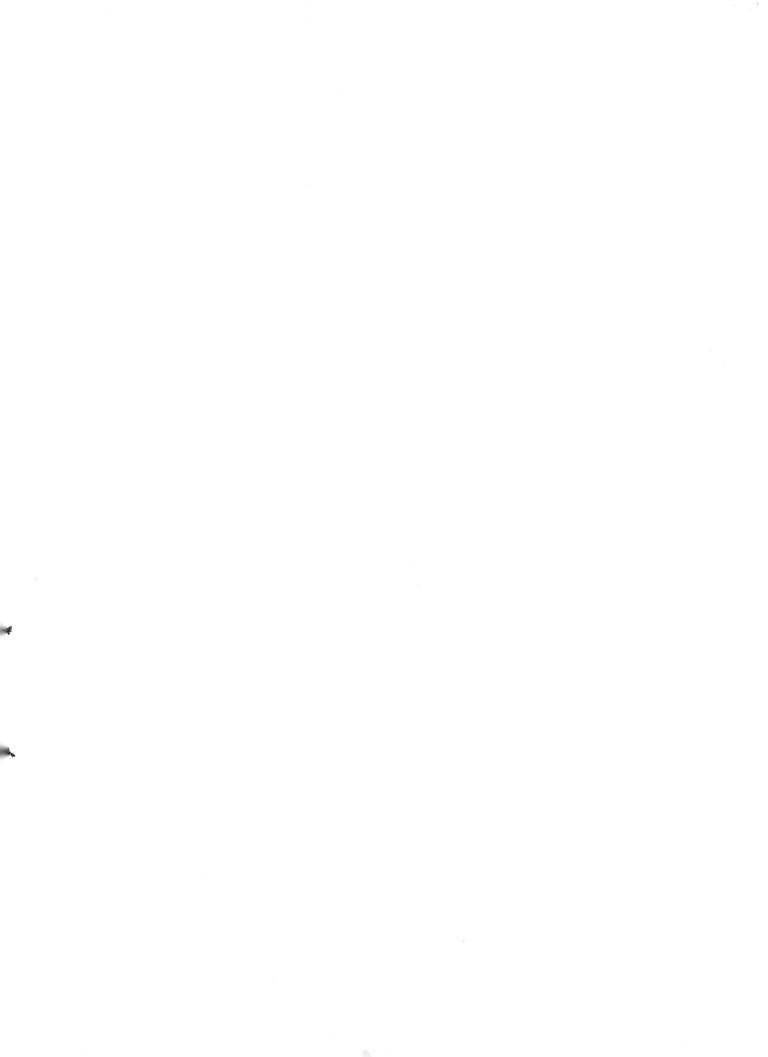

Congenital Cardiac Surgery

PART 1

Preoperative and Intraoperative Considerations

CHAPTER 1

The Cardiovascular History and Physical Examination

Clifford Chin, MD

Introduction

The clinical history is paramount in the diagnosis and management of pediatric cardiovascular disorders. It should not be replaced with ancillary tests such as echocardiography, and it should direct the clinician toward the appropriate studies after a careful and complete physical examination. The aim of this chapter is to highlight some important aspects of the medical history and physical examination.

History

The history may be broken into various components. The prenatal history can influence cardiac development (Tables 1–1 and 1–2). Among maternal disorders, diabetes and systemic lupus erythematosus are known to be risk factors for congenital heart disease in the offspring. Rates of congenital malformation for infants of diabetic mothers are at least three times higher than those for infants of nondiabetic mothers, and 40% of all perinatal deaths due to congenital malformations are found in such infants.[1] The absolute risk for cardiovascular system malformations among infants of diabetic mothers is 8.5 per 100 live births. Furthermore, those mothers who required insulin during the third trimester are almost 21 times more likely to have major cardiovascular system defects than infants of nondiabetic mothers.[2] Maternal connective tissue disease is associated with congenital heart block due to antibodies transmitted placentally.[3,4] The neonatal findings characterized by dermatologic, hematologic, and cardiac manifestations are linked to maternal antibodies to Ro (SS-A) and La (SS-B) antigens. Complete congenital heart block is the most frequent cardiac anomaly, occurring in <5% of pregnancies among women with anti-Ro or anti-La antibodies.

Family History

Congenital heart disease in the general population occurs in 8 per 1000 live births. The presence of congenital heart disease in a parent or sibling raises the risk to 3%. The incidence further increases to 9% when two family members are affected and may rise as high as 50% if congenital cardiac malformations are found in three affected family members.[5] The Baltimore-Washington Infant Study (BWIS) identified 4390 infants born with congenital heart disease between 1981 and 1989. The incidences of specific cardiac lesions were as follows: ventricular septal defect (VSD), 32%; pulmonic stenosis, 9%; secundum atrial septal defect (ASD), 7.7%; D-transposition of the great arteries, 4.6%; hypoplastic left heart syndrome, 3.8%; aortic valve stenosis, 2.9%; heterotaxy syndrome, 2.2%; pulmonary atresia, 1.7%; truncus arteriosus, 1.1%; L-transposition of the great arteries, 1.1%; Ebstein's malformation, 1%; tricuspid valve atresia, 0.7%; interrupted aortic arch, 0.7%; and single ventricle, 0.4%.[6]

Medical History

A history of cyanosis can be helpful to direct the clinician. The differential diagnosis may be narrowed by categorizing the case into cyanotic versus acyanotic heart disease (Figs. 1–1 and 1–2). Cyanosis is noted when the level of reduced hemoglobin is at least 5 g. The ability to detect cyanosis visually depends on the hemoglobin and hematocrit. Individuals with polycythemia appear cyanotic at higher levels of oxygen saturation compared with anemic patients. Tetralogy of Fallot is the prototypical lesion causing profound cyanosis. In the past, children and adolescents would report a history of squatting, especially after exercise or exertion. This type of history is no longer common, as these individuals often come to medical and surgical

TABLE 1–1.   Maternal Risk Factors

Factor	Malformation
Advanced age	Trisomy 21
Maternal congenital heart disease	Various
Diabetes mellitus	VSD, TGA, cardiomyopathy
Systemic lupus erythematosus	Congenital heart block
Phenylketonuria	ToF, VSD, coarctation, HLHS
Viruses (e.g., cytomegalovirus, herpesvirus, coxsackievirus B, parvovirus)	Teratogenic, myocarditis

HLHS = hypoplastic left heart syndrome; TGA = transposition of the great arteries; ToF = tetralogy of Fallot; VSD = ventricular septal defect.

TABLE 1–2.   Maternal Drug Exposures

Drug	Malformation
Diphenylhydantoin	Pulmonic stenosis, aortic valve stenosis
Trimethadione	VSD, ToF, TGA, HLHS
Thalidomide	ToF, truncus arteriosus
Lithium	Ebstein's anomaly of the tricuspid valve
Alcohol	VSD, ASD, PDA, ToF
Amphetamines	VSD, ASD, PDA, TGA
Birth control pills	VSD, ToF, TGA

ASD = atrial septal defect; PDA = patent ductus arteriosus. For other abbreviations, see Table 1–1 footnote.

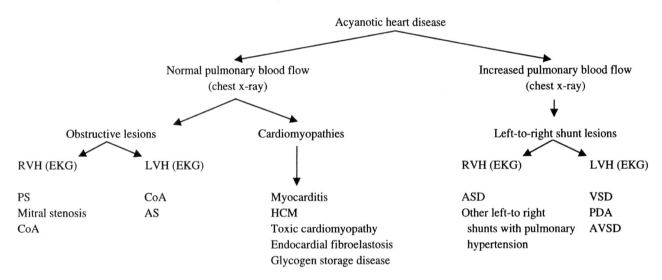

FIGURE 1–1.

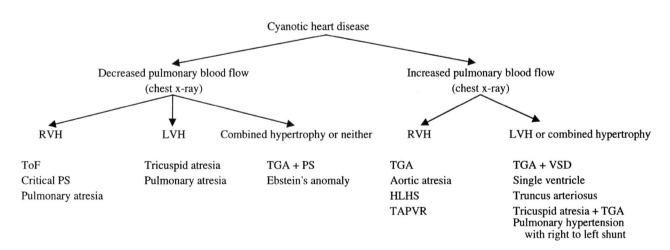

FIGURE 1–2.

attention within the first year of life. A hypercyanotic episode is usually seen in the infancy period, often after awakening in the morning or after feeding (i.e., exertion). One episode of hypercyanosis should prompt earlier surgical repair of this lesion.

Congestive heart failure (CHF) is defined as the inability of the heart to meet the metabolic demands of the body. VSD is a classic lesion that may cause CHF due to a large left-to-right shunt and hence pulmonary overcirculation. Important historical information that should be sought from the parents should include constant rapid breathing, especially while asleep, difficulty breathing while feeding, and tiring easily with feeds. These infants often do not gain significant weight despite optimal caloric intake. Older children may report an inability to keep up with peers or shortness of breath. Most infants with congenital heart lesions that result in significant left-to-right shunts can present with CHF. Furthermore, like adults with postmyocardial infarction, infants and children with cardiomyopathies will often complain or present with signs of heart failure. A fundamental difference between heart failure secondary to a left-to-right shunt versus a cardiomyopathy is that in congenital defects (e.g., VSD), the heart is often hyperdynamic.

The Physical Examination

The physical examination in a pediatric patient should include height, weight, and head circumference (in infants). Previous records of the patient's growth parameters are helpful to document growth failure. Individuals with significant heart disease may present with failure to thrive. Other noncardiac causes of growth failure need to be assessed as well. However, infants with poor weight gain (less than the fifth percentile for age) but with a normal head circumference may have a cardiac anomaly.[7]

Vital signs include the heart rate, respiratory rate, and four limb blood pressures. Similar to growth, these parameters are age related. Vital sign testing should be done while the child is at rest and comfortable. Especially in infants and small children, vital signs are best obtained while the child is in the parent's arms or lap. Many will attest to the difficulties in performing a physical examination in an upset child. Vital signs supportive of CHF include resting tachypnea and tachycardia. Appropriately sized blood pressure cuffs must be used. The width of the cuff bladder should be 125% to 155% of the diameter of the limb or 40% to 50% of the circumference.[5] The use of small blood pressure cuffs often yields falsely elevated blood pressure results. The lower extremity systolic blood pressure should be slightly higher compared with that of the arms. Discrepancy in the blood pressures should alert the clinician to possible coarctation of the aorta.

The emotional state of the child should dictate which system or body part to examine first. Often in an upset and crying child, the examiner moves from head to toe in a random fashion, taking advantage of periodic times when the child is calm to auscultate the heart. In otherwise quiet and comfortable patients, the cardiac exam should be performed last so that the other body systems are not overlooked. First, one inspects the mucous membranes and nail beds for signs of cyanosis. While doing so, estimates of perfusion can be made. Fingernail or toenail clubbing may be due to chronic arterial desaturation. Examination of the bulbar conjunctiva can identify those individuals with anemia. Sweating of the forehead in infants is another sign of CHF. Peripheral pulses should be palpated in all four extremities to detect a coarctation of the aorta. Absent, weak, or significant delay in femoral pulses compared with the radial or brachial pulse is highly suggestive of aortic coarctation.

Inspection of the thorax includes determination of symmetry. Significant left-to-right shunting from an ASD can cause thoracic asymmetry due to right ventricular enlargement. Palpation of the chest for heaves and lifts, as well as location of the point of maximal impulse, gives one an estimate of right or left ventricular enlargement. By convention, the presence of a thrill indicates at least a grade IV systolic murmur and therefore implies a significant cardiac defect. Examination of the neck is difficult in infants because of the short neck and presence of subcutaneous fat. Evaluation of the jugular veins in older children can reliably estimate the central venous pressure.

The abdomen should be palpated to identify hepatic situs. Furthermore, documentation of hepatic or splenic enlargement is useful in the evaluation for CHF, and serial examinations also give clues to the adequacy of CHF therapy.

Lastly, auscultation of the chest and back is performed. Individuals suspected of CHF may present with rales or decreased breath sounds due to pulmonary edema. Cardiac murmurs are usually easy to hear. The focus is placed on the presence and severity of the murmur, so that other parts of the cardiac examination are missed. One should first focus on the heart sounds (i.e., S1 and S2). The first heart sound is normally loudest at the cardiac apex and is due to closure of the mitral valve. Audible splitting of the first heart sound (both mitral and tricuspid valve closure) may be due to right bundle branch block. In a cyanotic child with a widely split first heart sound, suspect Ebstein's anomaly of the tricuspid valve. Closure of the aortic and pulmonic valves gives rise to the second heart sound. Normally, the aortic component of S2 precedes the pulmonic component. S2 becomes audibly split with inspiration. This phenomenon occurs due to variable filling of both the left and right ventricles. During inspiration, negative pressure is created in the thorax and aids in systemic venous return. Improved venous return yields an increase in right ventricular stroke volume, which manifests as an increased ejection time. The pulmonic component of S2 therefore separates from the aortic component. Fixed and wide splitting of S2 occurs in

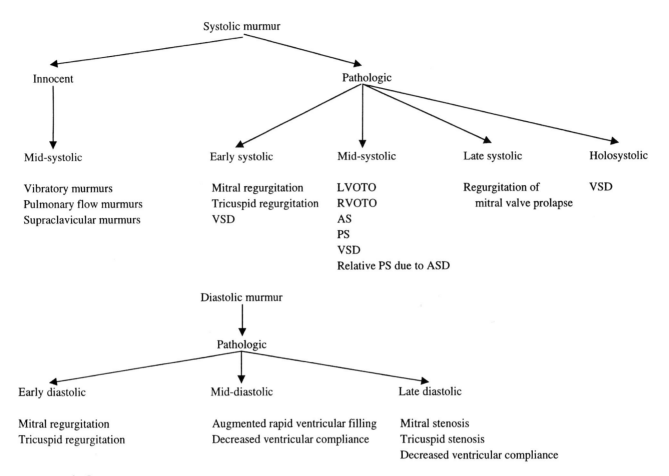

FIGURE 1–3.

left-to-right shunt lesions, most commonly due to an ASD. Intensity of the aortic or pulmonic components are useful aids to assess for aortic or pulmonic valve stenosis, respectively. Furthermore, audible systolic ejection clicks help to confirm the diagnosis. Finally, single second heart sounds in cyanotic infants may indicate transposition of the great arteries. In acyanotic individuals, the differential diagnosis includes severe pulmonic stenosis.

Heart murmurs are classified as systolic, diastolic, and continuous. Figure 1–3 shows the most common types of systolic and diastolic murmurs. Systolic murmurs can be early, mid, late, or holosystolic. Standard classifications range from grade I to VI; thrills are associated with murmurs of grade IV and above. Many cardiologists will claim that any murmur greater than grade III probably represents a pathologic process. Innocent murmurs are rarely above grade II. Diastolic murmurs often represent a pathologic process. Continuous murmurs are heard after surgical aortopulmonary shunts. Other sources of continuous murmurs include aortopulmonary collaterals, atrioventricular malformations, and patent ductus arteriosus in older infants and children.

Friction rubs are usually heard postoperatively due to small pericardial effusions. These sounds are harsh and gritty in nature and are ill timed to the cardiac cycle. Sudden absence of the friction rub in an ill child should alert the clinician to a worsening pericardial effusion.

The history and physical examination are important tools in the evaluation of children with suspected heart disease. After careful review, ancillary tests may be appropriate to delineate the nature of the heart lesion further. The time taken to perform these tasks also allows one to build rapport with the patient and family.

References

1. REECE EA, HOBBINS JC. Diabetic embryopathy: pathogenesis, prenatal diagnosis and prevention. *Obstet Gynecol Surv* 1986; 41:325–335.

2. BECERRA JE, KHOURY MJ, CORDERO JF, ERICKSON JD. Diabetes mellitus during pregnancy and the risks for specific birth defects: a population-based case-control study. *Pediatrics* 1990;85:1–9.

3. LITSEY SE, NOONAN JA, O'CONNOR WN, COTTRILL CM, MITCHELL B. Maternal connective tissue disease and congenital heart block. *N Engl J Med* 1985;312: 98–100.

4. LOCKSHIN MD, BONFA E, ELKON K, DRUZIN ML. Neonatal lupus risk to newborns of mothers with systemic lupus erythematosus. *Arthritis Rheum* 1988;31: 697–701.

5. PARK MK. *Pediatric Cardiology for Practitioners.* 2nd ed. Chicago: Year Book Medical Publishers; 1988.

6. FERENCZ C, RUBIN JD, LOFFREDO CA, MAGEE CA, eds. *Epidemiology of Congenital Heart Disease, The Baltimore-Washington Infant Study*, 1981–1989. Mount Kisco, NY: Futura; 1993.

7. ZUBERBUHLER JR. *Clinical Diagnosis in Pediatric Cardiology.* New York: Churchill Livingstone; 1981.

CHAPTER 2

Electrocardiographic Interpretation

Anne M. Dubin, MD

Introduction

Interpretation of the pediatric electrocardiogram (ECG) is challenging because normal values change with age. Table 2–1 summarizes normal values based on data published by Dauvignon et al.[1] and Walsh.[2] Pediatric ECGs should be read in a systematic fashion looking at rate, rhythm, axis, intervals, and waves.

Normal Electrocardiogram

Rate and Rhythm

The heart rate can be determined by measuring the interval between successive R waves on the ECG in sinus rhythm. The exact heart rate can be calculated by dividing the rate and rhythm (RR) interval in seconds into 60. Normal heart rate varies with age, increasing in the first 2 months of life and then slowly declining. Normal sinus rhythm can be defined as a rhythm in which each QRS complex is preceded by a P wave with a normal axis (upright in leads I and aVF).

Axis

The electrical axis is the direction of the predominant vector of a wave front in the frontal plane. This can be calculated for all three waves seen on ECG: P, QRS, and T waves. Several methods are used to determine axis. The hexaxial reference system will be described here. Using the system shown in Fig. 2–1, it is possible to determine a quadrant by looking at lead I and aVF. Once the quadrant is established, the frontal lead, which is most isoelectric, is identified. The mean QRS axis is perpendicular to this lead, in the previously identified quadrant. The heart shifts in the chest, and the left ventricle becomes the dominant ventricle with age. Thus, the QRS axis shifts from the right axis to the normal adult left axis. Abnormal axis deviation may be secondary to a conduction abnormality or hypertrophy, or (less commonly) to abnormalities of cardiac location or thoracic deformity.

P Wave

The P wave represents atrial depolarization. Abnormal morphology, amplitude, and duration may be indicative of right or left atrial enlargement.

PR Interval

The PR interval is measured from the beginning of the P wave to the initial deflection of the QRS complex. It represents atrioventricular (AV) nodal conduction. The normal PR interval is <0.16 in young children and 0.18 in adolescence. A prolonged PR interval may be secondary to AV nodal disease or trauma, cardiac medications, or increased vagal tone.

QRS Complex

The QRS interval reflects ventricular depolarization. The normal morphology is that of a small Q followed by a large R and small S in the left-sided leads (I, II, aVL, V4–6) whereas the right side shows a small R followed by a deep S wave (aVR, III, V1–3). Amplitude of the QRS complex can be helpful when determining hypertrophy. However, it is important to note that amplitude changes with age, and it is important to use the proper upper limit of normal. Duration of the QRS complex is also influenced by age. In normal infants, QRS width should be <0.08 seconds; in those older than 6 months, the QRS should be no wider than 0.10 seconds. Prolonged QRS complexes may be due to conduction abnormalities, medications, or ventricular hypertrophy.

QT Interval

The QT interval is measured from the beginning of the QRS complex to the end of the T wave. The longest interval in any lead should be measured. This interval is dependent on heart rate and thus, Bazett's[5] formula, which corrects for heart rate ($QT/\sqrt{RR}$), should be used to determine abnormalities. This rate-corrected interval (QTc) should be

TABLE 2–1. Normal Values[a]

	0–7 days	1 wk–1 mo	1–6 mo	6–12 mo	1–5 yr	5–10 yr	10–15 yr	>15 yr
HR/min	90–160 (125)	100–175 (140)	110–180 (145)	100–180 (130)	70–160 (110)	65–140 (100)	60–130 (90)	60–100 (80)
PR(II)	0.08–0.15 (0.10)	0.08–0.15 (0.10)	0.081.05 (0.10)	0.08–0.15 (0.10)	0.08–0.15 (0.12)	0.08–0.15 (0.12)	0.09–0.18 (0.14)	0.1–0.2 (0.16)
QRS	0.03–0.07 (0.05)	0.03–0.07 (0.05)	0.03–0.07 (0.05)	0.03–0.07 (0.05)	0.04–0.08 (0.06)	0.04–0.08 (0.06)	0.04–0.09 (0.07)	0.06–0.09 (0.08)
QTc	≤0.45	≤0.45	≤0.45	≤0.45	≤0.44	≤0.44	≤0.44	≤0.43
V1–Q	0	0	0	0	0	0	0	0
V1–R	5–25 (15)	3–22 (10)	3–20 (10)	2–20 (9)	2–18 (8)	1–15 (5)	1–12 (5)	1–6(2)
V1–S	0–22 (7)	0–16 (5)	0–15 (5)	1–20 (6)	1–20 (10)	3–21 (12)	3–22 (11)	3–13 (8)
V6–Q	0–1 (0.5)	0–3 (0.5)	0–3 (0.5)	0–3 (0.5)	0–5 (1)	0–5 (1)	0–3 (0.5)	0–2 (0.5)
V6–R	1–12 (5)	1–17 (7)	3–20 (10)	5–22 (12)	6–22 (14)	8–25 (16)	8–24 (15)	5–18 (10)
V6–S	0–9 (3)	0–9 (3)	0–9 (3)	0–7 (3)	0–4 (2)	0–4 (2)	0–4 (1)	0–2 (1)

[a]Values are ranges, with means in parentheses.

<0.45 seconds in infants and 0.44 seconds in children. Abnormalities of the QTc may be secondary to prolonged QT syndrome, a potentially fatal disorder, antiarrhythmic medications, other medications (antifungal agents and certain antibiotics), or metabolic abnormalities.

ST Segment

The ST segment is defined as the portion of the ECG between the end of the S wave and the beginning of the T wave. This is normally isoelectric. Elevations or depressions in the ST segment may be indicative of ischemia, inflammation, or hypertrophy. Early repolarization syndrome, a normal variant seen in adolescence, is characterized by elevation of the ST segment by 2–4 mm in the lateral and inferior leads.

T Wave

The T wave reflects repolarization of the ventricular myocytes. The T-wave amplitude is very variable in children. However, flattened T waves in several leads can be a sign of ischemia. The T wave should follow approximately the same axis as the QRS (i.e., within 60 degrees of each other).

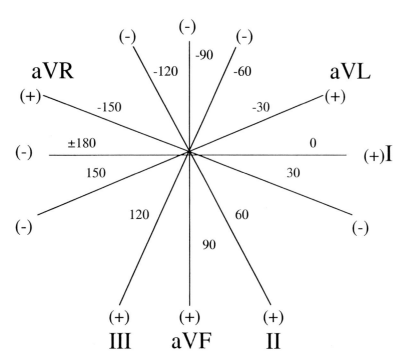

FIGURE 2–1. Hexaxial reference system for QRS axis determination.

U Wave

The U wave reflects the late repolarization of the His-Purkinje system. It is not always evident on the surface ECG. It should be of low amplitude (<50% of the T wave) and have the same polarity as the preceding T wave. When the U wave is abnormally tall (>50% of the T wave) and is immediately adjacent to the T wave, it should be included in the QT interval measurement. Abnormal U waves are seen with hypokalemia, long QT syndrome, and some anti-arrhythmic medications.

Chamber Hypertrophy

The ECG can be very useful in determining chamber enlargement and hypertrophy. However, even so, the ECG has only a 70% positive predictive value for determining chamber size in children.[3,4] Thus it is important to consider the clinical setting as well as the ECG when determining hypertrophy or enlargement.

Right Atrial Enlargement

Right atrial depolarization is reflected in the earliest portion of the P wave. The ECG criterion for right atrial enlargement is the presence of a peaked, tall (>0.3 mV) P wave in lead II. This may be accompanied by a biphasic or tall P wave in lead V1 (Fig. 2–2).

Left Atrial Enlargement

Left atrial depolarization is seen in the terminal portion of the P wave. The criteria for left atrial enlargement include a broad, notched P wave in lead II (>0.10–0.12 seconds) or a deep, slurred biphasic P wave in V1 (Fig. 2–3).

Biatrial Enlargement

Biatrial enlargement may be diagnosed when signs of both right and left atrial enlargement are seen on the ECG.

Right Ventricular Hypertrophy

Several criteria are necessary to determine right ventricular hypertrophy (RVH). These criteria are more sensitive than those worked out for left ventricular hypertrophy (LVH).

- *R Wave >98% in V1.* R-wave amplitude in lead V1 that is greater than the 98th precentile for age (Table 2–1) is a highly specific finding for RVH outside the neonatal period. However, it is somewhat less sensitive. There are children with RVH who have a normal R wave in V1.

- *S Wave >98% in V6.* An abnormally deep S wave in V6 (greater than the 98th percentile; see Table 2–1) is a highly sensitive indicator of RVH. It is often seen in patients with increased right ventricular pressure

secondary to chronic lung disease. This pattern, seen along with right atrial enlargement, is characteristic of cor pulmonale.

- *R/S Ratio in V1 or V6.* The R/S ratio is well established for various ages. If it is abnormally high in V1, or abnormally low in V6, this suggests RVH. However, it is rare to see an abnormal R/S ratio as an isolated finding. This criterion should therefore be applied in conjunction with other findings of RVH.

- *Abnormal T Wave.* The T-wave orientation changes with age. Normally, it is upright until 7 days of age. Between 1 week and adolescence it is negative and reverts to upright again in adolescence and adulthood. An upright T wave after 7 days of age is a sensitive indicator of increased right ventricular pressure. The sensitivity of this measure increases when R-wave amplitude is also taken into account.[5] Mild RVH manifests as a normal R-wave amplitude but an upright T wave. Moderate RVH is indicated by increased R-wave amplitude and an upright T wave, whereas severe RVH is associated with an increased R-wave amplitude and inversion of the T wave in a pattern indicative of strain.

- *QR in V1.* A QR pattern can also be indicative of RVH, especially when seen in conjunction with a tall R wave. It can also be seen with L-looping of the ventricles (abnormal septal depolarization) or anterior infarct (Fig. 2–4).

- *RSR' in V1.* An RSR' pattern can be associated with right ventricular volume overload, as seen in atrial septal defects, but it may also be a normal finding. It should be used to diagnose RVH only when the R' amplitude is large (Fig. 2–5).

- *Right Axis Deviation.* Right axis deviation alone is not a criterion for RVH, but it should be used to support other findings. A rare cause of right axis deviation in children is left posterior hemiblock.

Left Ventricular Hypertrophy

Compared with RVH, LVH is more difficult to predict by ECG, and thus multiple criteria should be met.

- *Voltage Criteria.* An R-wave amplitude greater than the 98th percentile in leads V5 and V6 and an S-wave amplitude greater than the 98th percentile in lead V1 have been used to predict LVH. Unfortunately, hypertrophy may be present with "normal" left-sided forces, and normal children may present with R waves in V5 and V6 that are above the 98th percentile.

- *T Wave Changes.* T-wave abnormalities have been found to be the most reliable indication of LVH. A strain pattern presents as inverted T waves in the inferior leads (II, III, aVF) and left precordial leads (V5, V6)

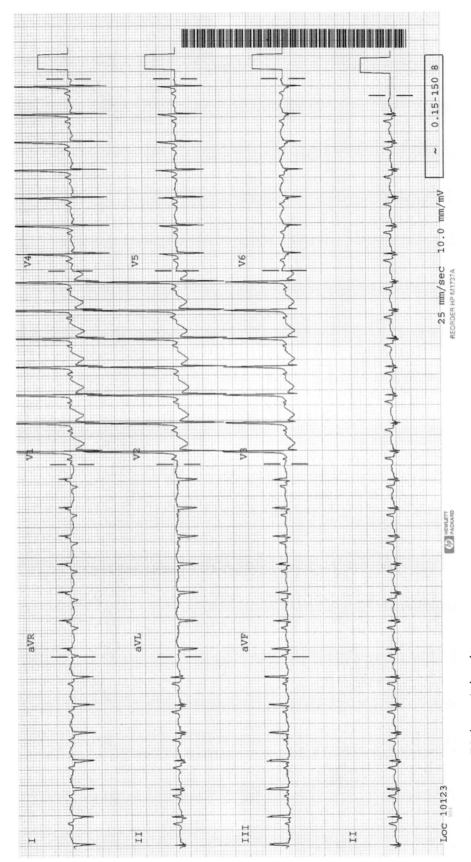

FIGURE 2–2.   Right atrial enlargement.

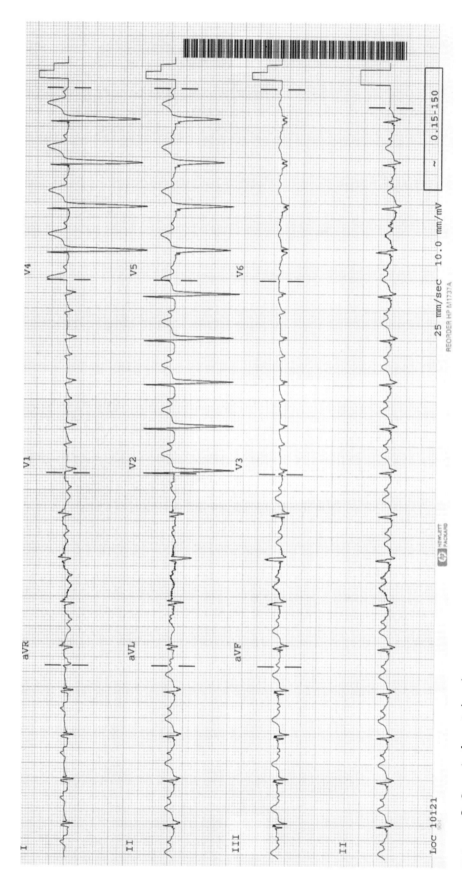

FIGURE 2–3. Left atrial enlargement.

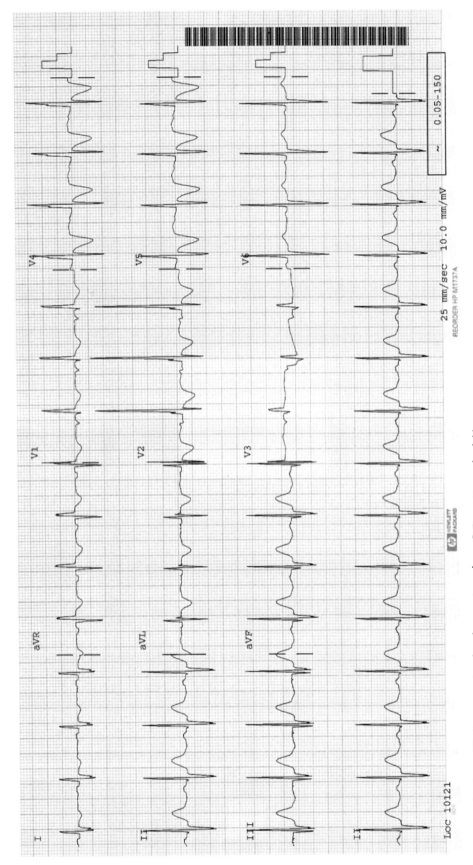

FIGURE 2–4. Right ventricular hypertrophy: QR pattern in V1.

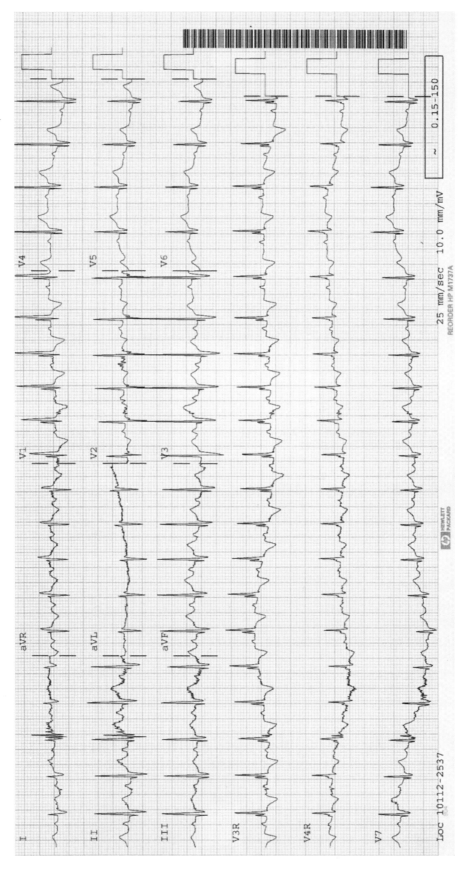

FIGURE 2–5.   Right ventricular hypertrophy: RSR′ pattern in V1, patient with ASD.

(Fig. 2–6). It may sometimes be associated with depression of the ST segment. T-wave inversion may also be a sign of ischemia or myocardial inflammation, and thus these causes must be ruled out prior to a diagnosis of left ventricular strain.

- *Left Axis Deviation.* Left axis deviation is supportive of the diagnosis of LVH, especially in infancy. Left anterior hemiblock may also cause left axis deviation.
- *Lateral Q Waves.* Abnormal Q waves in the lateral precordium (V5 and V6) result from abnormal position of the left ventricle or abnormalities of contraction in the left ventricle. A dilated volume-loaded left ventricle, such as is seen in aortic insufficiency or patent ductus arteriosus, tends to have a deep Q wave in the lateral leads. A hypertrophic left ventricle, which is seen with pressure loading, produces a small or absent Q wave.

Biventricular Hypertrophy

The diagnosis of biventricular hypertrophy can be made when abnormal voltage is found in both the right and left precordium. Usually, however, this is not seen because the abnormal vectors cancel each other. Large biphasic midprecordial voltages (the Katz-Wachtel criterion), are also seen with biventricular hypertrophy (Fig. 2–7).

Intraventricular Conduction Disturbances

Intraventricular conduction may be altered in one of two ways. There may be delay or block in the normal conduction system below the His bundle (right and left bundle branches, including the left anterior and posterior fascicle). An accessory pathway may bypass normal AV conduction, resulting in an abnormal QRS pattern.

Right Bundle Branch Block

Right bundle branch block (RBBB) results from delay in the right bundle branch. This causes delay in activation of the right ventricle, following the left ventricle. The resultant QRS complex is wide and has a characteristic morphology of a rapid initial deflection followed by a slurred slower portion of the QRS. This reflects the rapid depolarization of the left ventricle followed by the slower depolarization of the right ventricle through ventricular muscle. The criteria for complete right bundle branch are QRS above upper limits for age, in combination with normal initial forces and terminal conduction delay which is directed anteriorly and to the right (wide and slurred S in I, V5, and V6; slurred R in aVR, V1, and V2) (Fig. 2–8).

When the ECG demonstrates RBBB, it becomes impossible to determine RVH.[6] The usual markers of ischemia are also lost, as RBBB results in ST- and T-wave abnormalities.

Incomplete Right Bundle Branch Block

An RSR′ pattern in lead V1 with a normal or slightly prolonged QRS duration is commonly seen with an incomplete RBBB. However, this pattern of ventricular conduction may be seen in normal children as well. Further complicating matters, this pattern is commonly seen in right ventricular overload, such as in atrial septal defects.

Left Bundle Branch Block

Just as delay or block in the right bundle branch results in RBBB, delay or block in the main left bundle branch results in late activation of the left bundle and a QRS pattern of left bundle branch block (LBBB). The QRS is prolonged, slurred, and directed toward the left precordium. The criteria for LBBB include an abnormally prolonged QRS duration, absent normal initial forces (no Q waves in I, aVL, and V6), and notched, slurred QRS complexes directed leftward and posteriorly (QS or rS in V1 and a tall notched R wave in V6) (Fig. 2–9).

LBBB is uncommon in children but when present is the result of surgery on the left ventricular outflow tract. It may also be seen in hypertrophic cardiomyopathy and myocarditis. As with RBBB, it is difficult if not impossible to assess hypertrophy and ischemic changes when an LBBB is present.

Fascicular Block

The left bundle normally divides into two fan-like sheets of specialized conduction tissue: the anterior and posterior fascicles. Delay or block in either fascicle will result in a characteristic ECG pattern.

Left Anterior Hemiblock

Left anterior hemiblock results in sequential activation of the left ventricle. The posterior-inferior region of the left ventricle is activated prior to the anterior-superior region. This results in an abnormal QRS activation, with two sequential vectors: the initial forces are directed inferiorly and then spread in an anterior and superior fashion. This produces a marked left axis deviation (<30 degrees). The QRS is minimally or not prolonged.

This conduction abnormality is relatively rare in children. It may be seen in myocarditis, ischemia, or after cardiac surgery on the left ventricular outflow tract or ventricular septal defect closure. Tricuspid atresia and endocardial cushion defects have ECG findings consistent with left anterior hemiblock (leftward and superior axis).[7] However, these conditions do not have a true conduction defect but rather are related to the characteristic abnormal conduction system and heart position.

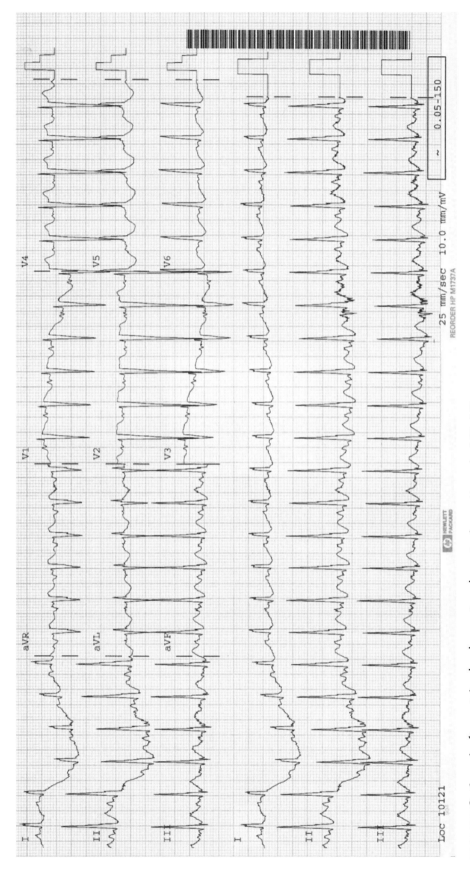

FIGURE 2–6. Left ventricular hypertrophy: strain pattern in V5–V6.

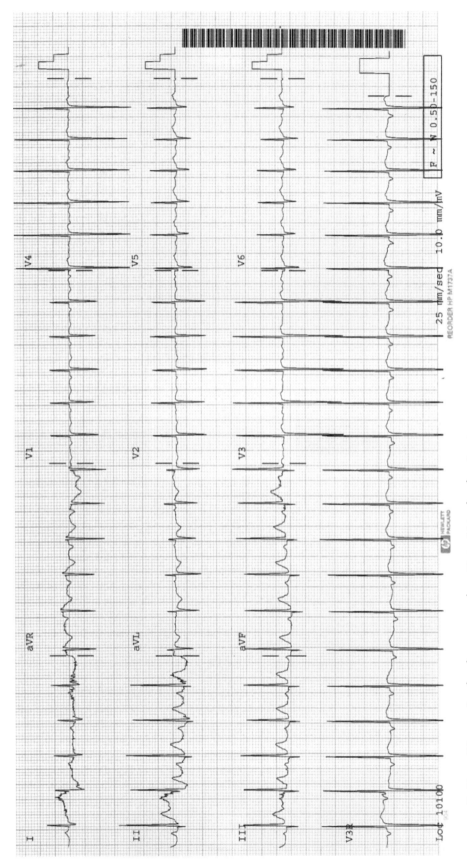

FIGURE 2–7.   Biventricular hypertrophy: Katz-Wachtel criteria.

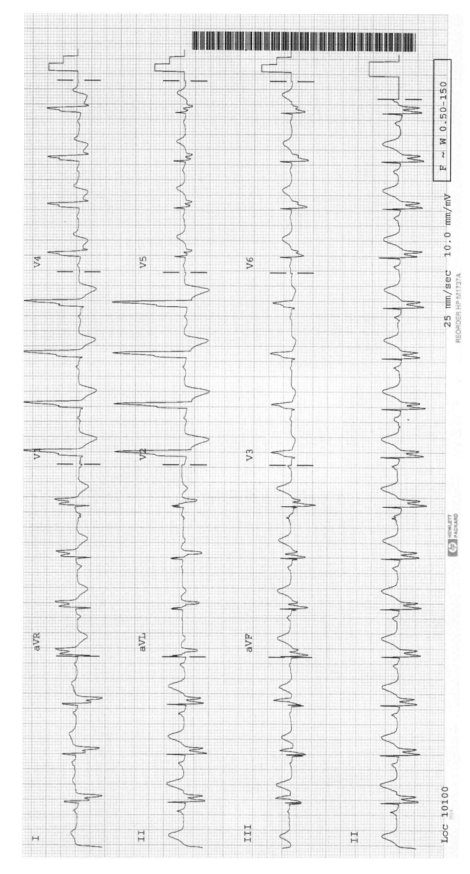

FIGURE 2-8. Right bundle branch block in patient following tetralogy of Fallot repair.

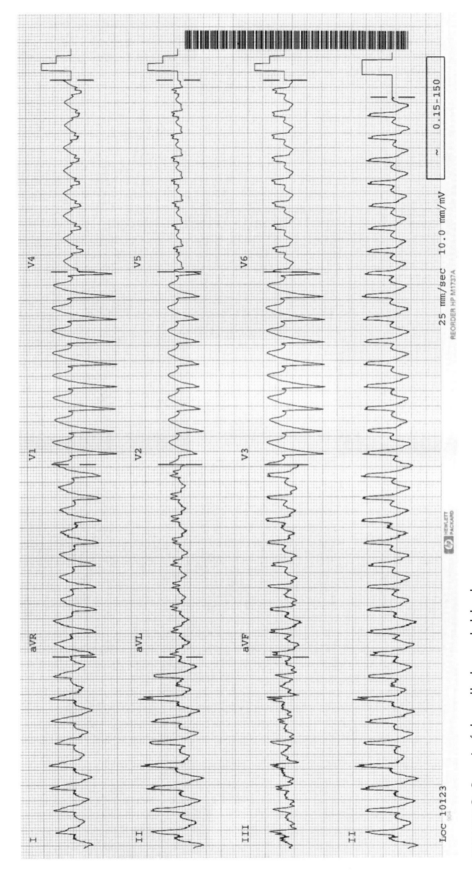

FIGURE 2-9.   Left bundle branch block.

Left Posterior Hemiblock

The activation sequence in left posterior hemiblock is the opposite of that seen with anterior hemiblock. The left ventricle depolarizes first in the anterior and superior region and then in the posterior and inferior portion. This produces an axis that is oriented rightward and inferiorly (120 degrees) with a normal QRS duration. Initial forces are directed superiorly (Q waves in II, III, and aVF). Left posterior hemiblock can be difficult to diagnose because most infants will have a rightward axis; the term should be reserved for a sudden change in axis between serial ECGs. It has been seen in association with surgical trauma and myocarditis.[7]

Bifascicular Block

RBBB in combination with left anterior hemiblock occurs most commonly following repair of tetralogy of Fallot (10% of such patients).[8] The ECG reflects the combination of these two conduction abnormalities. The initial forces, which in RBBB reflect the left ventricle, show a superior axis. The QRS complex reflects the characteristic terminal slurring of RBBB.

RBBB with left posterior hemiblock is extremely rare and difficult to diagnose by ECG. It is characterized by RBBB with initial rightward forces. Because most children who develop RBBB following surgery have preexisting RVH, it is extremely difficult to distinguish RBBB with left posterior hemiblock from preexisting RVH.

Rate-Dependent Aberrancy

In normal children functional bundle branch block may occur with the ventricular aberration of a tachyarrhythmia. However, rate-dependent bundle branch block is rare in children.[9]

Preexcitation

Preexcitation describes an abnormal depolarization of the ventricle prior to normal conduction through the His-Purkinje system. This takes place usually by an accessory connection between the two chambers.

Wolff-Parkinson-White Syndrome

Wolff-Parkinson-White syndrome describes early activation of the ventricle via an accessory pathway, which connects the atria directly to ventricular muscle. Conduction occurs across the normal conduction system (AV node and His-Purkinje system) as well as across the accessory pathway. The ECG has a characteristic appearance of a short PR interval and a wide QRS complex (Fig. 2–10). A delta wave or slurred upstroke of the QRS, indicating conduction from atrial to ventricular muscle, is pathognomonic of the syndrome. The terminal part of the complex may be wide or narrow depending on the degree of conduction via the AV node. Children who have this finding are subject to episodes of reciprocating atrioventricular tachycardia.

Mahaim

Mahaim fibers are defined as an accessory pathway originating in the AV node, His bundle, or proximal bundle branch and inserting into the right ventricular muscle. It will appear on a surface ECG as a normal PR interval with LBBB morphology. It too is a substrate for supraventricular tachycardia.

Pathologic Changes in the ST Segment and T Wave

Evaluating ST- and T-wave changes in the pediatric patient can be very difficult. Many pathologic changes can be relatively nonspecific. Several functional changes are also seen in adolescents, most notably early repolarization syndrome; this can be recognized by early J-point elevation, which can mimic pathologic ST-segment elevation.

Pericarditis and Pericardial Effusions

Pericarditis is the most common cause of ST-segment elevation in children. A series of changes occurs as pericarditis evolves. Initially the ST segment is elevated, with a normal T wave, thought to be secondary to subepicardial myocarditis. The ST segment then returns to normal, but the T wave becomes flattened and then inverted. Characteristically, these findings differ from ischemic changes in that they involve all leads. Pericardial effusions can result in diminished QRS voltages and electrical alternans (alternating QRS amplitude).

Myocarditis

Myocarditis usually results in flattened or inverted T waves and low-voltage QRS patterns. The QT interval may be prolonged. Atrioventricular block and intraventricular conduction delay may also be seen.

Ischemia

Myocardial ischemia is rarely seen in the pediatric population, but there are certain situations in which it must be considered, most notably Kawasaki's disease and congenital coronary artery abnormalities. Myocardial ischemia initially presents on the ECG as a distortion of the T wave that becomes tall and peaked in the leads near the affected myocardial segment. The ST segment may also be somewhat affected. If the ischemia is promptly reversed, these changes will resolve. If, however, ischemia persists, the myocardium will progress to the injury stage. This is seen on ECG as a deviation in the ST segments. The ST segments may be elevated or depressed depending on whether the injury is endocardial or epicardial. Reversal of ischemia may still reverse these changes. In 15 of 19 infants with patent ductus arteriosus, ST depression was evident in leads V1 and V2. These changes disappeared after ligation of the ductus and represented a marked imbalance in the

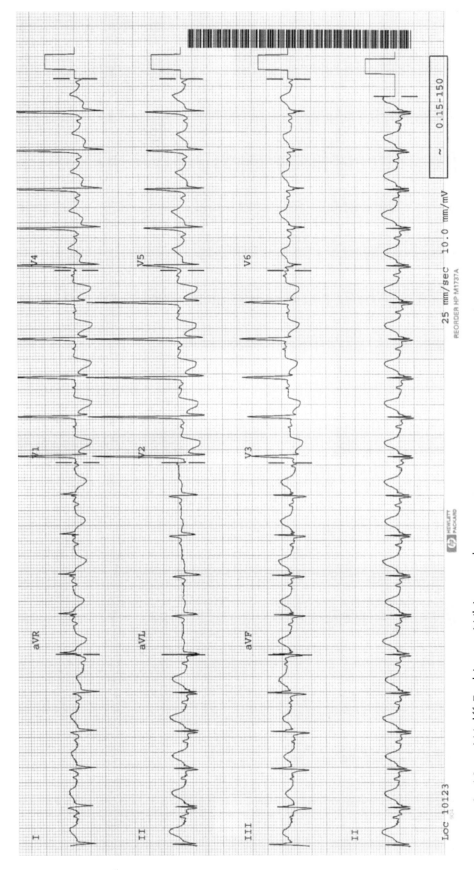

FIGURE 2–10.   Wolff-Parkinson-White syndrome.

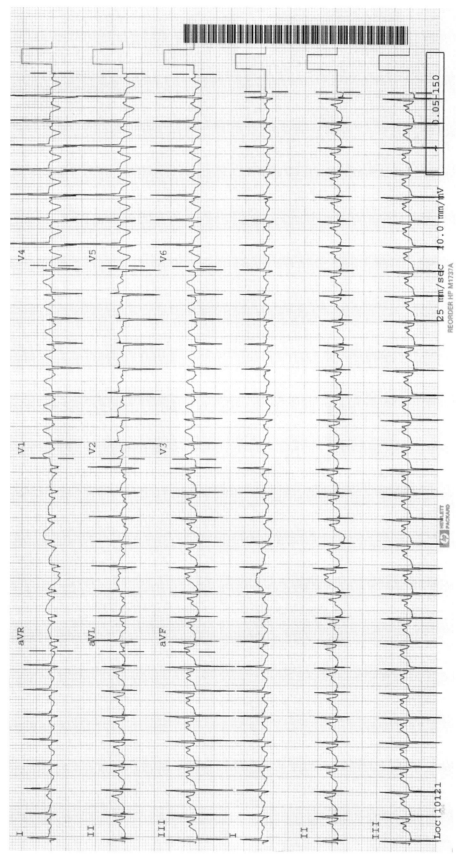

FIGURE 2–11. Anomalous left coronary artery from the pulmonary artery, deep Q waves in leads I and aVL.

myocardial oxygen supply-demand in the right ventricle.[10] Further injury will result in infarction, which is seen on ECG as a decrease in the R-wave voltage and appearance of Q waves facing the infarcted segment. Q waves in children are wide (>0.04) but may disappear as the child grows.

Myocardial ischemia in infancy is often related to congenital coronary abnormalities, the most common being anomalous origin of the left coronary from the pulmonary artery. These infants usually present with ECGs consistent with ischemia or infarction of the anterior and septal areas (distribution of the left anterior descending coronary artery). They have deep Q waves in leads I, aVL, and V3–V6. There is also loss of midprecordial R wave with a normal R wave in V1 and V6 (Fig. 2–11).

Kawasaki's disease is the most common acquired cause of myocardial infarction in pediatrics. The ECG initially shows low QRS voltages and nonspecific T-wave changes, which are typical of myocarditis. This may then progress to a myocardial infarction pattern.

Metabolic Disturbances

Electrolyte disorders may result in specific findings on the surface ECG, most notably imbalances in potassium, calcium, and magnesium.

Potassium Imbalance

Hyperkalemia results in high peaked T waves that are clearly abnormal at concentrations >7 mEq/L. However, this finding is not very specific or sensitive because normal children may have peaked T waves and those with hyperkalemia may not have peaked T waves. As the potassium level increases, the T waves become more peaked, and an intraventricular conduction delay results in a widened QRS along with PR prolongation. The resultant ECG resembles a sine wave or wide ventricular tachycardia. At concentrations of 9 mEq/L, arrhythmias occur, specifically atrial arrest, atrioventricular block, and ventricular fibrillation.

Hypokalemia lowers the T-wave amplitude. As potassium levels fall, a U wave becomes apparent, and the ST segment becomes depressed. Hypokalemia will enhance the arrhythmogenic effects of digoxin.

Calcium and Magnesium Imbalance

Hypercalcemia shortens the QT interval by shortening the ST segment. It also can affect the sinus node, with sinus rate slowing and sinoatrial block. Hypocalcemia lengthens the QT interval by prolonging the ST segment. A low magnesium level may enhance the effects of a low calcium level. In some infants correction of the ECG is only seen after both calcium and magnesium are corrected.

References

1. DAUVIGNON A, RAUTAHARJU PM, BOISSELLE E, et al. Normal ECG standards for infants and children. *Pediatr Cardiol* 1979;1:123–131.

2. WALSH EP. Electrocardiography and introduction to electrophysiologic techniques. In: Fyler DC, ed. *Nadas' Pediatric Cardiology.* Philadelphia: Hanley and Belfus; 1992:126.

3. ELLISON RC, FREEDOM RM, KEANE JF, et al. Indirect assessment of severity in pulmonary stenosis. *Circulation* 1977;56:15–20.

4. WAGNER HR, WEIDMAN WH, ELLISON RC, MIETTINEN OS. Indirect assessment of severity in aortic stenosis. *Circulation* 1977;56:20–23.

5. GARSON A. Recording the sequence of cardiac activity. In: *The Electrocardiogram in Infants and Children.* Philadephia: Lea & Febiger; 1983:19–99.

6. BROHET CR, STYNS M, ARRAUD P, BRASSEUR LA. Vectorcardiographic diagnosis of right ventricular hypertrophy in the presence of right bundle branch block in young subjects. *Am J Cardiol* 1978;42:602–612.

7. SCHATZ J, KRONGRAD E, MALM JR. Left anterior and left posterior hemiblock in tricuspid atresia and transposition of the great arteries. *Circulation* 1976;54:1010–1013.

8. GARSON A, MCNAMARA DG, COOLEY DA. Post-operative tetralogy of Fallot. In: Engle MA, ed. *Pediatric Cardiovascular Disease.* Philadelphia: FA Davis; 1981:407–430.

9. GARSON A. Supraventricular tachycardia. In: Cillette PC, Garson A, eds. *Pediatric Cardiac Dysrhythmias.* New York: Grune & Stratton; 1981:177–254.

10. WAY GL, PIERCE JR, WOLF RR, et al. ST depression suggesting subendocardial injury in neonates with respiratory distress syndrome and patent ductus arteriosus. *J Pediatr* 1979;95:609–611.

CHAPTER 3

Imaging of Congenital Heart Disease

Alvaro Huete, MD, Lina Sierra, MD, and Fernando R. Gutierrez, MD

Introduction

In the last decade, echocardiography has emerged as the centerpiece in the routine evaluation of patients with suspected cardiac disease. Conventional chest radiography still plays an important role in the initial assessment and follow-up of congenital heart diseases. Recent developments in computed tomography (CT) technology, including spiral CT and multidetector CT, have expanded the possible applications of this technique in the workup of mediastinal and cardiovascular anomalies. Magnetic resonance imaging (MRI) has dramatically evolved during the past two decades as a helpful problem-solving tool in cases with complex cardiac malformations, especially because of its multiplanar capability and high-contrast resolution.

Chest radiograph evaluation of patients with suspected congenital heart disease includes anteroposterior (AP) and lateral views of the chest in children younger than 1 year of age. In small infants, there is no significant difference in magnification between a supine AP view and an erect posteroanterior (PA) film. In this population of patients, supine AP views allow adequate immobilization. This is required to provide adequate positioning and limit motion artifact. The radiograph must be obtained at end inspiration during quiet respiration. In neonates, a frontal AP supine film is usually the only view obtained. A lateral film may be obtained with a cross-table or horizontal beam technique. Most children over 1 year of age can sit upright with support to obtain both the PA and lateral films. Children older than 3 years can be evaluated with an erect PA frontal film as well as a lateral view. Oral administration of barium to assess specific chamber enlargement no longer forms part of the routine evaluation of cardiac diseases with conventional radiography.

CT is the main cross-sectional imaging modality that utilizes ionizing radiation. The x-ray beams are collimated into thin sections of the human anatomy, allowing for a dramatic improvement in detection of attenuation differences between tissues and giving this technique improved contrast resolution. This can be further enhanced with the administration of intravenous iodinated contrast material, which expands the spectrum of attenuation differences due to differential uptake by various tissues. The advent of helical or spiral CT has revolutionized body imaging, decreasing scanning times and minimizing motion artifact and respiratory misregistration artifact. Faster scanning times have diminished the need for sedation in pediatric patients. Spiral CT, especially with the new multidetector scanners, allows contrast-enhanced studies to be performed during the period of peak vascular enhancement. The capability to perform retrospective two- and three-dimensional reconstructions from the helical data set of axially acquired images has allowed the development of high-quality CT angiographic techniques (CTA). Thorough evaluation of vascular anomalies of the chest is possible, including diseases of the thoracic aorta, thoracic veins, and pulmonary vasculature.

MRI has rapidly gained acceptance as a valuable tool in the evaluation of patients with congenital heart disease. It is especially useful in depicting the anatomy of complex cardiac malformations. MRI has direct multiplanar capability, which permits direct acquisition of images in the classic echocardiographic planes as well as the axial, sagittal, and coronal planes. MRI permits acquisition of images with superb contrast resolution without the need to use contrast material. High intrinsic contrast between the myocardium and flowing blood permits accurate depiction of the intracardiac anatomy.

Cardiac MRI protocols for the evaluation of heart anomalies are tailored to the specific questions posed by the referring physician. In general, both spin-echo sequences (SE) and gradient-recalled echo (GRE) or cine sequences are obtained. In simple terms, magnetic resonance (MR) images are obtained by stimulating protons within the body with a particular radiofrequency wave (pulse) under a magnetic field. The excited protons will return the energy deposited on them also as a radiofrequency wave (signal) that can be captured by the imaging system. The magnitude and phase of these waves or signals will ultimately determine image formation and contrast. Image contrast can therefore be altered by using different radiofrequency pulses and by modifications in the magnetic field strength over time and space (gradients). SE sequences are robust imaging techniques that allow depiction of flowing blood as dark signal (black blood imaging). These are slow and time-consuming techniques, but contrast resolution is unparalleled. GRE techniques are much faster; they permit acquisition of multiple images within a breath hold. Flowing blood is depicted as bright (white) signal intensity with respect to the hypointense myocardium. Its high sensitivity to dephasing artifact can be used to advantage in detection of areas with turbulent flow, which appear as foci of signal loss. This is very useful in the depiction of abnormal communications (shunts) and stenotic segments of the vascular circuit. Electrocardiographic (ECG) gating permits images to be obtained in both systole and diastole; these images can be reviewed in a cine-type mode. These capabilities, combined with the possibility of producing high-quality angiographic images with the use of intravenous gadolinium (Gd) contrast, have made MRI a premier tool in the postsurgical evaluation of complex congenital heart diseases.

In addition, flow-sensitive imaging techniques permit the measurement of flow expressed as either velocity or volume per unit of time. This MR technique is referred to as phase-contrast, phase-shift, or velocity-encoded cine (VEC). VEC thus allows accurate estimation of velocity profiles across a valve or any vascular structure, thereby providing quantitative measurements comparable to those provided by Doppler ultrasound. This MR technique allows quantitative measurement of valvular stenosis and regurgitation as well as noninvasive quantification of left-to-right shunts, thus making noninvasive "one-stop shopping" for congenital heart disease a possibility.

Currently the Food and Drug Administration (FDA) has approved three MR contrast agents for general use, all of which use the gadolinium ion as a paramagnetic metal species. Gadopentetate dimeglumine (Gd-DTPA) is an extracellular gadolinium chelate that is in clinical use in adults and in pediatric patients older than 2 years of age. Gd-HP-DO3A (gadoteridol) and Gd-DTPA-BMA (gadodiamide) are alternative nonionic compounds. After intravenous injection, these agents are distributed in the blood pool and extracellular fluid compartment and are rapidly excreted by glomerular filtration. These agents act as positive TI relaxation. The clinical dose of these agents is 0.1 mmol/kg, although high-dose trials with 0.3 mmol/kg with some agents have been used in particular clinical scenarios with improved enhancement. The use of approved

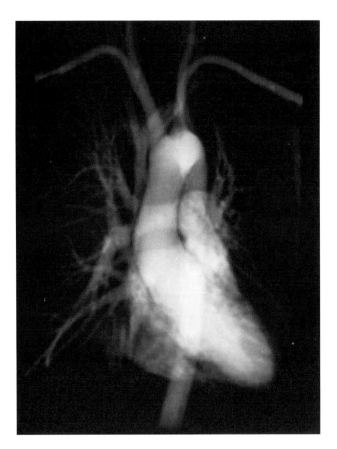

FIGURE 3–1. Coronal chest MRA with intravenous Gd demonstrating normal cardiovascular anatomy.

gadolinium chelates in combination with breath-hold techniques allows performance of magnetic resonance angiography (MRA) with excellent depiction of vascular structures in the mediastinum such as the aorta, pulmonary arteries, and pulmonary veins (Fig. 3–1).

Radiologic Anatomy

Although it is less critical in the initial diagnosis of congenital cardiac anomalies due to the emergence of echocardiography and other cross-sectional imaging techniques, routine evaluation of these patients continues to include standard PA and lateral views of the chest. An AP film may be the only examination obtained in younger infants and neonates. This technique provides a significant amount of information that, although it is nonspecific, can help narrow the differential diagnosis, especially when interpreted in conjunction with relevant clinical and physiologic information. Adequate knowledge of normal thoracic radiologic anatomy and common pitfalls is essential for correct interpretation of chest radiographs.

In the PA view, the upper right mediastinal contour is determined by the superior vena cava, and the lower right border by the right atrium. The left border of the mediastinum is determined by the aortic arch, main pulmonary artery, left atrial appendage, and the left ventricle from cephalad to caudad. The left atrial appendage is normally straight or concave. Of note is the fact that the ascending aorta and the right ventricle are not border-forming structures on the PA view. The lateral projection helps in assessing cardiac chamber size. Normally the right ventricle forms the anterior heart border occupying the lower third of the retrosternal space. Above this lies the retrosternal clear space, which in infancy is occupied by the thymus. After thymic involution, the right ventricular outflow tract and main pulmonary artery can be identified forming the upper portion of the cardiac silhouette. The posterior cardiac contour is formed by the left atrium superiorly, and the left ventricle in its lower half.

Evaluation of the Chest Radiograph

A systematic evaluation of the chest radiograph allows a complete analysis of pertinent anatomic and physiologic findings commonly associated with congenital cardiac lesions. The approach includes evaluation of radiographic technique, situs, heart location, size and specific chamber enlargement, pulmonary vascularity, and great vessel position and size.

Technique

Adequate technique is essential to avoid misinterpretation of chest radiographs. Films should be scrutinized for proper centering, without angulation or rotation. Adequate use of technical parameters is essential to avoid overexposure, as this may produce decreased lung opacity, which can mimic decreased lung vascularity. Films should be obtained during inspiration. Small lung volumes may give a false impression of cardiomegaly and increased lung vascularity. With adequate inspiration, the dome of the diaphragm is at the level of the anterior sixth rib.

Situs

Situs refers to the distribution of asymmetric organs in the body following a particular pattern. Spatial relationships between certain organs remain constant in normal conditions. Thus the liver, inferior vena cava (IVC), right atrium, and trilobed lung are located on the same side of the body. The descending aorta, left atrium, stomach, spleen, and bilobed lung are on the opposite side. Both chest and abdominal radiographs, as well as cross-sectional imaging such as ultrasound, CT, or MRI, can provide information about the situs and thus of the probability of coexistent cardiac disease. The tracheobronchial tree anatomy is a useful parameter to detect normal right and left lungs. The morphologic right lung is recognized by the presence of three lobes and is supplied by a pulmonary artery that runs in front of the

short, right main bronchus (eparterial). The morphologic left lung is bilobed and is perfused by an artery that arches above the corresponding elongated left main bronchus (hyparterial). The situs may be solitus (normal), inversus, or ambiguus.

Situs solitus is the normal alignment of the right atrium, inferior vena cava, liver, and trilobed lung on the right side of the body. The expected incidence of congenital heart disease in these cases is less than 1% if associated with levocardia.

Situs inversus refers to a mirror image of the normal thoracic and abdominal situs. The trilobed lung, right atrium, and liver are on the left, and the bilobed lung, left atrium, stomach, and spleen are on the right. This abnormality affects 0.01% of the general population and has up to a 5% incidence of congenital cardiac malformations, most commonly corrected transposition of the great arteries.

Situs ambiguus is a rare condition in which the abdominal and atrial situs is indeterminate. Situs ambiguus suggests the presence of a heterotaxy syndrome, either asplenia or polysplenia. These are complex developmental syndromes characterized by symmetric development of normally asymmetric organs within the trunk, abnormal relationships between abdominal organs, and the presence of congenital cardiac anomalies. Whenever discordance between the cardiac apex and the situs is seen, a heterotaxy syndrome must be suspected.

In asplenia there is a tendency toward bilateral right-sidedness. This may be confirmed by detecting bilateral eparterial bronchus on plain films or cross-sectional imaging. Associated findings include a symmetric or transverse liver, midline stomach, and cardiac apex malposition. This syndrome is almost invariably associated with complex cardiac anomalies in patients who are usually cyanotic during the neonatal period. Polysplenia is characterized by a tendency toward bilateral left-sidedness. These patients have a decreased incidence of congenital heart disease compared with asplenia patients (10%), usually of moderate complexity and acyanotic. These include atrial septal defect (ASD) (84%), ventricular septal defect (VSD) and partial anomalous pulmonary venous return (40%). Many patients may present in adult life. Plain film indicators of polysplenia include bilateral hyparterial bronchi, variable hepatic position, malposition of the stomach, and thickened paravertebral stripes from a dilated azygos vein due to a high frequency of interrupted IVC with azygos continuation. Cross-sectional imaging frequently demonstrates multiple splenules in the right upper quadrant.

Heart Position

Cardiac position depends not only on embryogenetic factors intrinsic to heart development such as cardiac looping, but also on thoracic extracardiac factors such as skeletal, pulmonary, pleural, and diaphragmatic lesions. The heart is normally just to the left of midline. Congenital dextroposition refers to a heart of normal configuration but displaced toward the right hemithorax. This most commonly occurs in scoliosis, pulmonary agenesis or hypoplasia, and diaphragmatic hernia.

The normal orientation of the cardiac apex toward the left is referred to as levocardia. If the cardiac apex points toward the right, dextrocardia is present. In the presence of situs solitus, dextrocardia is a marker for significant increase in the incidence of congenital heart disease, up to 95%. In situs inversus, dextrocardia signals the presence of a mirror image position of thoracic organs, with only a 3% to 5% incidence of cardiac malformations.

Heart Size

Evaluation of the cardiac size is often difficult in young infants due to the presence of a large thymus. The thymus is located in the anterior mediastinum, in front of the heart and great vessels. The thymic parenchyma is soft and is normally compressed and deformed by the overlying ribs and costal cartilages. This can be recognized on the frontal film by an undulating lateral contour of the gland. The lateral view will confirm that the soft tissue density seen on the PA film is located in a retrosternal location and corresponds to the thymus.

Cardiothoracic ratios are usually unreliable in young children. Expiratory films make the heart appear large. The lateral view can be helpful in assessing cardiac size. If the posterior cardiac border does not extend beyond an imaginary line drawn down the anterior margin of the trachea, cardiomegaly can be excluded.

Cardiac Chamber Assessment

Specific heart chambers may enlarge because of either volume overload or increased resistance distally to blood flow (pressure overload). An accurate assessment of individual chambers frequently is not possible in infants, and in these cases evaluation of pulmonary vascularity combined with clinical data is more helpful in the interpretation of chest radiographs.

The right atrium forms the normal right cardiac border on the frontal view. Right atrial enlargement causes a bulge of the right heart contour. It is frequently associated with right ventricular enlargement. Volume overload in atrial left-to-right shunts or in cases of endocardial cushion defect will present with right atrial enlargement. The right atrium can become markedly dilated and is commonly the underlying anatomic culprit in cases of massive cardiomegaly, such as Ebstein's anomaly and pulmonary atresia with an intact septum.

The right ventricular cavity only contributes to the cardiomediastinal contour on the lateral film, normally contacting the lower half to third of the sternum. Nevertheless, when right ventricular dilation is present, posterior displace-

ment of the left ventricle and counterclockwise rotation of the heart occur. The left cardiac border will straighten, and uplifting of the cardiac apex will be present on the frontal film. A typical example occurs in tetralogy of Fallot. On the lateral film there will be filling in of the retrosternal clear space and posterior displacement of the left ventricle.

The left atrium is not a border-forming structure on the frontal film, although in a third of normal children the right border of the left atrium may be seen projecting to the right of the spine behind the right atrium as a normal radiographic finding. The left atrial appendage is normally flat or concave. Outward bulging of this segment reflects left atrial enlargement. A dilated left atrium can also manifest as dorsal bulging of the upper posterior cardiac border on the lateral film. When moderate to severe, elevation and posterior displacement of the left main stem bronchus may be seen. Left atrial enlargement from volume overload is present in left-to-right shunts, including VSD and patent ductus arteriosus (PDA). Mitral stenosis or insufficiency may also produce left atrial dilation.

Left ventricular enlargement is most frequently due to dilation. Left ventricular hypertrophy usually does not cause radiologic enlargement of the ventricular cavity unless some degree of dilation is also present. Typical signs of enlargement include increased convexity of the left heart border and an inferiorly displaced apex. This may sometimes be difficult to differentiate from right ventricular enlargement. The lateral view may be helpful, as the posterior heart border may be displaced behind the inferior vena cava shadow with left ventricular enlargement. One can exclude right ventricular dilation as a cause for this displacement if there is normal contact between the anterior heart border and the sternum, signaling a normal-sized right ventricle. Left ventricular dilation can be seen in cases of myocardial dysfunction, mitral or aortic valve regurgitation, and PDA, the only isolated left-to-right shunt with volume overload of the left ventricular cavity.

Pulmonary Vascularity

Evaluation of the status of the pulmonary vasculature is the most critical step in the categorization of patients with congenital heart disease. Pulmonary blood flow may be normal, increased, or decreased.

Normally, pulmonary vessels taper gradually from the hila to the periphery. On erect films, lower lobe vessels are more prominent than vessels located in upper lung zones. On supine films this zonal difference disappears, and vessel distribution is uniform throughout upper and lower lobes. The size of the peripheral pulmonary arteries can be assessed using the arterial-bronchial index, comparing the size of an artery seen end on with the adjacent bronchus. Normally, the diameter of the artery and accompanying bronchus is the same. Comparison of the diameter of the right interlobar pulmonary artery and the trachea has also been used to evaluate pulmonary blood flow. Throughout childhood, the diameter of the trachea at the level of the aortic arch is equal to that of the right interlobar pulmonary artery.

Shunt vascularity or pulmonary plethora is characterized by uniform enlargement of the central pulmonary arteries, the parenchymal arteries, and the intrapulmonary veins. The entire pulmonary circuit is subject to volume overload. The normal tapering and branching pattern of vessels is preserved. There is no vascular redistribution or cephalization of flow as occurs in cases of passive congestion. Of importance is the fact that vessel-lung interface is sharp in cases of shunt vascularity. Haziness and indistinctness of vascular markings signal the presence of peribronchovascular interstitial edema and pulmonary venous hypertension.

Pulmonary venous hypertension is characterized by the development of vascular redistribution and pulmonary edema. The severity of pulmonary venous hypertension correlates with the radiographic findings. Initially, on erect films, vascular redistribution appears due to increased resistance to blood flow in dependent regions of the lung. Upper lung zone vessels appear more prominent, reaching equal size than lower zone vessels. On supine images of the chest, redistribution produces increased flow to both upper and lower lung zone vessels that are closer to the anterior chest wall, and thus cephalization is not evident. In these cases, differentiation from shunt vascularity may be difficult. With increasing venous hypertension, interstitial edema accumulates in peribronchial and perivascular spaces, producing indistinct vascular markings. Interlobular septal thickening, manifesting as Kerley B lines, and subpleural edema, manifesting as fissural thickening, are also markers of interstitial edema. When pulmonary venous wedge pressures exceed 30 mm Hg, alveolar edema ensues, manifesting as airspace opacification.

Shunt vascularity and pulmonary venous hypertension are usually associated with a secondary increase in pulmonary arterial pressures. Pulmonary arterial hypertension may become the dominant physiologic abnormality in cases with long-standing left-to-right shunts due to a reactive increase in pulmonary arteriolar resistance. Radiographically, these cases are characterized by a discrepancy in the size between central pulmonary arteries, which are markedly enlarged, and peripheral vessels, which are decreased in number and size, producing a "pruned tree" appearance.

Decreased lung vascularity is the hallmark of obstructive lesions of the right ventricle or outflow tract with an associated right-to-left shunt. The main pulmonary artery is usually small or absent, and parenchymal vessels are diminished in number and size. Care must be taken not to misinterpret the decrease in lung vessels as lung hyperlucency.

Other less frequent patterns of abnormal blood flow include asymmetric flow, usually seen in cases of unilateral pulmonary artery stenosis and unilateral palliative shunts to the pulmonary circulation (e.g., Blalock-Taussig shunt). Systemic collateral flow is most frequently seen in severe cases of pulmonary artery stenosis or atresia and manifests radiographically as irregular and disorganized vessels with an unusual branching pattern. If a marked profusion of collateral vessels is present, the radiographic appreearance may be misinterpreted as increased pulmonary blood flow or even interstitial lung disease.

Great Vessels

The main pulmonary artery is a normal border-forming structure along the upper left mediastinal border. Normally, it is of equal or less size than the adjacent aortic knob, although in adolescent females, it may be slightly larger. Enlargement of the main pulmonary artery occurs in left-to-right shunts, pulmonary arterial hypertension, and pulmonary valvular stenosis. In this last case, due to the direction of the blood jet through the stenotic valve, the left pulmonary artery is also enlarged, with the right pulmonary artery remaining normal in size. A small or concave pulmonary artery segment along the left mediastinal border suggests the presence of either decreased flow through the pulmonic valve, as seen in cases of right ventricular ouflow obstruction, or malalignment of the pulmonary artery, as seen in transposition of the great vessels.

The position of the aortic arch is most frequently determined by visualization of the aortic knob itself. This is easy in older children, but in infants, the overlapping thymic shadow may obscure the aortic knob. In these cases, the location of the arch may be inferred by the impression on the lower tracheal air column by the arch, or identification of the descending aorta, as the thoracic aorta descends on the same side of the arch in most cases. A right aortic arch is a common variant. When associated with an aberrant left subclavian artery, the incidence of cardiac malformations is low. On the lateral film, anterior bowing of the tracheal air column is seen. If mirror image branching is present, no anterior displacement of the trachea will be present on the lateral view, and the incidence of cyanotic congenital heart disease will be high, most frequently truncus arteriosus, tetralogy of Fallot, pulmonary atresia with VSD, and double outlet right ventricle.

Classification of Congenital Heart Disease

Although many anatomic, physiologic, and pathologic classifications of congenital cardiac anomalies exist, the imaging evaluation is based on a combined clinical and radiographic approach. The basis of the interpretation of imaging studies, particularly conventional radiographs, is the presence or absence of cyanosis and the radiologic appearance of the pulmonary vasculature.

Acyanotic Anomalies with Increased Pulmonary Blood Flow

Ventricular Septal Defect　VSD is the most common congenital heart disease except for bicuspid aortic valve. Although most commonly an isolated abnormality, in up to 20% of cases it may accompany other cardiac and aortic anomalies. The most common anatomic variant, and the one associated with classic roentgenographic findings, is the perimembranous type (80%).

The radiographic presentation in VSD is dependent on the magnitude of the left-to-right shunt. Small shunts of less than 50% (2:1) present with normal chest radiographs. With larger defects and shunts, there is volume overload of the pulmonary circulation, from the central pulmonary arteries to the peripheral intraparenchymal branches. This produces enlargement of the main pulmonary artery segment along the left mediastinal contour, as well as hilar branches. The peripheral arteries are also increased in diameter and visible to the outer margin of the lungs, in close contact with the pleural surface. This appearance has been termed *shunt vascularity* or *pulmonary plethora* and implies the diffuse enlargement of the entire pulmonary arterial system, from the main pulmonary artery to the distal subsegmental branches. There is an associated increase in pulmonary venous return, and thus the veins are also increased in caliber.

In young infants, especially those younger than 2 years of age, precise chamber assessment on chest radiography is difficult due to the overlying thymic shadow. In these instances VSD will present with nonspecific cardiomegaly in 75% of cases. Associated shunt vascularity in an acyanotic child suggests the diagnosis of left-to-right shunt (Fig. 3–2).

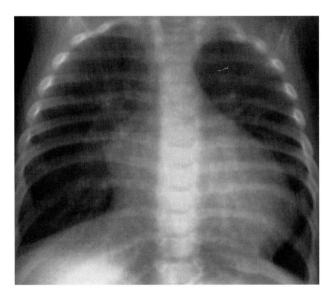

FIGURE 3–2.　Frontal radiograph of a 7-month-old male with a ventricular septal defect. Note moderate cardiomegaly and increased pulmonary vascularity.

The volume overload induced by the shunt increases the amount of blood return to the left atrium, which is enlarged, and constitutes the hallmark of VSD. This sign is usually best recognized in older children as a double density along the right heart border on the PA view or as elevation and posterior displacement of the left main stem bronchus on the lateral film. The left ventricle may be normal, slightly dilated, or hypertrophied. The excess volume produces right ventricular enlargement, which appears as increased surface of contact of the anterior heart border with the sternum. The right ventricle is not a border-forming structure on the frontal film, but enlargement of this cavity, especially if moderate to severe, may produce counterclockwise heart rotation with elevation of the cardiac apex, which can appear more rounded. The right atrium and aorta are not affected by the shunt and thus are normal.

In long-standing left-to-right shunt, reactive changes may occur in distal pulmonary arterioles with ensuing pulmonary arterial hypertension. The peripheral pulmonary vessels decrease in number and in size. There is an abrupt transition compared with the central vessels, which are markedly enlarged. This combination produces an appearance resembling a pruned tree. As with other chronic left-to-right shunts with Eisenmenger physiology, significant right chamber enlargement is present.

Another associated finding, although not specific, may be bilateral pulmonary hyperinflation, usually mild to moderate, secondary to decreased lung compliance. This may also be seen in other left-to-right shunts.

MRI can depict the different portions of the interventricular septum so that proper anatomic classification can be established (inlet, muscular, perimembranous, outlet). Although standard axial images are the workhorses in the identification of these defects, other orthogonal images as well as oblique views can provide further anatomic detail in the same fashion as cineangiocardiography. Cine MRI techniques are crucial not only in the identification of smaller defects, but also in determining the direction of blood flow across a defect, and even in the calculation of the shunt fraction. The most common type of ventricular defect can be identified by close inspection of the area just below the crista supraventricularis. The presence of a septal "aneurysm" associated with a closing VSD can also be identified if present, if contiguous thin sections are obtained through the area in question. As previously mentioned, the VEC technique allows calculation of left-to-right shunt.

Atrial Septal Defect　ASD accounts for approximately 10% of congenital heart disease and is the most frequent shunt lesion in adults. The most common anatomic defect is the ostium secundum type, located at the level of the fossa ovalis. This lesion accounts for most isolated ASDs and is the prototype of the classic radiologic findings. An ostium primum defect, the mildest form in the atrioventricular canal spectrum, may have similar characteristics.

Patients with a small ASD have normal heart size and pulmonary vascularity. The typical changes occur at shunts of moderate size and are determined by volume overload of the right atrium, which receives part of the pulmonary venous return through the septal defect plus the systemic return via the superior and inferior vena cava. This excess volume is then passed along to the right ventricle and pulmonary vascular bed. Right atrial enlargement manifests as prominence of the right lower heart border. As the right ventricle increases in size, there is filling of the retrosternal space. This right chamber enlargement may rotate the heart toward the left. These findings are most clearly appreciated in older children. Shunt vascularity is present with dilation of the main pulmonary artery segment, the central hilar branches, and the peripheral segmental arteries. Although the left atrium is exposed to increased volume, it does not dilate, as a significant fraction of the venous return is shunted quickly toward the right atrium. This is the primary distinguishing characteristic of ASD compared with other left-to-right shunts and is reliable as long as there is no superimposed mitral regurgitation (Fig. 3–3).

In long-standing shunt there is a progressive elevation of the pulmonary vascular resistance and development of pulmonary arterial hypertension, with discordance between massively enlarged central pulmonary arteries and strikingly attenuated peripheral branches. This is uncommon in childhood and is usually detected in untreated adolescents or young adults with chronic ASD.

Attention must be paid to the venous circulation when ASD is suspected radiographically due to the known association with partial anomalous pulmonary venous return. Abnormal, dilated venous channels such as a left superior

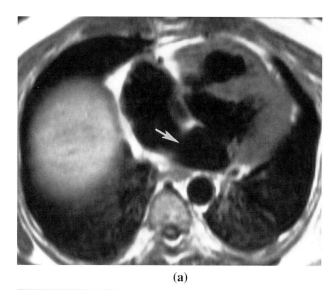

(a)

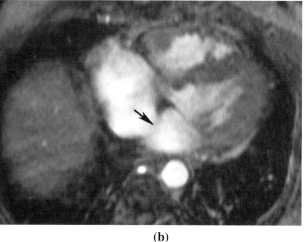

(b)

FIGURE 3–4. Axial T1-weighted (*a*) and cine (*b*) MRI of a moderate-size ASD. Note abrupt termination of atrial septum with communication between atrial chambers (arrow).

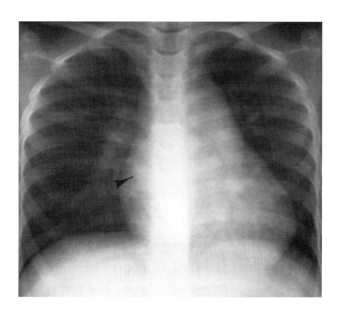

FIGURE 3–3. ASD. Frontal radiograph of a 2-year-old patient with an ASD. Note shunt vascularity and normal sized left atrium (arrowhead).

vertical vein or a common right vessel (Scimitar) may be identified, signaling the presence of a partial aberrant venous return.

Although echocardiography is the imaging modality of choice, MRI can provide additional information regarding the size, location, and magnitude of the shunt. Particular case must be taken not to confuse lack of signal in the septum as a result of a fossa ovalis with an actual defect. In general, a patent foramen ovale will have tapered borders around the edges of the fossa ovalis, whereas a septal defect will exhibit blunt or abrupt termination of the septum (Fig. 3–4). In patients with increased pulmonary arterial pressure as a result of the long-standing left-to-right shunt, high signal intensity may be visible in the central pulmonary arteries on SE images from turbulent flow. On GRE images, dephasing and signal loss may be evident (Fig. 3–5).

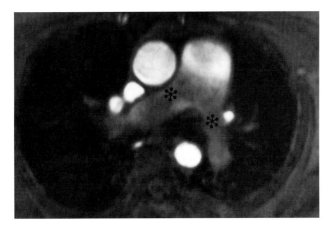

FIGURE 3–5. Pulmonary arterial hypertension. Cine MR at the level of the central pulmonary arteries shows low signal at the level of the proximal right and left branches (asterisk) as a result of sluggish flow.

Patent Ductus Arteriosus PDA is a common congenital anomaly. The ductus arteriosus is a vessel that extends from the proximal left pulmonary artery to the descending aorta, just distal to the origin of the left subclavian artery. After birth there is functional closure of the ductus by 24 hours of age, and anatomic closure is achieved in over 90% of cases after 2 months. A patent ductus can thus be considered abnormal after the first trimester of life. Although seen in term infants, the incidence of PDA increases substantially with low birth weight, neonatal asphyxia, congenital infections, and chromosomic abnormalities.

As pulmonary resistance decreases in the first hours of life and systemic pressures increase, there is shunting of blood from the aorta into the pulmonary vascular bed. As the pressure gradient is significant in both diastole and systole, there is continuous left-to-right diversion of blood throughout the cardiac cycle.

If the shunt is small, no roentgenographic abnormalities will be seen. With moderate-to-large PDA, there is increased pulmonary vascularity or plethora, with dilation of central and peripheral pulmonary arteries (Fig. 3–6). The pulmonary veins, left atrium, and ipsilateral ventricle are also exposed to overcirculation of blood and become enlarged. As opposed to other left-to-right shunts, the ascending thoracic aorta and aortic arch receive the increased cardiac output and consequently become dilated in patients with PDA. This sign is best seen in older children who do not have their mediastinal contours obscured by the thymus. If the defect is untreated, pulmonary vasoconstriction ensues, and pulmonary resistance overcomes systemic resistance with development of Eisenmenger's physiology and right heart enlargement. Calcification in the region of the aortopulmonic window may be identified, signaling either

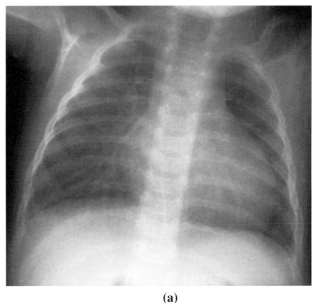

(a)

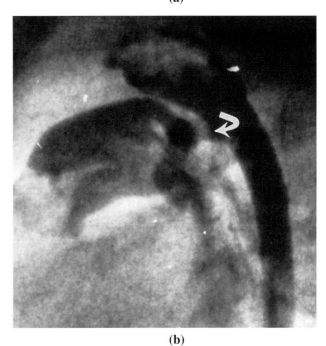

(b)

FIGURE 3–6. A 3-month-old girl with PDA. (*a*) Frontal radiograph shows mild increase of pulmonary vessels particularly at the bases. (*b*) Lateral aortogram on same patient demonstrating a moderate size PDA (arrow).

a closed ligamentum arteriosus or a patent ductus, although ligamentum closure calcification is more punctate versus a "railroad track" appearance of a calcified ductus. This is more common in adult patients.

The classic findings of PDA, or any left-to-right shunt, are at best subtle in newborn infants; PDA usually manifests as cardiomegaly with increased vascularity. Vessel

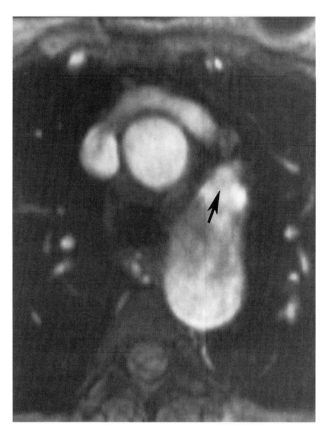

FIGURE 3–7. Large PDA. Axial GRE MR image just below the aortic arch demonstrating a large tubular communication (arrow) between the proximal descending aorta and main pulmonary artery.

indistinctness and pulmonary parenchymal haziness may represent superimposed pulmonary edema and congestive heart failure, a frequent manifestation of PDA in premature infants.

On MRI, a patent ductus can be seen as a tubular connection between the proximal descending aorta and the connection between the main and left pulmonary arteries (Fig. 3–7). GRE images are more sensitive in the identification of a patent ductus on MRI than standard SE images, particularly small ones. In addition, thin-section images must be obtained so that a small defect will not go undetected. One of the drawbacks of MRI, particularly in older patients, is its inability to visualize calcium within the wall of a PDA, a finding that may have surgical implications. CT, with its great ability to detect calcium, is better suited to characterize the wall of a PDA if calcium is suspected.

Atrioventricular Canal This spectrum of malformations is also referred to as endocardial cushion defects, because they affect structures derived from the embryologic

endocardial cushion, which includes the atrioventricular septum and portions of both atrioventricular valves, mainly the septal leaflets. This is the most common clinically diagnosed cardiac anomaly in Down's syndrome.

Anomalous development of the endocardial cushion produces a spectrum of abnormalities of the atrioventricular septum, including ostium primum ASD, high VSD, and a common atrioventricular canal, as well as associated anomalies of the mitral and tricuspid valves (clefts).

The radiologic findings depend on the complexity of the malformation. An isolated ostium primum defect has similar physiology to an ostium secundum ASD, that is, a left-to-right shunt, although mitral insufficiency may also be present. The heart size may be normal or only mildly enlarged, and if chamber assessment is possible, right atrial and ventricular enlargement can be seen. As with any left-to-right shunt, the presence of shunt vascularity depends on the amount of blood overcirculation.

A complete atrioventricular canal is characterized by a large interventricular communication and thus is commonly symptomatic in early infancy, usually during the first year of life. These infants may have radiographic evidence of concomitant congestive heart failure. There is moderate to marked cardiomegaly, with significant enlargement of the right atrium determined by both left atrium to right atrium and left ventricle to right atrium shunting. These patients may have a prominent left atrium due to associated mitral insufficiency as a result of a cleft anterior mitral valve leaflet. Pulmonary artery enlargement and pulmonary plethora are present.

Additional thoracic abnormalities may be seen in cases with associated trisomy 21, including a second manubrial ossification center and 11 pairs or ribs. If these findings are seen in conjunction with a large left-to-right shunt, an atrioventricular canal must be suspected.

MRI, particularly with the addition of GRE images, can be utilized in selected cases in which (due to the inability to obtain a proper echocardiographic acoustic window because of chest deformities, scar, or associated lung hyperinflation) additional information is needed for further characterization of the anatomy of the defect as well as the presence and quantification of mitral regurgitation.

Cyanotic Anomalies with Decreased Pulmonary Blood Flow

Tetralogy of Fallot Tetralogy of Fallot (ToF) constitutes the most common congenital cyanotic heart malformation of childhood. The hallmarks of this anomaly include 1) severe right ventricular outflow hypoplasia and obstruction, 2) large perimembranous VSD, 3) overriding aorta, and 4) right ventricular hypertrophy. The two main components that determine the physiology, and thus the radiologic findings, are the right ventricular outflow obstruction and the subaortic VSD. As the severity of the right infundibular obstruction increases so does the right-to-left shunt, thus increasing cyanosis.

The malalignment or anterior displacement of the ventricular septum is the initial determinant of the infundibular stenosis, although frequently the degree of right ventricular outflow obstruction is compounded by associated stenosis of the pulmonic valve, pulmonary trunk, right or left pulmonary arteries, or peripheral pulmonary vessels.

In most cases the heart size is within normal limits. However, there is evidence of right ventricular dilation and hypertrophy. On the PA film there is uplifting of the cardiac apex, and the left heart border has a more rounded appearance than usual. This is due to counterclockwise rotation of the heart and posterior displacement of the left ventricle induced by right ventricular enlargement. On lateral views, there is increased contact between the heart and the anterior chest wall. Right infundibular stenosis manifests as an absent or concave main pulmonary artery segment. The combination of a diminutive or absent pulmonary artery and an uplifted cardiac apex leads to the characteristic boot-shaped heart (Fig. 3–8)

The size and number of visible central and peripheral pulmonary vessels is determined by the amount of blood entering the pulmonary vascular bed, either directly through the right infundibulum or indirectly via systemic collaterals. The presence of collateral bronchial circulation is associated with severe pulmonic stenosis or atresia and can be recognized as unusually shaped pulmonary parenchymal vessels with a disorganized branching pattern. This may even mimic interstitial lung disease and be a cause of rib

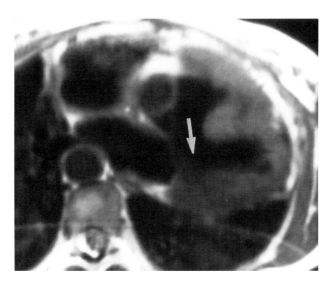

FIGURE 3–9.   Axial MRI SE image of an infant with Tetralogy of Fallot. Severe right ventricular hypertrophy and a subaortic VSD (arrow) are clearly depicted. Note right-sided aorta.

notching in older children. These are radiographically evident in only a minority of ToF patients, less than 5%.

Most frequently, the pulmonary vascularity is diminished, with diffuse decrease in caliber of the parenchymal arterial branches. This may be an asymmetric finding either because of superimposed pulmonary branch stenosis (usually the left pulmonary artery) or because of a previous palliative shunt into one pulmonary artery.

A right aortic arch is present in 25%–40% of patients with ToF. Most of these cases have mirror image branching of the supraaortic vessels. The aortic root is anteriorly positioned due to lack of support from a malaligned crista supraventricularis and thus is overriding the VSD. This leads to dilation of the ascending aorta secondary to volume overload from the sum of the pulmonary venous return and a significant portion of the systemic return that is shunted through the large VSD.

Although echocardiography is generally sufficient in the noninvasive evalution of ToF, MRI has proved very useful: not only does it help to clarify the intracardiac anatomy (Fig. 3–9), but, more importantly, it can serve as adjunct in the evaluation of the size and branching pattern of the pulmonary arteries for surgical mapping. GRE images obtained in multiple planes can exclude the presence of peripheral stenosis and determine the confluence of the right and left branches as well as the presence, location, and size of bronchial collaterals, information that may be crucial for proper surgical planning. The use of gadolinium helps to depict the vasculature in better detail, obviating the need for traditional angiographic studies (Fig. 3–10). In infants who

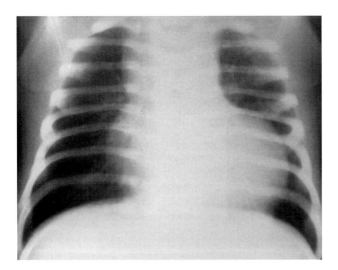

FIGURE 3–8.   Tetralogy of Fallot. Frontal radiograph of a 6-month-old patient with cyanosis. The pulmonary vascularity is diminished, and the pulmonary outflow tract appears concave. In addition, some uplifting of the cardiac apex is suggested.

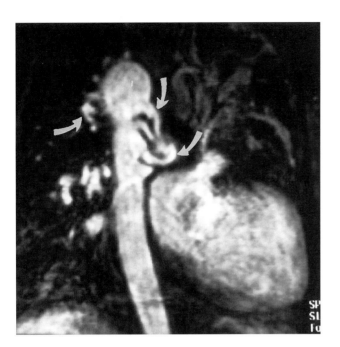

FIGURE 3–10. Thoracic MRA with Gd demonstrating multiple large bronchial collaterals (arrows) feeding pulmonary circulation in another patient with severe infundibular stenosis.

have respiratory distress (and if adequate sedation is not advisable, thus precluding MRI), helical CT can be performed more quickly, usually only requiring restraint for a few minutes and providing similar anatomic information. Contrast-enhanced helical CT can be as accurate as angiocardiography in revealing aortopulmonary collaterals and stenotic or nonconfluent pulmonary branches. In addition, the patency of palliative shunts as well as definitive repair can also be evaluated with helical CT (Fig. 3–11). In summary, whether as a complementary tool or as a definitive means of diagnosis, these two cross-sectional methods can be applied very effectively in patients with right-sided obstructive lesions in which precise pulmonary arterial anatomy is required.

Pulmonic Atresia with Ventricular Septal Defect
This malformation forms part of a spectrum of anomalies in which the pulmonary vascular system is disconnected from the right ventricle. No forward blood flow is possible between the right ventricular chamber and the main pulmonary artery. When a VSD is present, the entire cardiac output exits through the aortic valve into the thoracic aorta. This abnormality may be considered a severe form of ToF. It is also known as pseudotruncus.

These patients usually have a hypoplastic or absent main pulmonary segment with associated abnormalities of the left and right pulmonary arteries and intraparenchymal branches, producing a complex pattern of pulmonary

arterial arborization. The blood flow reaches the lung either by a PDA or aortopulmonary collaterals. If they are predominantly ductus dependent, these infants may become severely symptomatic upon ductus closure. If the child survives the first months of life, there is gradual enlargement of collaterals, usually originating from the descending aorta and connecting with the pulmonary arteries at the hila.

The radiographic findings mimic ToF (Fig. 3–12). The heart size is usually normal overall, with signs of right ventricular enlargement, including uplifting of the cardiac apex. The main pulmonary artery segment is absent, and the hilar vessels are diminutive. The lungs appear severely underperfused, but this may be an asymmetric finding due to unequal development between the right and left pulmonary artery and the presence of large systemic to pulmonary artery collaterals. This is a distinguishing feature from ToF, which presents with a much more homogeneous decrease in size and number of visible pulmonary parenchymal vessels. If aortopulmonary collaterals are prominent, their large caliber and disorganized branching pattern may occasionally give the lung a plethoric appearance.

The ascending aorta is prominent in pulmonic stenosis with VSD since all the systemic and venous return exits the heart through the aortic root. The incidence of right aortic arch is greater than in ToF, present in one-third to one-half of cases.

Similarly to ToF, MRI can be crucial in the evaluation of the pulmonary arteries to determine size and continuity and to identify number and size of bronchial collaterals. As before, the use of Gd can dramatically improve the visualization of smaller vascular structures not well seen on SE or GRE images.

Ebstein's Anomaly   An inferior displacement of the effective tricuspid annulus is the embryologic culprit in the origin of Ebstein's malformation. The malposition of the tricuspid ring is associated with redundancy of the tricuspid valvular apparatus and adherence to the proximal right ventricular wall. The inflow portion of the right ventricle thus presents with altered architecture and is described as "atrialized," leading to a decrease in size of an inferiorly located functional right ventricular chamber. The hemodynamic consequence of this altered anatomic configuration is tricuspid regurgitation accentuated by the decreased right ventricular myocardial contractility. The morphologic end result is right atrial and right ventricular enlargement. A patent foramen ovale is usually present.

The classic hemodynamic features described above may vary widely, depending on the severity of tricuspid regurgitation, the amount of functional right myocardium, and the presence and size of the ASD. Newborns with the obstructive form of Ebstein's malformation usually present early with severe cyanosis, massive cardiomegaly due to right atrial enlargement, and marked decrease in pulmonary blood flow.

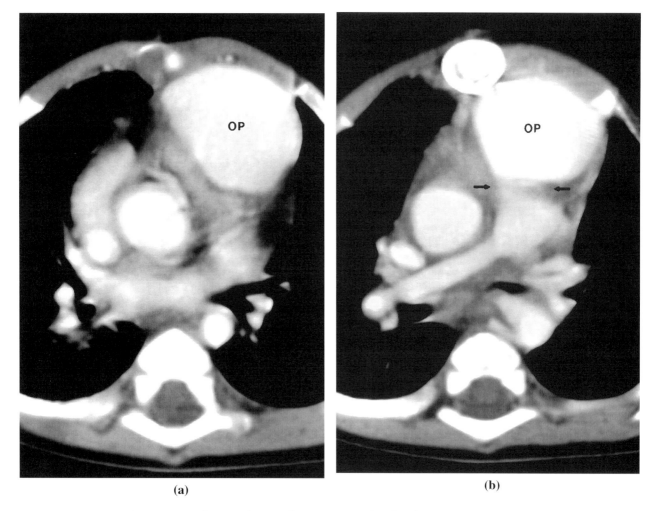

(a)   (b)

FIGURE 3–11.   Contrast-enhanced CT of a patient who had
recently undergone total repair of a ToF. Note large outflow patch
(OP) (*a*); at a higher level (*b*), the distal anastomotic site to the
pulmonary artery can be seen (arrows).

Patients with the nonobstructive form of Ebstein's
anomaly may have minimal symptoms and present in late
childhood. The classic radiographic feature is massive cardiomegaly, with a globular configuration of the heart. This is
also referred to as "box-like" or "funnel-like" cardiomegaly.
There is increased curvature of the right heart contour reflecting right atrial enlargement, and rotation of the heart
into the left chest secondary to right ventricular dilation.
There is an increased zone of contact between the anterior
heart border and the sternum on the lateral projection, with
posterior displacement of the left ventricle toward the spine
due to right ventricular dilation. The main pulmonary artery
segment is small and may be concave. The pulmonary vascularity may be normal or decreased, depending on the size
of the right-to-left shunt through the ASD (Fig. 3–13).

MRI has been used in a complementary role in the
evaluation of Ebstein's anomaly, particularly with the use
of GRE images that can depict the displaced, sometimes

tethered tricuspid valve as well as tricuspid insufficiency.
Phase-contrast images can be used to determine the regurgitant fraction across the tricuspid valve.

Cyanotic Anomalies with Increased Pulmonary Blood Flow

*Transposition of the Great Arteries   Complete trans-
position of the great vessels,* also known as *D*-transposition
of the great arteries (*D*-TGV), is the most common anomaly
in the group of cardiac malformations characterized by a
discordant ventriculoarterial connection. It has a marked
male predominance and is the most common congenital
heart disease to manifest with cyanosis in the first 24 hours
of life.

With *D*-TGV, the systemic and pulmonary circulations
are in parallel rather than in series. This is secondary to
discordant connection between the ventricles and the great

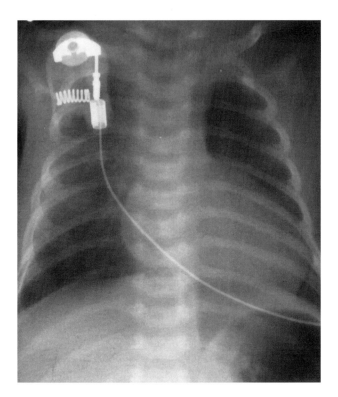

FIGURE 3–12. Frontal chest radiograph of newborn with pulmonary atresia and intact ventricular septum. Note decreased pulmonary vascularity and cardiomegaly.

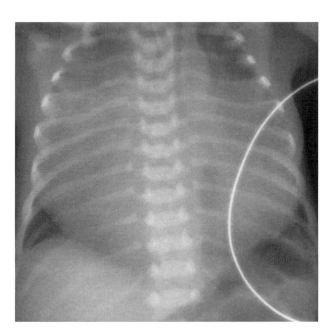

FIGURE 3–13. Ebstein's malformation. Severe cardiomegaly and diminished vascularity are readily evident on this frontal radiograph of a newborn with severe cyanosis.

arteries so that the aorta arises totally or predominantly from the right ventricle, and the pulmonary artery arises completely or in large part from the left ventricle. An obligatory connection between both circuits, including a patent foramen ovale, ASD, VSD, PDA, or systemic collaterals to the pulmonary arteries, must be present for this malformation to be compatible with life. A combination of these may be present.

Radiographically, *D*-TGA has been grouped with congential cardiac lesions presenting with increased pulmonary flow. For historical reasons it will be included in this section of anomalies; however, due to surgical repair in the first weeks of life, this is now rarely seen. Pulmonary blood flow is most frequently normal, and the appearance of pulmonary plethora may actually represent congestive heart failure due to elevated left atrial pressures.

Classic roentgenographic findings in *D*-TGV are seen in less than half of cases. It is important to note that a normal chest radiograph does not exclude the diagnosis. The abnormal arrangement of the great vessels, with the aortic root most frequently located anterior and to the right of the main pulmonary trunk, combined with a decrease in size of the thymic shadow in hypoxemic patients, produces narrowing of the superior mediastinum. This narrow mediastinal pedicle produces a configuration of the heart that has been described as an "egg-on-its-side" or "egg-on-a-string." There is lack of visualization of the main pulmonary artery segment and the abnormally oriented aortic arch on the left. Finally, the spatial orientation between the left ventricle and the main pulmonary artery produces an apparent asymmetry in pulmonary blood flow, with the right pulmonary artery being larger and slightly higher than the left.

As noted, these findings may be quite variable depending on the age of presentation and associated lesions. Pulmonary blood flow may be decreased, normal, or increased (if there is a large VSD with no associated pulmonic stenosis). The vascular pedicle is typically narrow, but, depending on the orientation of the great vessels, it may appear normal. Palliative surgery such as an atrial septostomy may improve oxygenation and account for regrowth of thymic tissue, which can mask a narrow pedicle.

Patients with *congenitally corrected transposition* of the great arteries or *L*-TGV have a functionally corrected anomaly. In addition to transposition of the great vessels, there is inversion of the ventricles with the morphologic left ventricle on the right side and the morphologic right ventricle on the left side. The ventriculoarterial discordance is balanced by the simultaneous presence of atrioventricular discordance. Infrequenlty this anomaly is isolated, and patients remain asymptomatic. Most commonly there are associated lesions that lead to symptoms in the first year of life, most frequently VSD and pulmonic stenosis. Other associated anomalies include left atrioventricular valve insufficiency and heterotaxy syndromes.

The classic radiographic findings include dextrocardia with normal atrial situs and an abnormal convexity along the left upper heart border, explained by the malposition of the ascending aorta. The pulmonary trunk is usually inapparent since it is located posterior to and to the right of the aortic root. In about a third of cases the ascending aorta is obscured by other mediastinal structures and cannot be completely outlined. The heart size and pulmonary vascularity are variable depending on the presence and size of a VSD and right ventricular outflow tract obstruction.

Transposition complexes and the ventriculoarterial relationship in regard to ventricular morphology, location, and the presence/absence of a VSD (and its relationship to the respective semilunar valves) can be adequately evaluated with MRI due to its noninvasive nature and multiplanar capabilities. MRI and CT have been found helpful in postoperative patients (Mustard, Senning, Switch operations) in which suspected complications can be evaluated in a noninvasive fashion (Fig. 3–14). The intrinsic advantage of MRI over CT is its superior ability to detect flow abnormalities, particularly in the different portions of the intraatrial baffle. This feature allows depiction of leaks or stenosis.

Tricuspid Atresia   Tricuspid atresia (TA) corresponds to a group of malformations in which there is no antegrade

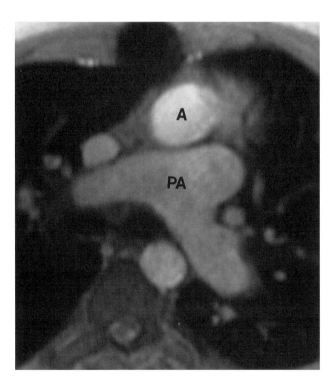

FIGURE 3–14. Axial cine MR image of a patient with *D*-transposition of the great vessels status post Senning repair. Note ascending aorta (A) anterior and to the right of the pulmonary artery (PA).

filling of the right ventricle from the right atrium due to agenesis of the tricuspid valve. It is frequently associated with a hypoplastic right ventricle. In most cases there is a normal atrioventricular connection. As ASD, either a patent foramen ovale (80%), an ostium secundum, or an ostium primum, must be present for blood to flow toward the left side of the heart. The cardiac output then reaches the pulmonary vascular tree through either a VSD or a PDA. Approximately 70% to 75% of patients with TA have a normal ventriculoarterial connection. Thus, in most cases, although a VSD is frequently present, the pulmonary blood flow is almost always decreased, due to hypoplasia of the right ventricle and outflow tract. The exception includes the 20% of patients with a discordant ventriculoarterial connection (complete or *D*-TGV), in which the left ventricle connects with the pulmonary artery and most of the cardiac output enters the pulmonary circulation directly. These patients have a clinical behavior similar to that of patients with TGA. In rare cases of patients with normally positioned great vessels, the VSD may be large enough to produce shunt vascularity if the right ventricular hypoplasia is not severe. In summary, the physiologic and radiographic findings in TA depend on the relationship of the great arteries with the ventricles, the presence and size of the VSD, and the status of the pulmonic valve.

In cases with normal ventriculoarterial connections, the heart size is usually normal. As the left ventricle sustains both systemic and pulmonic flow (via either a VSD, a PDA, or systemic to pulmonic collaterals), left ventricular dilation and/or hypertrophy ensues, with increased convexity of the left heart border and an elevated apex. There is variable enlargement of the right and left atrium. The hypoplastic pulmonary artery is not identified, and this is expressed as a flat or concave main pulmonary artery segment along the left heart border. The lung is oligemic, with decreased caliber and number of parenchymal pulmonary vessels.

The presence of decreased lung vascularity, overall normal-sized heart, small or absent pulmonary artery, and prominence of the left heart contour in a cyanotic patient are overlapping features between cases of TA and ToF. In infants, when precise chamber assessment is difficult, clinical and ECG findings usually orient toward the correct diagnosis, as TA patients frequently present with cyanosis in the immediate postnatal period, with associated signs of left ventricular overload on ECG. In older patients, chamber evaluation is useful. In ToF cases, the left heart border is usually more rounded, and there are signs of right ventricular enlargement on the lateral film. Patients with TA have normal contact between the right ventricle and the sternum, with dorsal displacement of the lower posterior cardiac contour on the lateral film, signaling left ventricular enlargement. Cross-sectional imaging, whether MRI or CT, can demonstrate not only the absence of the right atrioventricular valve, but also the presence of abundant fat in the right atrioventricular groove (Fig. 3–15).

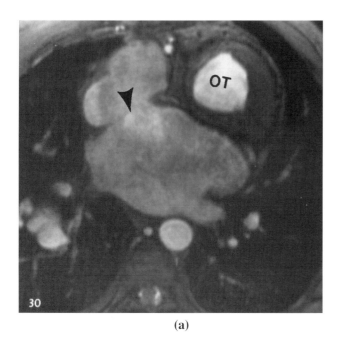

(a)

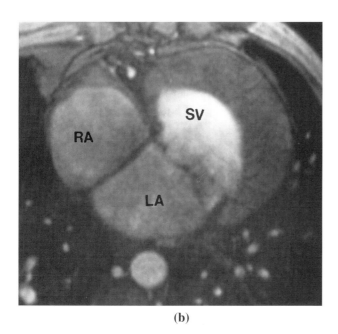

(b)

FIGURE 3–15. Tricuspid atresia and univentricular heart. (*a*) A large interatrial communication is seen (arrowhead) on this axial cine MR image. A single muscular infundibulum (OT) is seen anteriorly. (*b*) At a lower level, the atretic tricuspid orifice is evident in front of the right atrium (RA). Note single atrioventricular valve separating left atrium (LA) from univentricular chamber (SV).

Single Ventricle This malformation, which is also referred to as univentricular heart, is a rare anomaly in which both atria connect with only one ventricular chamber. There is variability in the number of atrioventricular valves connecting with the ventricular cavity as well as the ventricular morphology itself. The most common variant is a single ventricle with left ventricular configuration and an associated rudimentary right ventricle located anteriorly. There is almost always a VSD connecting the main and rudimentary ventricular chambers. These patients usually have a discordant ventriculoarterial connection, and thus the dominant left ventricle supports the pulmonary artery and the rudimentary right ventricle the aorta.

The radiographic findings are quite variable due to the spectrum of abnormalities and the associated lesions, including pulmonic stenosis. Patients without pulmonic stenosis demonstrate cardiomegaly, enlarged central pulmonary arteries, and increased lung vascularity. These patients usually present in early infancy with cyanosis and clinical evidence of congestive heart failure. When stenosis of the main pulmonary artery is present, there is preferential flow through the aorta with decreased lung vascularity, mimicking severe ToF. In selected cases, MRI can be provide additional valuable anatomic detail (Fig. 3–15*b*).

Truncus Arteriosus In this uncommon anomaly the cardiac output passes through a single ventriculoarterial valve into a common vascular channel, the truncus, which then gives origin to the aorta and pulmonary arteries in various arrangements. Thus there is only one great artery originating from the heart that supplies the systemic, coronary, and pulmonary circulations. There is always a large VSD. Due to the relatively large pressure gradient between the high-resistance systemic vascular bed and the low-resistance pulmonary circuit, there is preferential flow toward the lung, which appears plethoric.

In the most common morphologic variant, there is a small pulmonic trunk arising posteriorly from the truncus and giving origin to left and right pulmonary arteries (type I). In type II, the pulmonary arteries arise separately from the truncus (there is no main pulmonary artery). *Pseudotruncus* refers to absence of pulmonary arteries, with the pulmonary vascular supply originating from systemic collaterals arising from the descending aorta. A third of patients present with a right aortic arch with mirror image branching (Fig. 3–16).

Clinically, these patients present in early infancy with cyanosis and congestive heart failure. The radiographic signs include cardiomegaly and increased or shunt vascularity. The association with a right aortic arch suggests the diagnosis. A prominent truncus or ascending aorta may be noted as well as an enlarged left atrium when chamber assessment is possible. In older patients, signs of reactive pulmonary hypertension may be seen, with discordance in the

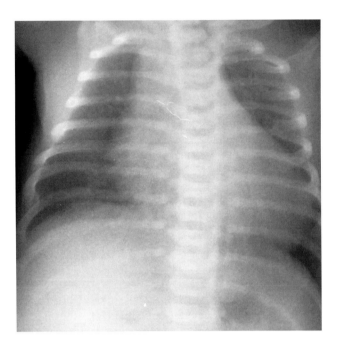

FIGURE 3–16. Truncus arteriosus. Frontal chest radiograph demonstrating cardiomegaly, increased pulmonary vascularity, and right paraspinal density representing a right aortic arch.

size of enlarged central pulmonary vessels and diminutive parenchymal vascular channels.

As in other cyanotic congenital heart defects, the noninvasive combination of two-dimensional echocardiography and MRI can be helpful, particularly when additional information regarding ventriculoarterial connections is needed.

Total Anomalous Pulmonary Venous Return   This anomaly is present when there is agenesis or underdevelopment of the embryologic common pulmonary vein. The pulmonary veins connect with other venous structures that normally form part of the systemic venous return system such as the superior vena cava (SVC), azygos vein, right atrium, or umbilical vitelline system.

Depending on the site of connection between the pulmonary common channel and the systemic vessel or chamber, total anomalous pulmonary venous return (TAPVR) is divided into four types; the most common (50%) is the supracardiac or type I, in which pulmonary venous return converges into a paramediastinal left vertical vein. This vascular channel drains into the left brachiocephalic vein and then into the SVC. It is seldom obstructed (less than 10%). In type II TAPVR, the anomalous drainage is into the right atrium or coronary sinus. Type III includes abnormal communication with the portal venous system through a vascular channel that descends behind the left atrium and penetrates the diaphragm to join the portal vein, ductus

venosus, hepatic veins, or IVC. This variant is almost always obstructed, mainly due to constriction at the level of the diaphragmatic hiatus and the increased resistance of the hepatic sinusoids, as well as the length of the anomalous vascular channel. Type IV is a mixed type.

An ASD is needed for survival, and major right-to-left shunting is usually present. The pulmonary overcirculation produces enlarged pulmonary vessels and right cardiac chambers. If there is obstruction to venous return, increased pulmonary hydrostatic pressure is transmitted to the capillary bed, and secondary pulmonary hypertension with pulmonary edema ensues.

The radiographic findings depend on the location of the anomalous draining vein and whether obstruction is present. In TAPVR type I the upper mediastinum is widened due to the presence of an enlarged left vertical vein and a dilated SVC, producing a "snowman" or "figure or eight" configuration of the cardiomediastinal silhouette. On lateral projection a pretracheal density may be observed accounting for the presence of the left vertical vein. The body of the "snowman" is produced by an enlarged right atrium due to volume overload. The right ventricle is also enlarged, as in any moderate to large left-to-right shunt. Increased pulmonary flow is evident as shunt vascularity.

With cardiac-type TAPVR, the radiologic findings mimic a large left-to-right shunt at the atrial level. The anomalous vessel is not seen on chest radiograph.

The vast majority of infracardiac TAPVRs are obstructed. Pulmonary overcirculation is not possible, and thus the cardiac silhouette is normal in size. Severe pulmonary edema due to pulmonary venous hypertension is frequently present. This appearance may simulate hyaline membrane disease. Most patients with TAPVR type III present clinically in the first 24 hours of life with progressive hypoxemia.

Double Outlet Right Ventricle   This is a condition in which more than one and a half of the great vessels (aorta and pulmonary artery) originate from the right ventricle. This condition represents a spectrum of severity, which will depend on the location and relationship of the aorta and pulmonary artery to a VSD, which is typically present.

Plain radiographs are nonspecific, and the appearance will depend on the degree of left-to-right shunt and the presence or absence of pulmonary stenosis. In many cases the radiographic findings will be similar to those described in VSD.

Cross-sectional imaging will help depict the exact location of the vessels as well as the size and relationship of the VSD (Fig. 3–17). The side-by-side relationship of the great vessels to each other as well as their relationship to the VSD can be ascertained effectively. For this purpose, sagittal and coronal images should be prescribed in addition to axial views. As is the case in the evaluation of other shunt lesions, GRE images are important for the

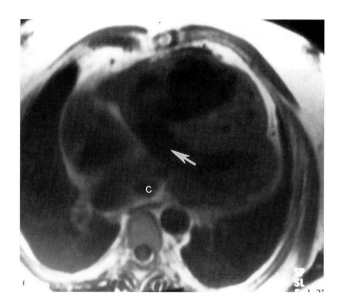

FIGURE 3–17. Type I double outlet right ventricle. A subaortic VSD (arrow) is seen on this axial SE image. Of incidental note is a left-sided superior vena cava (c) as it drains into the coronary sinus.

visualization of flow characteristics as well as to calculate associated valvular stenosis by the presence of "dark jets."

Acyanotic Anomalies with Normal Pulmonary Blood Flow

Coarctation of the Aorta This refers to congenital narrowing of the aorta. The most common type is the adult or postductal variant, which is a short, discrete stenosis at the level of the ductus immediately beyond the origin of the left subclavian artery. These patients are usually asymptomatic but may have upper extremity hypertension. In up to 50% of cases a bicuspid aortic valve may be present. The diffuse type is less common and corresponds to a segmental narrowing between the left subclavian artery and the ductus. Also known as the infantile type, it is frequently associated with intracardiac left-to-right shunts and commonly presents with congestive heart failure in early infancy.

The radiographic findings in infantile coarctation include cardiomegaly and shunt vascularity secondary to left-to-right shunt. Superimposed congestive heart failure and pulmonary edema may be seen if there is a critical stenosis (Fig. 3–18).

The adult-type coarctation is associated with the "classic" radiographic findings. The heart size is usually not enlarged, but a left ventricular configuration exists. The ascending aorta is frequently dilated as well as the transverse portion. The aortic knob, which is the radiologic correlate for the transverse thoracic aorta distal to the subclavian artery, is inconspicuous. A "figure of three" configuration

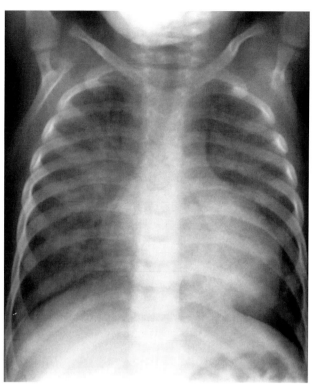

FIGURE 3–18. Frontal chest radiograph of a 2-year-old patient with coarctation of the aorta. Note redistribution of blood flow and bilateral pulmonary edema as evidenced by indistinctness of perihilar vessels and diffuse cardiomegaly.

of the proximal descending aorta may be noted. This is produced by dilation of the origin of the subclavian artery (the upper part of the figure three), the stenotic area of the thoracic aorta (the waist of the figure three), and poststenotic dilation of the descending aorta (the lower part of the figure three). The "reverse three sign" refers to the indentation of these same vessels on the barium esophagogram.

Radiographic signs of arterial collateralization are present in the context of a significant pressure gradient. These include areas of pressure erosion with sclerotic margins in the undersurface of the posterior third through eighth ribs. This is known as rib notching and is explained by dilation of intercostal arteries that serve as a collateral pathway between the internal mammary arteries and the descending aorta distal to the stenosis. The first two intercostal arteries originate from the thyrocervical trunk (which arises from the ascending aorta proximal to the coarctation) and do not function as collaterals. The lowermost intercostal arteries arise from the descending aorta, distal to the stenosis, and thus are not available to serve as collateral vessels. Rib notching is usually seen in children over the age of 6 years and is most frequently bilateral. Unilateral rib notching may be present on the left side if there is an anomalous origin of the right subclavian artery, arising from the poststenotic segment of the aorta. Rarely, rib notching may be confined to the right ribs if the coarctation is proximal to the origin of the left subclavian artery. Associated occlusion or stenosis of either subclavian artery may also account for unilateral rib notching. It is important to remember that rib notching is not specific for coarctation, and that rib erosions can be seen with any process that produces enlargement of the components of the intercostal bundle including veins and nerves (e.g., nerve sheath tumors in neurofibromatosis and venous collaterals in SVC syndrome). The dilated internal mammary arteries, which give rise to the tortuous intercostal collaterals, project as irregular wavy opacities behind the sternum on the lateral chest radiograph.

Both CT and MRI are well suited for the noninvasive evaluation of coarctation of the aorta. MRI has been found effective not only in the initial evaluation of coarctation of the aorta, but also in the follow-up after treatment. To depict all the necessary anatomic details of the lesion, axial images should be complemented with axial and oblique parasagittal views using thin collimation (Fig. 3–19). Additional information about the size of the aortic arch should be included in the study, to exclude the tubular arch hypoplasia sometimes seen in the infantile form of the disease. Although "jetting" across the stenotic area can be used to quantitate degree of obstruction across the lesion on GRE images, other methods have been tested with better results (Fig. 3–20). VEC MRI has recently been utilized to determine the actual pressure gradient across the coarcted segment. This technique, in combination with gadolinium-enhanced studies if necessary for better evaluation of collateral vessels, is a noninvasive alternative to classic angiography in the preoperative evaluation of coarctation of the aorta (Fig. 3–21). In addition, associated bicuspid aortic valve with resultant stenosis can be assessed with the above-mentioned techniques of GRE and VEC and a gradient calculated if necessary.

Pseudocoarctation refers to tortuosity and elongation of the distal aortic arch. The transverse aorta is redundant, which leads to bucking, usually without a stenotic segment and thus without a pressure gradient between the ascending and descending aorta. On the frontal view, a spheroid density or "second aortic arch" can be seen forming the upper left mediastinal contour. No rib notching or other signs of collateralization should be seen in isolated pseudocoarctation.

Aortic Stenosis Congenital aortic stenosis may occur at the valvular, supravalvular, or subvalvular levels. The most common type is valvular, accounting for up to 75% of the total. This occurs most frequently in a bicuspid aortic valve, which is the most common congenital cardiac anomaly. In most cases, this malformation is asymptomatic, although there is increased incidence of significant aortic stenosis in adult life. Up to 50% of all bicuspid valves may

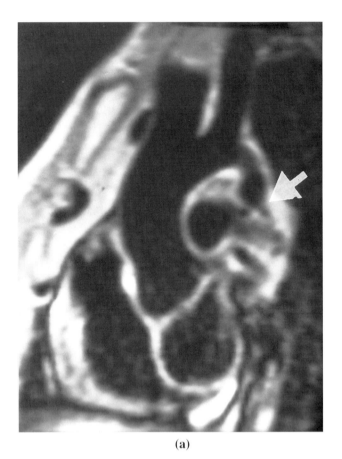

(a)

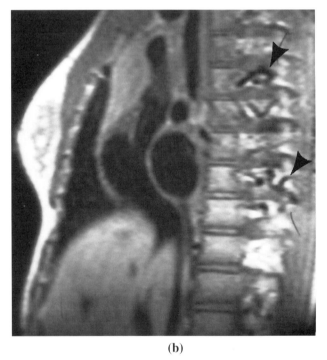

(b)

FIGURE 3–19. (*a*) Left anterior oblique SE MRI sequence of a high-grade aortic coarctation (arrow). (*b*) Image to the right of (*a*) demonstrating abundant paraspinal collateral vessels (arrowheads).

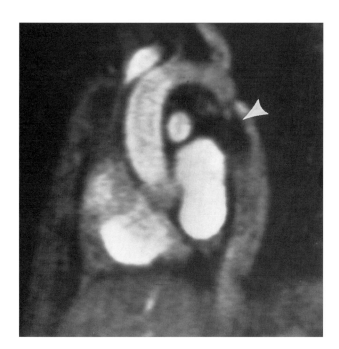

FIGURE 3–20. Left anterior oblique GRE MR image of a high-grade coarctation in another patient showing a jet of flow void (arrowhead) distal to the coarcted segment during systole.

be stenotic by age 40 years. In 10% of cases it will present in early infancy, being referred to as critical aortic stenosis, predominantly affecting boys. It may be associated with coarctation and PDA.

Radiographically, most patients with aortic stenosis have a normal heart appearance. Left ventricular hypertrophy may manifest as uplifting of the cardiac apex on the AP view and posterior displacement of the heart border behind the IVC on the lateral film. As the valvular cross-sectional area decreases, the high-velocity blood "jet" produces poststenotic dilation of the ascending aorta, with a normal transverse and descending aorta (Fig. 3–22). Ascending aorta dilation is usually not present in subvalvular or supravalvular stenosis. Infants with critical stenosis present with congestive heart failure due to acute ventricular dysfunction, and pulmonary edema is the main radiographic finding.

Aortic valve calcification, if present, particularly in older patients, can be readily depicted with CT and poststenotic dilation distal to the valve evaluated. VEC cine MR has the intrinsic advantage of being able to calculate the pressure gradient across the valve, as previously mentioned.

Pulmonary Valvular Stenosis Congenital pulmonary valvular stenosis is a common anomaly, frequently associated with other cardiac abnormalities. When isolated, it is usually due to commisural fusion of the pulmonary cusps. The right ventricle reacts with compensatory concentric

hypertrophy to this outflow obstruction, most patients being mildly to moderately symptomatic.

Valvular pulmonic stenosis should be considered when radiographic findings demonstrate a dilated main pulmonary artery segment with normal pulmonary parenchymal vascularity. These patients have normal pulmonary artery pressure and blood flow. There is poststenotic dilation of the main pulmonary artery and the left pulmonary artery. The right pulmonary artery is usually normal in caliber. This is related to the orientation of the high-velocity blood "jet" through the stenotic valve, which is directed predominantly toward the left side. Unless a critical stenosis is present, pulmonary vascularity is normal. The heart size is frequently normal, although signs of right ventricular enlargement may be seen in severe cases, such as increased convexity of the left heart contour and diminution of the retrosternal clear space.

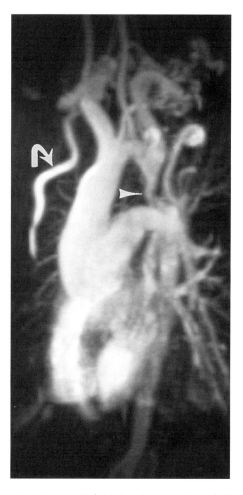

FIGURE 3–21. Gd MRA image in a left anterior oblique projection illustrating severe coarctation of the aorta (arrowhead). Large collateral vessels are also identified, including a large internal mammary vessel (curved arrow).

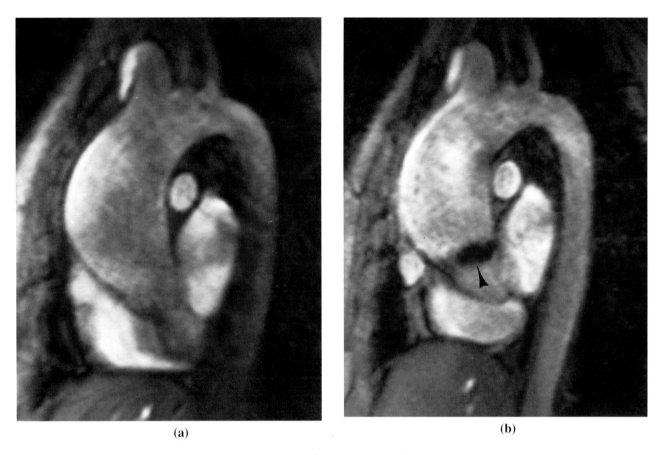

(a)   (b)

FIGURE 3–22a.   Aortic valvular stenosis. Left anterior oblique GRE MR images in diastole (*a*) demonstrating enlargement of the ascending aorta as a result of poststenotic dilation. During systole (*b*), an area of flow void is generated at the level of the valve (arrowhead) as a result of high-velocity turbulent flow.

Although CT can demonstrate enlargement of the main and left pulmonary artery, sparing the right branch, GRE images can provide additional information by demonstrating "jetting" or flow voids across the stenotic valve. Similarly to the application for aortic stenosis, VEC MR can be used to calculate pulmonary valve gradients.

Aortic Arch Anomalies and Vascular Rings

The most common congenital malformation of the aortic arch is a *left aortic arch with an aberrant right subclavian artery*. The right subclavian artery arises distal to the left subclavian artery and crosses the mediastinum toward the right behind the esophagus, producing a characteristic posterior oblique indentation on barium esophagogram. Less frequently, the right subclavian artery may cross between the trachea and the esophagus. The origin of the aberrant vessel may be dilated, producing a structure known as a diverticulum of Kommerell. The vast majority of these patients are asymptomatic, and there is no significant increase in the incidence of associated cardiac malformations.

The most common type of right arch anomaly is a *right aortic arch with an aberrant left subclavian artery,* resulting from interruption of the left arch between the left common carotid and left subclavian artery. It is the second most common cause of vascular ring after a double aortic arch, which is completed by the left ligamentum or ductus arteriosus. It has a higher incidence of intracardiac defects (up to 12%) than the normal population, most commonly ToF and intracardiac septal defects. Although most patients have a complete vascular ring, only a minority of them develop compression symptoms. Radiographic findings include a right impression on the tracheal air column from a right arch, an anterior tracheal indentation on the lateral view, and a posterior impression on the esophagus on barium swallow from the aberrant left subclavian artery. This indentation may be broad if there is a diverticulum at the origin of the aberrant vessel. These findings are identical in cases of a double aortic arch, and MRI, CT, or angiography may be needed to clarify the diagnosis.

The second most common right arch anomaly is a *right aortic arch with mirror image branching.* In the absence of situs inversus, this lesion has a high incidence of associated congenital heart disease, most frequently ToF. This configuration is due to interruption of the embryonic left arch distal to the left ductus arteriosus. The first vessel originating from the arch is the left innominate artery. The right common carotid and right subclavian arteries follow. Chest radiographs demonstrate a right arch and descending aorta. Because there is mirror image branching, no vascular structure crosses the mediastinum, and there are no abnormal impressions on the trachea or esophagus. No vascular ring is present. These patients are almost invariably symptomatic from associated severe cardiac malformations.

The third most common right arch anomaly is a *right aortic arch with an isolated left subclavian artery,* due to double interruption of the arch between the left common carotid and left subclavian arteries and immediately distal to the left ductus. The left subclavian artery is thus separated from the arch and connected to the left pulmonary artery via a ligamentum or ductus arteriosus. This produces a congenital subclavian steal syndrome as the left subclavian artery derives its blood supply from the vertebral artery. Radiographically, a right arch is present, but no retroesophageal component is noted on barium esophagograms. No vascular ring is present. Most of these cases are associated with ToF.

Double aortic arch is the most common cause of a true vascular ring, surrounding both the trachea and the esophagus. Although usually asymptomatic, it is the most common cause of a symptomatic vascular ring, predominantly manifesting with tracheal compression symptoms including stridor, dyspnea, and recurrent pneumonia. Most cases occur in isolation, but congenital cardiac anomalies may coexist. The configuration of the ring depends on many variables including the size and patency of the anterior components (bilateral aortic arches), as well as the location of the common descending aorta. Most commonly the right arch is larger and located more cephalad, crossing posterior to the trachea and esophagus to join the left arch. In 75% of cases the descending aorta is located on the left. The lateral chest film may show anterior bowing of the trachea from the right arch. A smaller anterior tracheal indentation may also be noted. Barium swallow demonstrates that the posterior tracheal impression is actually a large, posterior retroesophageal indentation caused by the right arch. Overall, the radiographic findings are frequently indistinguishable from a right aortic arch with an aberrant left subclavian artery. Cross-sectional imaging may help differentiate between both entities (Fig. 3–23).

Pulmonary sling refers to an anomalous origin of the left pulmonary artery arising from the right pulmonary artery. It does not correspond to an arch anomaly but is included in the causes of symptomatic vascular rings. The left pulmonary artery crosses above the right main stem bronchus and between the trachea and esophagus toward the left hilum. The distal trachea and carina are usually displaced to the left. Airway stenosis or tracheomalacia may occur at the level of vascular compression. Radiologic findings include asymmetric lung inflation, caudad position of the left hilum, and anterior displacement of the lower trachea. Barium esophagogram frequently demonstrates anterior indentation on the midesophagus.

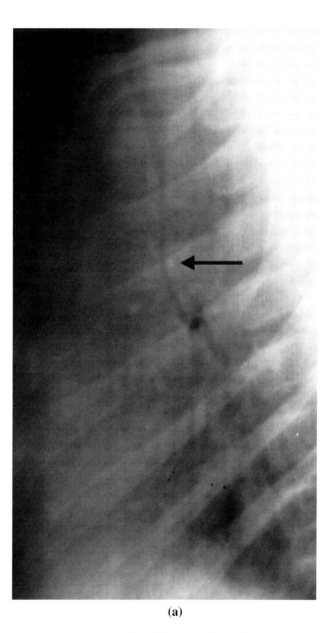

(a)

FIGURE 3–23a. Double aortic arch. (*a*) Lateral chest radiograph shows vascular impression indenting the posterior wall of the trachea (arrow) in this infant with dyspnea. (*b*) Contrast-enhanced CT in another patient with a double aortic arch. Note one arch (R) to the right side of the trachea at a slightly higher level than the left arch (L; right) before coming together as the descending aorta (D).

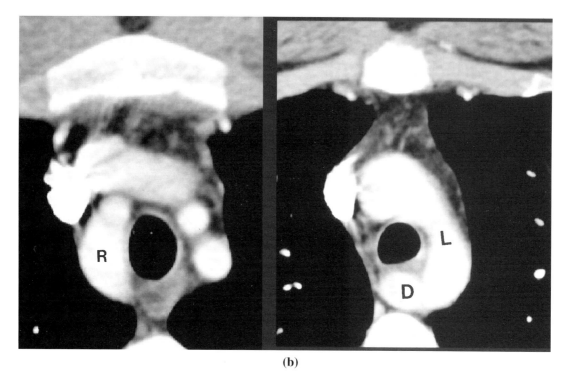

(b)

FIGURE 3–23*b*.   (Continued)

Although the combination of plain films and barium esophagogram is generally sufficient to establish the diagnosis of a vascular ring, cross-sectional imaging can provide additional information regarding vascular branch detail as well as information regarding the lung parenchyma due to airway obstruction. As in other conditions previously described, for those infants with respiratory distress and in whom sedation may pose some risks, CT may be a safer alternative, for it can be performed faster, only requiring infant restraint for a few minutes, rather than the 30 to 45 minutes required for MR scanning.

Suggested Readings

BARON MG. Plain film diagnosis of common cardiac anomalies in the adult. *Radiol Clin North Am* 1999;37:401–420.

BOXERMAN JL, MOSHER TJ, MCVEIGH ER, ATALAR E, LIMA JA, BLUEMKE DA. Advanced MR imaging techniques for evaluation of the heart and great vessels. *Radiographics* 1998;18:543–564.

CROWLEY JJ, OH KS, NEWMAN B, LEDESMA-MEDINA J. Telltale signs of congenital heart disease. *Radiol Clin North Am* 1993;31:573–582.

DE ROOS A, ROEST AA. Evaluation of congenital heart disease by magnetic resonance imaging. *Eur Radiol* 2000;10:2–6.

DIDIER D, RATIB O, LERCH R, FRIEDLI B. Detection and quantification of valvular heart disease with dynamic cardiac MR imaging. *Radiographics* 2000;20:1279–1299.

FAYED LM, BOXT LM. Chest film diagnosis of congenital heart disease. *Semin Roentgenol* 1999;34:228–248.

HOPPE UC, DEDERICHS B, DEUTSCH HJ, THEISSEN P, SCHICHA

H, SECHTEM U. Congenital heart disease in adults and adolescents: comparative value of transthoracic and transesophageal echocardiography and MR imaging. *Radiology* 1996;199:669–677.

KAWANO T, ISHIL M, TAKAGI J, et al. Three-dimensional helical computed tomographic angiography in neonates and infants with complex congenital heart disease. *Am Heart J* 2000;139:654–1660.

KERSTING-SOMMERHOFF BA, SEELOS KC, HARDY C, KONDO C, HIGGINS SS, HIGGINS CB. Evaluation of surgical procedures for cyanotic congenital heart disease by using MR imaging. *AJR* 2000;155:259–266.

REBERGEN SA, NIEZEN RA, HELBING WA, VAN DER WALL EE, DE ROOS A. Cine-gradient echo MR imaging and MR velocity mapping in the evaluation of congenital heart disease. *Radiographics* 1996;16:467–481.

SOTO B, KASSNER EG, BAXLEY WA. *Imaging of Cardiac Disorders. Vol 1: Congenital Disorders.* Philadelphia: JB Lippincott; 1992:69–254.

STARK DD, BRADLEY WG. *Magnetic Resonance Imaging.* 3rd ed. St. Louis: CV Mosby; 1999:257–275.

STRIFE JL, BISSET GS III, BURROWS PE. Cardiovascular system. In: Kirks DR, ed. *Practical Pediatric Imaging. Diagnostic Radiology of Infants and Children.* 3rd ed. Philadelphia: Lippincott-Raven; 1998:511–618.

STRIFE JL, SZE RW. Radiographic evalution of the neonate with congenital heart disease. *Radiol Clin North Am* 1999;37:1093–1107.

WESTRA SJ, HILL JA, ALEJOS JC, GALINDO A, BOECHAT MI, LAKS H. Three-dimensional helical CT of pulmonary arteries in infants and children with congenital heart disease. *AJR* 1999;173:109–115.

CHAPTER 4

Introduction to Echocardiography

David N. Rosenthal, MD

Introduction

Over the past decade, echocardiography has emerged as the premier imaging modality for children with congenital heart disease. Although cardiac catheterization remains the diagnostic gold standard and continues to offer greater accuracy than echocardiography for hemodynamic measurements, echocardiography provides a level of accuracy that is more than sufficient for most clinical settings, and does so noninvasively. With echocardiography, one may obtain precise imaging of the internal cardiac structures and the great vessels, evaluate cardiac performance, and estimate chamber pressures and valve gradients with considerable accuracy. At the same time, the limitations of echocardiography must be acknowledged and understood to make the best use of the technique. The aim of this chapter is to provide the foundation necessary to properly interpret and utilize the information echocardiography can provide.

History

In Sweden in 1954, Edler and Hertz first recorded the motion of cardiac structures (the mitral valve) using ultrasound.[1] In the United States, Joyner and Reid were the first to use ultrasound to examine the heart in 1963.[2] Shortly thereafter, Feigenbaum et al. introduced echocardiography into clinical practice, with the ultrasonic recognition of a pericardial effusion.[3] Tajik and colleagues introduced tomographic imaging of the heart (sector scanning) in 1977.[4] Also in the 1970s, the application of Doppler techniques to cardiac imaging extended echocardiography from a pure imaging modality to one that also allowed hemodynamic measurements. This greatly extended the importance of echocardiography. In the 1980s, transesophageal echocardiography became widespread, bringing echocardiography into the operating room.

Physics and Instrumentation

This section will introduce the reader to certain fundamental principles of ultrasound as it relates to imaging the heart and will also introduce modern imaging equipment. For those whose interests lie elsewhere, this section may be omitted, but an understanding of these principles is often of use for understanding how best to obtain the desired information using ultrasound and how to reconcile conflicting information from diverse imaging techniques.

Clinical ultrasound imaging employs ultrasound in the frequency range of 1 to 12 MHz. The basic principle is that of reflective imaging. The target structure is illuminated by an ultrasound source. Some of the ultrasound waves striking the target are scattered, some are transmitted, and other waves are reflected. The reflected waves are collected and analyzed with respect to timing and intensity. From this information, the target is reconstructed and displayed pictorially. It is important to note that the received signal undergoes extensive processing prior to display, including filtering and differentiating. Thus, despite its pictorial nature, the ultrasound image is not a literal representation of the target.

Reflection of ultrasound occurs at tissue interfaces, with the intensity of reflection proportional to the change in ultrasound transmission between the adjacent structures. For example, the endocardial edge is an excellent ultrasound reflector, since the ultrasound transmissivity of blood and myocardium are quite different. Thus, in echocardiography, the endocardial surface appears as a distinct line. On the other hand, the difference in ultrasound transmissivity between thrombus and myocardium is small, and thus there is usually no such clear distinction between the edge of a thrombus and the myocardial surface. It is also essential for image formation that a structure be sufficiently illuminated by ultrasound to generate a strong reflection. Lung tissue contains many tissue-air interfaces, which are strong ultrasound reflectors and allow little ultrasound to pass. Thus, the distal pulmonary arteries cannot be well visualized by ultrasound, since they are effectively shielded from ultrasound illumination.

All ultrasound imaging is governed by the tradeoff between tissue penetration and image resolution. This situation arises because a reflector must be at least one-fourth the wavelength of the ultrasound beam.[5] Thus, the shorter the wavelength of the ultrasound, the greater the theoretical resolution of the system. On the other hand, tissue penetration is proportional to wavelength. As a practical matter, a frequency of 2 MHz corresponds to a resolution of 1 mm.[5] This issue explains the superior image quality that can be obtained in pediatric imaging, as opposed to adult imaging in which longer wavelengths are generally needed for penetration.

Since ultrasound is a reflective imaging technique, it differs fundamentally from such modalities as angiography, computed tomography, or magnetic resonance imaging. These latter methods gather information based on the volume of the structure being imaged, whereas echocardiographic data emerge from the edges of the structures. For this reason, ultrasound excels in such realms as the visualization of a cardiac valve (which, for imaging purposes, is "pure edge"), whereas it is less efficient in distinguishing normal myocardium from tumor.

In addition to measuring the intensity of the reflected signal to reconstruct an image, it is also possible to measure the ultrasound frequency of the reflected signal. By exploiting the **Doppler effect,** first described by Christian Johann Doppler in 1842, one can calculate the velocity of the ultrasound target. This is the basis of Doppler echocardiography. Doppler echocardiography is typically used to determine the velocity of blood flow at various locations in the heart and vasculature. This is possible because red blood cells are good ultrasound reflectors; it is worthwhile because of the implications of the Bernoulli principle. In its full form, the Bernoulli principle describes the relationship between pressure drop and flow velocity. By using a small number of assumptions, the Bernoulli principle can be used to relate instantaneous blood flow velocity to instantaneous pressure gradient as, for example, in aortic stenosis.[6] The relationship states:

$$\text{pressure (mm Hg)} = 4 \times \text{velocity (m/sec)}^2.$$

Because of this, Doppler has become a routine component of echocardiography, and echocardiography in turn has become a complete physiologic probe rather than just a static imaging tool.

Modern echocardiography equipment combines these two applications of ultrasound into a multimodality imaging tool. From reflected intensity data, an "ice-pick" view of the heart can be constructed, in which one-dimensional spatial information is displayed on the y-axis with time on the x-axis. This is known as **M-mode echocardiography** (Fig. 4–1A). Historically, this was the first cardiac application of ultrasound. It is chiefly of interest today as a means

of estimating cardiac function. By combining multiple scan lines (each of which corresponds to a single "ice-pick"), a two-dimensional image of the heart can be built. These data are displayed in near real time and are known as sector scanning (Fig. 4–1B). This is the fundamental means of viewing cardiac anatomy using echocardiography.

Doppler data can also be collected and analyzed in several ways. Roughly analogous to the one-dimensional nature of M-mode is spectral Doppler. In this modality, the user selects a single region of interest. The velocity information corresponding to this region is displayed as positive and negative velocities displayed on the y-axis, with time displayed on the x-axis (Fig. 4–1C). By convention, positive velocities represent movement toward the transducer, whereas negative velocities are movement away from the transducer. Corresponding to the sector scan is color flow Doppler. In this modality, individual lines of Doppler information are built up into a two-dimensional velocity map. To assist in interpreting this information, the map is displayed superimposed on the sector scan, with each velocity represented by a different color (Fig. 4–1D).

In virtually all modern ultrasound platforms, the send-and-receive functions are combined into a single ultrasound transducer. The transducer consists of multiple related elements that function as a phased array, with software control of beam forming and focusing, steering, and receiving. Most systems operate at multiple frequencies simultaneously in order to obtain a versatile compromise between resolution and penetration. In addition, most systems offer a number of different transducers to choose from, each of which has a different range of frequencies. To optimize image quality, the operator should possess a detailed knowledge of the equipment, as transducer design entails a number of trade-offs between the competing requirements of sector scanning and Doppler scanning. In addition, the system offers a number of user-customizable settings that can have a considerable impact on the image quality. For these reasons, ultrasound imaging is heavily operator dependent, more so than most imaging techniques.

Assessment of Cardiac Anatomy

The fundamental approach to understanding cardiac anatomy from an echocardiographic standpoint is based on the framework of segmental analysis of the cardiac structures, an approach that was popularized by Robert Anderson[7] and Richard Van Praagh.[8] Despite diverse systems of nomenclature, this approach is remarkably consistent across the spectrum of pediatric cardiologists. In its simplest form, segmental analysis is a recognition that all hearts have certain basic components, each of which has certain characteristic elements. Each of the basic components of the heart is identified and named according to its internal structure, rather than by its location. Thus, a right atrium remains a right atrium by virtue of possessing the

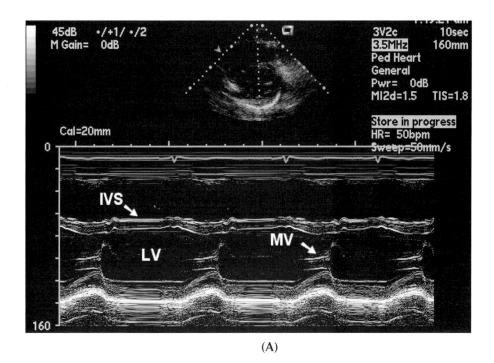

(A)

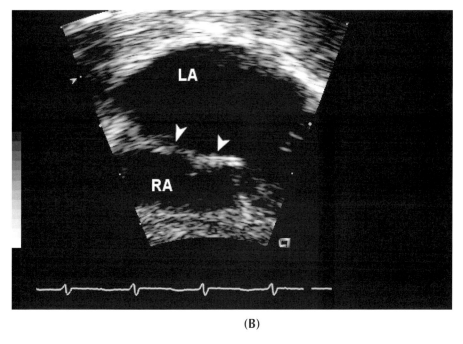

(B)

FIGURE 4–1. *A)* M-mode tracing of left ventricle. The motion of the septum, mitral valve, and left ventricular free wall are visualized in this image, in which time is displayed on the abscissa, and depth on the ordinate axis. The dotted cursor on the reference image depicts the imaging plane. IVS = interventricular septum; LV = left ventricular cavity; MV = mitral valve leaflets. *B)* This is an example of a 2d sector image, which is built up from multiple single scan lines. LA = left atrium; RA = right atrium; arrowheads indicate the atrial septum.

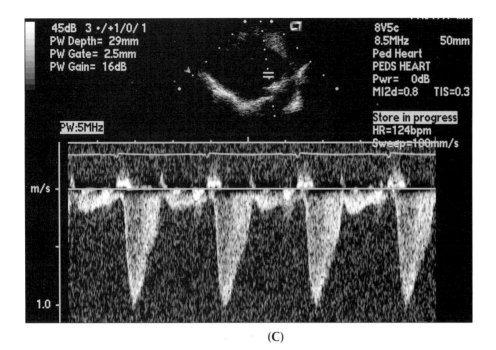

(C)

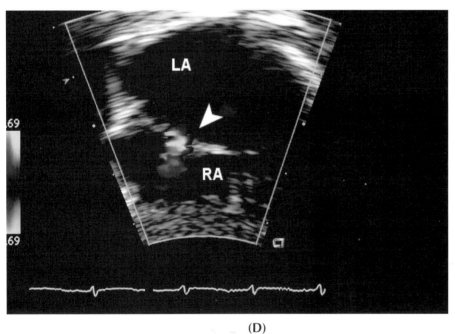

(D)

FIGURE 4–1. (Continued) *C)* In this Doppler image, the abscissa represents time (as it does in Figure 4.1a, the M-mode), and the ordinate demonstrates the velocity of the blood signal at the given timepoint. In this case, the signal is below the baseline, indicating flow away from the ultrasound transducer. *D)* In this image, colorflow mapping is illustrated. In this modality, the instantaneous blood flow velocity is converted to a color scheme (indicated by the color bar at screen left), and superimposed on the 2d scan. LA = left atrium; RA = right atrium; arrowhead indicates flow across the atrial septum.

orifice of the coronary sinus and the mouth of the inferior vena cava, regardless of where it may be found. For a detailed description of the segmental approach to anatomy, the reader is referred to Anderson et al.[7] and Van Praagh.[8] Echocardiography lends itself well to the segmental approach, because of its ability to demonstrate internal cardiac landmarks clearly. The mainstay of echocardiographic assessment of cardiac anatomy is the two-dimensional sector scan, with further contributions from color flow mapping.

For transthoracic echocardiography, a number of standard windows have been described, each of which has multiple views. Taken together, these constitute a complete echocardiographic evaluation.

The first one is the **subcostal window,** obtained from the abdomen, just below the right costal margin. From this window, a number of views can be obtained (Fig. 4–2). First, a cross section of the abdomen demonstrates the location of the abdominal aorta and inferior vena cava as they cross the diaphragm. Tilting cephalad, a long-axis view of the heart is obtained. This is optimal for evaluation of ventricular morphology and for visualization of the ventricular septum, which is perpendicular to the ultrasound beam from this plane. Shifting the imaging plane to the right demonstrates the atrial septum to good advantage. Together, these views are helpful in assessing the existence of defects of septation. With further anterior angulation, the outflow tracts of both ventricles are seen, first the left and then the right. Additionally, the inflow of the superior vena cava is well visualized. With rotation of the transducer, a coronal imaging plane is defined that shows the right ventricular outflow tract. When the transducer is angulated posteriorly in this plane, the right atrium with inflow from both cavae is displayed.

The second standard window is the **parasternal window,** obtained from the left parasternal location. In the long-axis view of the heart, the imaging plane is aligned along the axis of the heart (Fig. 4–3). With right and inferior angulation, this view demonstrates the anatomy of the tricuspid valve and right atrium as well as the inflow portion of the right ventricle. Angling more posteriorly demonstrates the mitral valve, the body of the left ventricle, and the proximal aorta. Further angulation toward the left brings the pulmonary arteries into view. Rotating the transducer to a perpendicular orientation generates a family of short-axis views. Toward the apex of the heart, the papillary muscles of the left ventricle are seen, and their morphology can be readily assessed. As the transducer is directed more toward the base of the heart, the chordae tendinae come into view, followed by the mitral valve leaflets. Finally, a view of the right ventricle is obtained. Inflow and outflow tracts, including the proximal pulmonary arteries as well as the right ventricular body, can be seen. Furthermore, in this view, the aortic valve is well visualized.

The third standard window is the **apical window** (Fig. 4–4). From the apex of the heart, the four-chamber view can be obtained, demonstrating all four cardiac chambers and showing the architecture of the atrioventricular valves. The morphology of the ventricles can usually be well visualized from this view, and the muscular septum is also easily seen. The atrial septum is remote from the transducer in this view and parallel to the ultrasound beam, so it is not visualized effectively from this window. With anterior angulation, the left ventricular outflow tract comes into view, allowing for assessment of the subaortic region. It is generally difficult to visualize the right ventricular outflow tract from this window.

Finally, the fourth and final window is via the **suprasternal notch.** This window is used to visualize the aortic arch and proximal superior vena cava (Fig. 4–5). With appropriate angulation and transducer manipulation, it is possible to detail the anatomy of the aortic arch accurately, including the proximal head vessels. It is especially important to establish this anatomy from transthoracic echocardiography in those patients who are referred for surgery, as it is often impossible to visualize this area well from intraoperative transesophageal echocardiography.

Using these views, and modifying them as circumstances dictate, an experienced echocardiographer can build up a three-dimensional model of the cardiac anatomy. It is possible to perform a complete segmental analysis of the cardiac connections in the vast majority of patients. In addition, one can assess chamber size, integrity of the atrial and ventricular septa, dimensions of virtually any intracardiac structures, valve leaflet morphology, and size of the great vessels, to name just a few possibilities. Figures 4–6 to 4–8 illustrate several common lesions and their echocardiographic appearances.

It is not always possible to obtain adequate quality transthoracic images. Access to the chest wall may be limited, or acoustic windows may be poor. In these circumstances, it is possible to perform echocardiography via a probe passed into the esophagus (**transesophageal echocardiography** [TEE]). This technique generally provides excellent image quality, particularly of the posterior structures of the heart. However, especially for small children, TEE requires significant sedation and is associated with significant, albeit rare, complications.

Intraoperative TEE is most valuable as an adjunct to cardiac surgery, where it can provide much useful information without interfering with the conduct of surgery. Using TEE, the cardiologist and surgeon can assess the quality of the surgical repair in a timely fashion such that significant residual defects can be corrected while the patient is still in the operating room. Although data have been published concerning the frequency with which TEE provides useful information (i.e., rate of surgical revision), these data are highly specific to the practices of individual centers and may not generalize well. The usefulness of intraoperative TEE ultimately depends on the relationship of the cardiac surgeon and the cardiologist and their ability to communicate effectively.

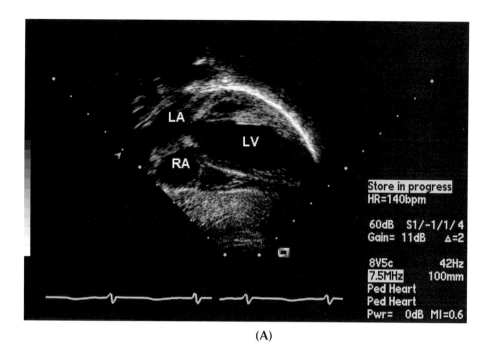

(A)

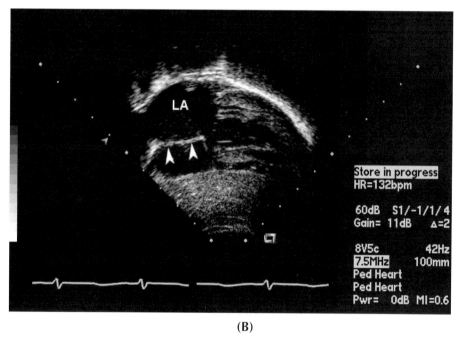

(B)

FIGURE 4–2. Subcostal images are shown, in several common planes. Panel A shows the long axis of the left ventricle to good advantage. Panel B, which is a more rightward plane of insonation, demonstrates the atrial septum and both atria. In Panel C, the imaging plane is more anterior, bringing the superior vena cava and ascending aorta into view. LA = left atrium; RA = right atrium; LV = left ventricle; arrowheads indicate atrial septum; SVC = superior vena cava; Ao = ascending aorta.

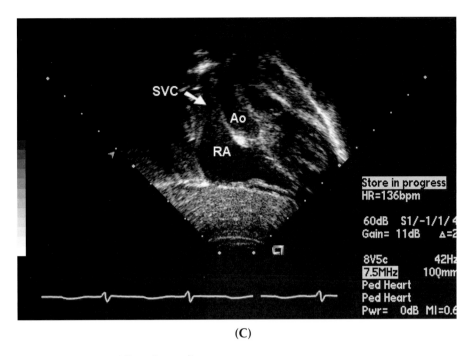

(C)

FIGURE 4–2. (Continued)

Assessment of Cardiac Function

Global cardiac systolic function reflects the interplay of preload, afterload, and contractility.[9] For research purposes, it may be informative to isolate these factors, but for clinical care, it is often sufficient to summarize them in a single index of cardiac function. Echocardiography is uniquely well suited to the measurement of cardiac function because of its noninvasive nature, which makes serial measurements over time feasible. Several different approaches have been developed for measuring ventricular systolic function using echocardiography, the most commonly employed being **fractional shortening** and **ejection fraction.**

Fractional shortening is determined using M-mode echocardiography (Fig. 4–9). It is calculated by the equation: FS = (LVIDD − LVIDS)/LVIDD. The normal values in children range from 0.28 to 0.44.[10] The chief sources of measurement error are likely to be poor alignment of the M-mode cursor along the short axis of the heart and alteration of the ventricular shape. In addition, the measurement varies with afterload, preload, and heart rate. Therefore, this index has theoretical limitations. Nevertheless, fractional shortening has proved to be a useful clinical index.

Ejection fraction can be estimated using two-dimensional echocardiography. A number of algorithms have been devised for this task. The American Society of Echocardiography recommends the use of the modified Simpson's method, which is based on segmentation of the left ventricle into a number of disks and summing the volume of the disks.[11] This technique is superior to M-mode measurements, since fewer assumptions about the shape of the ventricle are made. However, two-dimensional echocardiographic estimations are technically more demanding, requiring high-quality images of the left ventricle with good delineation of the endocardial surface. Studies have shown an acceptable accuracy for echocardiographic estimations of ejection fraction compared with angiography.[12,13]

From a theoretical standpoint, ejection fraction and shortening fraction are confounded by the same issues, so there is no reason to prefer one over the other on this basis. Ejection fraction is more directly comparable to data obtained from magnetic resonance imaging or nuclear imaging techniques, but fractional shortening can be mathematically transformed to ejection fraction for this purpose. Unfortunately, both of these indices are limited to the evaluation of the *left* ventricle because of its simpler geometry. Since the right ventricle has a more complex shape, there are as yet no simple ways to assess right ventricular systolic performance despite its importance in congenital cardiac lesions. A qualitative assessment of the right ventricle is usually all that can be obtained. Additionally, it should be acknowledged that these techniques are limited to the assessment of *systolic* ventricular performance and are not suited for an accurate index of diastolic performance.

Assessment of Valvular Function

With the application of Doppler techniques, it is possible to assess valvular function using echocardiography. It should be stated at the outset that physiologic data should always be correlated to anatomic data as a means of internal validation. In addition, the physical state of the patient can have a significant impact on the results of Doppler evaluation.

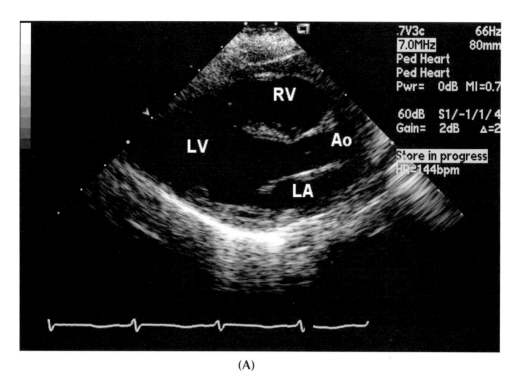

(A)

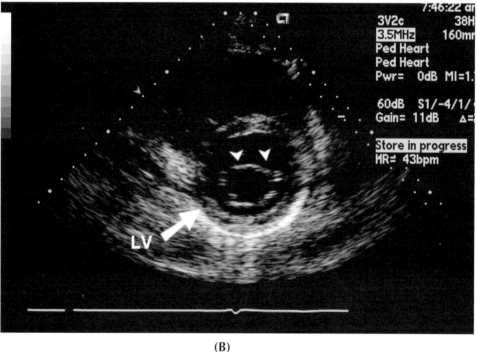

(B)

FIGURE 4–3. This figure illustrates some of the imaging planes which can be obtained from the parasternal window. Panel A is the long axis view of the left ventricle, showing the mitral valve, ascending aorta and a small section of the right ventricle as well. Panel B demonstrates the short axis view of the left ventricle at the level of the mitral valve. LV = left ventricle; RV = right ventricle; Ao = ascending aorta; LA = left atrium; arrow shows left ventricle; arrowheads indicate mitral valve leaflet.

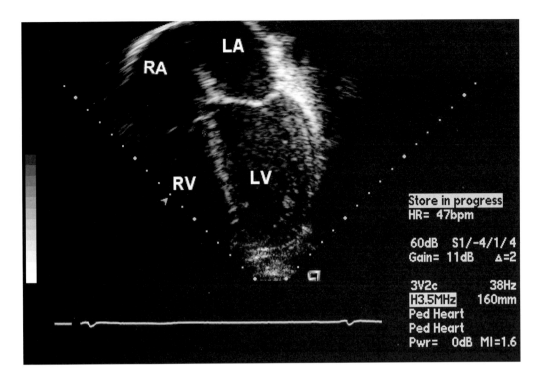

FIGURE 4–4. Apical four-chamber view of the heart is shown. Additional apical views can be obtained with anterior and posterior angulation of the transducer. LA = left atrium; RA = right atrium; LV = left ventricle; RV = right ventricle.

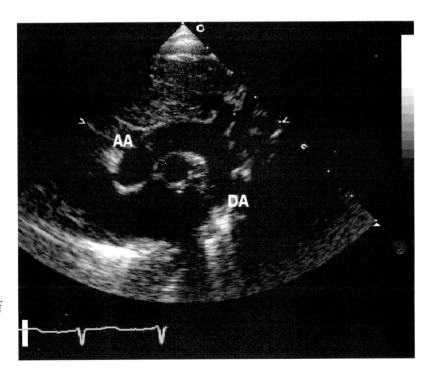

FIGURE 4–5. Example of a suprasternal view. In this case, the transducer is angulated along the plane of the aorta, demonstrating a long segment of the ascending aorta, and aortic arch. AA = ascending aorta; DA = descending aorta.

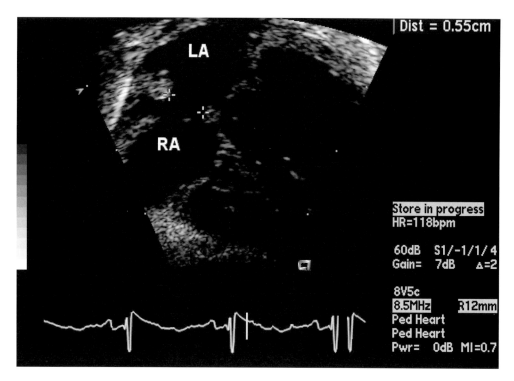

FIGURE 4–6. This parasternal image demonstrates an atrial septal defect, characterized by an absence of the reflection normally caused by the atrial septum. The edges of the defect are indicated by the electronic calipers, applied during the study to estimate the size of the defect. LA = left atrium; RA = right atrium.

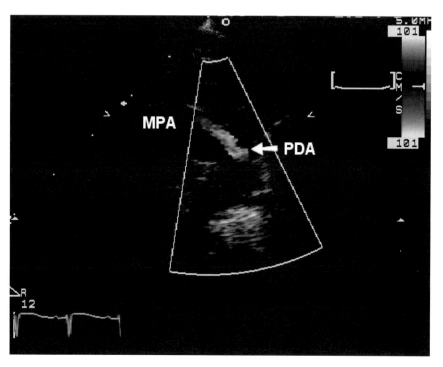

FIGURE 4–7. Echocardiography is commonly employed to detect the presence of a patent ductus arteriosus. In this image, the main pulmonary artery is shown, with color flow mapping illustrating the retrograde flow into the pulmonary artery via the ductus. MPA = main pulmonary artery; PDA = patent ductus arteriosus.

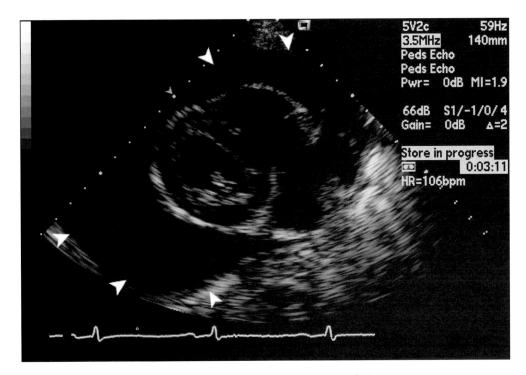

FIGURE 4–8. This 2d image of the heart, obtained from the parasternal window, demonstrates a very large pericardial effusion surrounding the heart. The effusion appears dark since it does not have any ultrasound reflectors. Arrowheads indicate the border of the effusion.

FIGURE 4–9. This tracing illustrates the use of M-mode to measure fractional shortening. The internal dimension of the heart at end-diastole is indicated by LVIDD, and at end-systole by LVIDS. The measurement is easily made, but as discussed in the text, has important limitations.

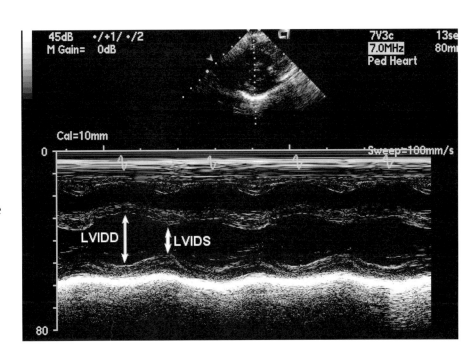

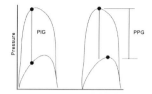

FIGURE 4–10. This diagram illustrates the difference between peak-to-peak pressure gradients (PPG, measured by catheterization), and peak instantaneous pressure gradients (PIG, measured by echocardiography). The two curves represent pressure traces obtained in any 2 sites. Although the PIG and PPG are related, the PIG, shown in the left, can occur at any time in the cardiac cycle and is the moment at which the pressure difference between the two sites is greatest. The PPG, on the other hand, does not actually occur at any point in time, but is created by substracting the peak pressure in one site from that in the other.

Valvular stenosis is assessed using **spectral Doppler.** Most commonly, the mean velocity and peak velocity are measured and converted to pressure equivalents by the application of the Bernoulli equation. Thus, a peak and mean transvalvular gradient can be determined. Physiologically, the mean pressure gradient is the same quantity as the mean pressure gradient measured in the catheterization laboratory. However, the peak pressure gradient measured echocardiographically is the *peak instantaneous pressure gradient,* irrespective of when in the cardiac cycle this occurs. In contrast, the catheterization measurement typically utilized is the *peak-to-peak pressure gradient* (Fig. 4–10). This gradient does not exist physiologically but is a convention that has been correlated to many years of clinical experience; it is therefore considered the gold standard for valvular stenosis estimations. Because these echocardiographic and catheter-based techniques measure different phenomena, the correlation between the two is imperfect. However, numerous clinical studies have confirmed that this correlation is good, so it is rarely necessary to obtain catheterization measurements for diagnostic purposes.

In addition to measuring pressure gradients, the effective valve area can be calculated as a means of estimating the severity of valvular stenosis. This estimation is somewhat more cumbersome but has the advantage of accounting for differences in flow, which do not affect valve area calculations but do alter pressure measurements. The calculation is based on the continuity equation and requires the measurement of transvalvular flow at another site.[14] It correlates very well with catheterization-derived data.

In contrast to the excellent methods available for assessment of valvular stenosis, it is comparatively more difficult to judge the severity of valvular regurgitation. It should be noted that this is true for invasive as well as noninvasive methods. To arrive at a reliable estimation of regurgitation, it is necessary to evaluate diverse data including two-dimensional images, spectral Doppler traces, and color flow mapping.

For aortic insufficiency, the length of the color flow map of the regurgitant jet has been shown to correlate poorly with angiographic assessment of regurgitation, whereas the width or cross-sectional area of the jet correlates better with angiography.[15] The flow pattern in the descending aorta should be examined for evidence of flow reversal (indicative of severe regurgitation). The size of the left ventricle should be evaluated as an indirect indicator of the extent of regurgitation. This latter measure is predictive of postoperative outcome in adult patients. By combining these factors, a semiquantitative determination of the degree of severity can be made.

The evaluation of mitral insufficiency is performed in a similar manner, also incorporating the size of the left atrium into the final determination. For right-sided valves, the process is analogous.

Conclusions

Echocardiography is one of the basic tools used for the assessment of patients with congenital heart disease, providing both anatomic and physiologic data. When properly employed, the echocardiogram should provide definitive management data in the vast majority of patients.

References

1. EDLER I, HERTZ CH. The use of ultrasonic reflectors for the continuous recording of the movements of heart walls. *Kunliga Fysiografiska Saliskapets I Lund Forhandlingar* 1954;24:1–19.

2. JOYNER CR, REID JM. Applications of ultrasound in cardiology and cardiovascular physiology. *Prog Cardiovasc Dis* 1963;5:482–497.

3. FEIGENBAUM H, WALDHAUSEN JA, HYDE LP. Ultrasound diagnosis of pericardial effusion. *JAMA* 1965;191:711–714.

4. TAJIK AJ, SEWARD JB, HAGLER DJ, MAIR DD, LIE JT. Two-dimensional real-time ultrasonic imaging of the heart and great vessels: technique, image orientation, structure identification, and validation. *Mayo Clin Proc* 1978;53:271–303.

5. FEIGENBAUM H. *Echocardiography.* 3rd ed. Philadelphia: Lea & Febiger, 1994:3.

6. HATLE L, ANGELSEN B, TROMSDAL A. Noninvasive assessment of aortic stenosis by Doppler ultrasound. *Br Heart J* 1969;3:284.

7. ANDERSON RH, BECKER AE, FREEDOM RM, et al. Sequential segmental analysis of congenital heart disease. *Pediatr Cardiol* 1984;5:281–287.

8. VAN PRAAGH R. The segmental approach clarified. *Cardiovasc Intervent Radiol* 1984;7:320–325.

9. LLOYD TR, DONNERSTEIN RL. Afterload dependence of echocardiographic left ventricular ejection force determination. *Am J Cardiol* 1991;67:901.

10. GUTGESELL HP, PAQUET M, DUFF DF, et al. Evaluation of left ventricular size and function by echocardiography. Results in normal children. *Circulation* 1977;56:457–462.

11. SCHILLER NB, SHAH PM, CRAWFORD M, et al. Recommendations for quantitation of the left ventricle by two-dimensional echocardiography. *J Am Soc Echocardiogr* 1989;2:358.

12. FOLLAND ED, PARISI AF, MOYNIHAN PR, et al. Assessment of left ventricular ejection fraction and volumes by real-time, two-dimensional echocardiography. A comparison of cineangiographic and radionuclide techniques. *Circulation* 1979;60:760–766.

13. SILVERMAN NH, PORTS TA, SNIDER AR, et al. Determination of left ventricular volume in children: echocardiographic and angiographic comparisons. *Circulation* 1980;62:548–557.

14. SKJAERPE T, HEGRENAES L, HATLE L. Noninvasive estimation of valve area in patients with aortic stenosis by Doppler ultrasound and two-dimensional echocardiography. *Circulation* 1985;72:810–818.

15. PERRY GJ, HELMCKE F, NANDA NC, BYARD C, SOTO B. Evaluation of aortic insufficiency by Doppler color flow mapping. *J Am Coll Cardiol* 1987;9:952–959.

CHAPTER 5

Cardiac Catheterization, Angiography, and Interventional Procedures

Jeffrey A. Feinstein, MD, MPH, and Phillip Moore, MD

Introduction

Cardiac catheterization has long been, and remains today, a critical component in the evaluation and management of children with congenital heart disease. The role of cardiac catheterization, however, has changed dramatically since its initial use in the 1940s. As a result of advances in two-dimensional and color flow Doppler echocardiography and the development of magnetic resonance imaging (MRI), the number of patients requiring cardiac catheterization solely for diagnostic purposes has decreased dramatically. One could therefore reasonably expect a corresponding decrease in the total number of cardiac catheterizations performed yearly. This, however, has not occurred. Concurrent advances in pediatric cardiac surgery enabling palliation and/or definitive repair of previously fatal congenital cardiac defects have dramatically increased the number of children and adults requiring long-term follow-up, including cardiac catheterization. In addition, the development over the last 15 years of transcatheter therapeutic procedures has increased the overall number of patients requiring catheterization; this has changed the case mix so that interventional procedures now account for nearly half of all catheterizations at large centers. Thus catheterization plays a larger and more therapeutic role in the care of children and adults with congenital heart disease.

Indications

The decision to perform a cardiac catheterization is based on a number of ever-changing factors. As recently as the 1960s, cardiac catheterization in newborns was felt to be so risky that some sick infants were sent to surgery without a catheterization in an attempt to improve overall survival. Today cardiac catheterization is very safe, with an associated mortality of <0.5% even in neonates; therefore procedural risk is not a factor in determining whether a catheterization is done.

In general, diagnostic catheterization is needed if the data for a complete diagnosis or clinical decision making are unattainable by noninvasive methods. Because of the advances in echocardiography and magnetic resonance imaging, nowadays diagnostic catheterization is performed most often to assess the structure and physiology of the pulmonary arterial and venous bed, which are poorly assessed noninvasively. The wealth of diagnostic information obtainable during cardiac catheterization is summarized in Table 5–1. In preoperative patients, the surgeon's judgment as to the adequacy of the noninvasive data weighs heavily on the decision to catheterize. Common indications for interventional catheterization include aortic or pulmonary valve stenosis, coarctation of the aorta, collateral vessels, patent ductus arteriosus, and peripheral pulmonary artery stenosis. Sample cardiac catheterization guidelines for diagnostic and interventional procedures are presented in Table 5–2. Obviously these guidelines will vary based on individual/institutional preferences and catheterization resources/therapeutic techniques available.

Precatheterization Assessment and Preparation

Adequate preparation prior to entering the catheterization lab, including a complete history (both cardiac and noncardiac) and physical exam, is crucial to the overall success of the procedure. Details of previous operations and interventional procedures are invaluable for precatheterization planning. Review of previous cardiac catheterization

TABLE 5–1. Information Obtained by Cardiac Catheterization

Anatomy
  Define morphology, position, and relationships of the cardiac segments (systemic and pulmonary
  veins, atria, atrioventricular valves,
  ventricles, outflow tracts, and great vessels)
  Delineate obstructions

Hemodynamics
  Quantitate cardiac output and pulmonary flow (directly by thermodilution or indirectly by Fick method)
  Quantitate intracardiac and extracardiac shunts
  Calculate relative pulmonary/systemic flows (Q_p/Q_s ratio)
  Calculate pulmonary and systemic vascular resistances
  Measure cardiac pressures including obstruction gradients
  Assess cardiac function
  Systolic (pump) function, qualitatively
  Diastolic (relaxation) function, quantitatively (end-diastolic pressure)

Therapeutic trial
  Monitor cardiac or vascular responses to drugs (delivered systemically or locally via inhalation)
  Monitor transcatheter maneuvers simulating postoperative or postinterventional conditions

Other
  Electrophysiologic evaluation (±therapy)
  Endomyocardial biopsy

data and cineangiograms will assist in preparing for the catheterization and will prevent duplication of previous efforts, thereby speeding the procedure and reducing the amount of contrast used.

Usual laboratory studies include hemoglobin, hematocrit, a coagulation profile for patients on anticoagulants, and a urine pregnancy test for females of childbearing age. Additional blood work (for example, a renal panel for patients with preexisting kidney disease) should be obtained as the medical history dictates. Patients undergoing interventional procedures or a transseptal approach to the left atrium or who may need transfusion for other reasons will have a type and cross sent with their precatheterization blood work as well. Diagnostic studies obtained in the precatheterization workup should include an echocardiogram and, depending on the diagnosis, may include an electrocardiogram (ECG), chest x-ray, lung perfusion scan, electron beam computed tomography, or MRI.

Support for the patient during catheterization is determined by the precatheterization assessment of the patient's clinical condition, as well as the type of procedure to be performed. Decisions regarding the need for endotracheal intubation, intravenous (IV) placement, inotropic support, prostaglandin infusion, or anesthesia assistance should all be made long before the patient reaches the catheterization lab.

Premedication, Sedation, and Pain Management

Adequate premedication serves to decrease patient anxiety, facilitate parental separation, comfort the patient, and allow proper positioning and preparation for the catheterization. As a general rule, premedication of neonates and infants is usually accomplished without sedatives or narcotics. IV lines may not be necessary for all diagnostic catheterizations; therefore premedication must sometimes be given orally.

Diphenhydramine is one of the most commonly used premedicating agents because it works not only as a mild sedative but serves to decrease the likelihood of infrequent but serious allergic reactions to contrast. Additional premedication may include chloral hydrate, meperidine HCl compound (meperidine HCl, promethazine HCl, chlorpromazine), pentobarbital, ketamine, or diazepam. Local anesthetic is used before percutaneous access is attempted and consists of topical anesthetic cream (Emla: 2.5% lidocaine and 2.5% prilocaine) applied at the time of premedication followed by injection at the access site (1% lidocaine). Sedation during the procedure is accomplished using a combination of sedative/hypnotic and narcotics tailored to each patient's needs. Pentobarbital, midazolam, fentanyl, and morphine are the most commonly used medications for this purpose. When using these drugs, careful monitoring of the patient's respiratory and hemodynamic status is mandatory. Trained personnel and resuscitation equipment must be available at all times to respond immediately to respiratory or cardiac depression.

The catheterization lab nursing staff can provide monitoring and sedation for most patients. An occasional patient may be difficult to sedate or may require a deeper level of sedation, necessitating airway management by an anesthesiologist with either a laryngeal mask or endotracheal intubation. Endotracheal intubation and general anesthesia serve to provide a secure airway for patients who are critically ill or who are undergoing a high-risk procedure. In addition, children requiring transesophageal echocardiography during interventional procedures will require endotracheal intubation for safety and comfort. In some patients, deep sedation with a continuous infusion of propofol and spontaneous breathing with a laryngeal mask airway may allow more accurate hemodynamic assessment than that afforded by positive pressure ventilation with inhalation anesthesia, which may alter baseline vascular tone and cause myocardial depression.

Vascular Access

It has been said, "Access may be the hardest part of the catheterization procedure." Regardless of the size of the patient or the type of catheterization, great care should be taken to obtain access in the most atraumatic fashion. Minimizing

TABLE 5–2. Indications and Guidelines for Cardiac Catheterization

Lesion	Diagnostic	Interventional
Anomalous pulmonary venous return	Occasionally: delineate venous anatomy or evaluate pulmonary venous obstruction	No
Atrial septal defect	No	Device closure (therapeutic option)
Aortic stenosis (valvar)	Assess peak systolic gradient and aortic regurgitation if noninvasive clinical data do not correlate	Balloon valvuloplasty (treatment of choice)
Coarctation of the aorta	Occasionally: delineate anatomy and presence of collaterals	Balloon dilation ± stenting Native (therapeutic option) Recoarctation (treatment of choice)
Complete AV canal	Occasionally: define additional ventricular septal defects or assess pulmonary hypertension	No
Single ventricle (preshunt/band)	Occasionally: assess pulmonary artery anatomy, pressures, and resistance	No
Single ventricle (pre-Glenn/Fontan)	Yes: assess pulmonary artery anatomy, pressures, and resistance; ventricular end diastolic pressures	Coil embolization of collateral vessels, balloon pulmonary arterioplasty, recoarctation dilation
Hypoplastic left heart syndrome (preoperative)	No	Creation of an unrestrictive interatrial communication
Mitral stenosis	Measure transmitral gradient when contemplating repair	Balloon valvuloplasty
Patent ductus arteriosus	No	Transcatheter closure (treatment of choice in all but premature infants)
Patent foramen ovale	No	Device closure in selected patients (stroke/ transient ischemic attack, cyanotic right-to-left shunt)
Pulmonary atresia/intact ventricular septum	Define right ventricle size, coronary anatomy, pulmonary architecture, collateral anatomy	Occasionally valve performation/ balloon dilation
Pulmonary stenosis (peripheral)	Delineate pulmonary artery anatomy	Balloon angioplasty (treatment of choice)
Pulmonic stenosis (valvar)	No	Balloon valvuloplasty (treatment of choice)
Tetralogy of Fallot (ToF)	Occasionally: define coronary anatomy and peripheral pulmonary artery anatomy	Palliative balloon valvuloplasty (controversial)
Tetralogy of Fallot with pulmonary atresia	Define coronary and pulmonary artery anatomy and evaluate aortopulmonary collaterals	Embolization of collaterals, balloon valvuloplasty, pulmonary artery angioplasty
Transposition of the great arteries	Occasionally: delineate coronary anatomy	Preoperative palliation—balloon atrial septostomy
Ventricular septal defects	Occasionally: assess pulmonary hypertension in older patients	Device closure—muscular ventricular septal defects (investigational therapeutic option)

damage to these vessels is critical because they are often needed for repeat catheterizations and for central lines during or after cardiac surgery. The specific number and site of vessels accessed will be determined by the planned catheter course and specific information needed.

Venous access is nearly always obtained, whereas arterial access is used more stringently, especially in newborns and infants. Venous access may be obtained "from below" (the heart) by using the femoral, umbilical, or hepatic veins to reach the inferior vena cava or "from above" by using the internal jugular or subclavian veins to reach the superior vena cava. In newborns, arterial access is usually via the

femoral or umbilical arteries. In the older infant and child, the femoral arteries are most often used, although in rare instances the brachial or axillary arteries have been used. In nearly all patients, access is obtained percutaneously using a modified Seldinger (i.e., over the wire) technique, although in some rare instances a cutdown approach may be required. Using a beveled needle, the anterior wall of the vessel is punctured, and when blood return is seen, a soft-tipped wire is placed through the needle into the blood vessel. Once the wire is confirmed by fluoroscopy to be in the intended blood vessel, either a catheter or a sheath with a hemostatic valve is placed over the wire into the blood vessel. The wire is then removed. Sheaths are always placed in the vein and are used in the artery if (1) multiple catheter exchanges are expected, (2) simultaneous blood pressure recording with an indwelling catheter is needed or, (3) the operator feels the additional width of the sheath is unlikely to increase the risk of pulse loss.

The umbilical vessels are usually patent up to a week after birth and have the advantage of preserving the femoral vessels. Catheter manipulations from the umbilical vein and artery are often more difficult than those from the femoral approach. In older patients, the femoral vein is the first choice for venous access. For patients who have undergone cavopulmonary anastomosis (the Glenn shunt or hemi-Fontan), additional access via the internal jugular or subclavian vein is required to evaluate the pulmonary arteries. For patients requiring access "from below" who have bilaterally obstructed femoral veins, transhepatic catheterization has now been shown to be safe and effective.[1] The reader is referred elsewhere for step-by-step descriptions on obtaining access for each of the above-mentioned sites.[2]

Catheters and Equipment

Catheters, which are long, thin plastic tubes with one or more holes at the end, come in many sizes, shapes, and materials. In general, there are three categories of catheters based on their structure and function: (1) angiographic, (2) directional, and (3) balloon tipped. All can be used to measure pressures within the heart. Angiographic catheters typically have multiple holes at the tip to allow rapid injection of contrast for angiography. Directional catheters generally have a single end hole and are made out of stiff materials such as woven Dacron to provide excellent torque control (i.e., "steerability"). They come in a variety of preformed shapes to allow manipulation into very tortuous vascular structures. Balloon-tipped catheters have much softer shafts and thus less torque control, but with the balloon inflated they will tend to follow the course of blood flow. Examples of commonly used catheters are shown in Fig. 5–1. Not all catheters are available in all sizes, but commonly used arterial catheters come as small as 3 French; the smallest commonly used venous catheter is 4 French. It should be emphasized that all catheters can be used in both the arterial and venous circulation depending on where the catheter needs to go and what it will be used for once it gets there.

Another important tool used for catheterization is the guidewire. Guidewires come in various sizes and have various properties. Those used for coronary interventions may be as small as 0.010 inches; those commonly used for congenital heart disease are as "large" as 0.038 inches. Guidewires are placed within catheters to improve maneuverability. Standard guidewires have one soft end and one stiff end. On some wires, the soft end is "J" shaped, prevent-

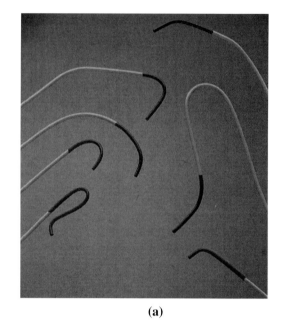

(a)

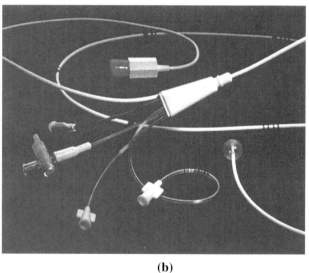

(b)

FIGURE 5–1. Commonly used catheter types. *(a)* Diagnostic catheters are available in a variety of shapes. (Reproduced with permission from Cook, Inc.); *(b)* Balloon tipped, flow-directed catheters may be used for angiography, measurement of pulmonary capillary wedge pressure, or thermodilution cardiac output measurement. A Swan-Ganz catheter is pictured. (Reproduced with permission from B. Braum Medical, Inc.)

ing the end, if advanced without the protection of a catheter, from disrupting the endothelium or perforating the vessel or heart. The ends of these wires can also be shaped by hand to help direct a catheter to the desired destination. "*Torque*" wires, as their name suggests, have very stiff shafts and are highly maneuverable. These wires also have exceedingly soft and floppy distal ends, making their use in probing for chambers or vessels quite safe. *"Tip-deflecting wires"* have a trigger-like handle at the proximal end, which, when pulled, curves the distal end of the wire. The harder the trigger is pulled, the tighter the radius of the curve on the distal end of the wire.

As mentioned above, sheaths are used predominantly to facilitate catheter entry and exchange, which minimizes vessel injury. These sheaths are usually 5 to 11 cm in length. Long sheaths (25 to 90 cm) are now being used with increasing frequency. The most common use for the long sheath is for the transseptal approach to the left heart. With the growth of interventional procedures, long sheaths are now more commonly used for stent implantation, device placement, and to maintain distal access in complicated pulmonary artery dilations. In addition, long sheaths are often placed across the tricuspid valve into the right ventricle to guide the bioptome for endomyocardial biopsies.

Data Collection

As shown in Table 5–1, a great deal of information is available from catheterization. It is therefore imperative to know what information is needed to ensure that a directed and complete catheterization is performed. Data that can be measured directly include cardiac output, intracardiac and intravascular pressures, and oxygen saturations. Data that can be derived include cardiac output (when not measured directly), pulmonary flow, systemic and pulmonary vascular resistances, and quantification of shunts. Interpretation of hemodynamic data is important not only for catheterization lab personnel but for those managing intensive care patients as well. Peripheral and intracardiac lines, often present in intensive care unit patients, provide access to pressure and saturation data that can be used to assess a patient's hemodynamic status to determine the optimal management.

Pressure Measurements

A fluid-filled catheter system connected to a mechanical membrane transducer is the most common system used for measuring intracardiac pressures during catheterization. Intravascular pressure waves are transferred through the fluid column, causing membrane movement that is converted into electrical signals. These signals are sent to a recording device that displays them on a monitor and/or prints them on paper. In newer labs the data are recorded digitally for future reference. The transducer membranes are able to detect small pressure changes with a rapid response time to differentiate the multiple components of the atrial, ventricular, and arterial pressure waves. The attenuation (i.e., magnification) of the waveforms can be altered to allow accurate analysis. When comparing pressure measurements, those that are made simultaneously are considered the "gold standard." Often, simultaneous measurements are not possible or feasible. In that case, pull-back measurements are the next best thing. These measurements are made in very close time proximity and, as the name implies, are obtained as the catheter is pulled back from one chamber to the next. If no pullback data are available, the measurements most closely approximated in time are compared.

When a right heart catheterization is performed, pressures are usually measured in the right atrium, right ventricle, pulmonary arteries, and pulmonary capillary wedge position (PCW), an estimation of left atrial pressure. A catheter in the PCW occludes antegrade flow in the pulmonary artery segment, creating a continuous fluid column from the left atrium through the capillary bed to the catheter tip. This allows transmission of the left atrial pressure to the catheter without directly entering the left atrium. This measurement accurately represents the left atrial pressure only if no obstructions exist between the catheter and the left atrium (i.e., no pulmonary venous obstruction). Assuming no mitral level obstruction exists, the PCW can be an accurate representation of the left ventricular end-diastolic pressure as well. Pressure measurements obtained during a complete left heart catheterization include the left atrium, left ventricle, and ascending and descending aorta. The left heart measurements can either be obtained retrograde via the femoral artery or antegrade via either a pre-existing or a created communication in the atrial septum. Normal pressure measurements in children are shown in Fig. 5–2 and sample pressure tracings in Fig. 5–3.

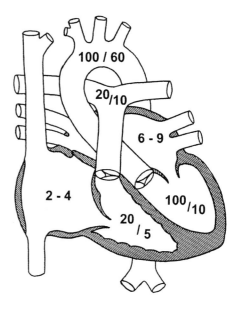

FIGURE 5–2. Normal pressure data in children. Adapted with permission from Congenital Heart Disease: A Diagrammatic Atlas, Mullins CE, Mayer DC, eds. John Wiley & Sons, Inc.

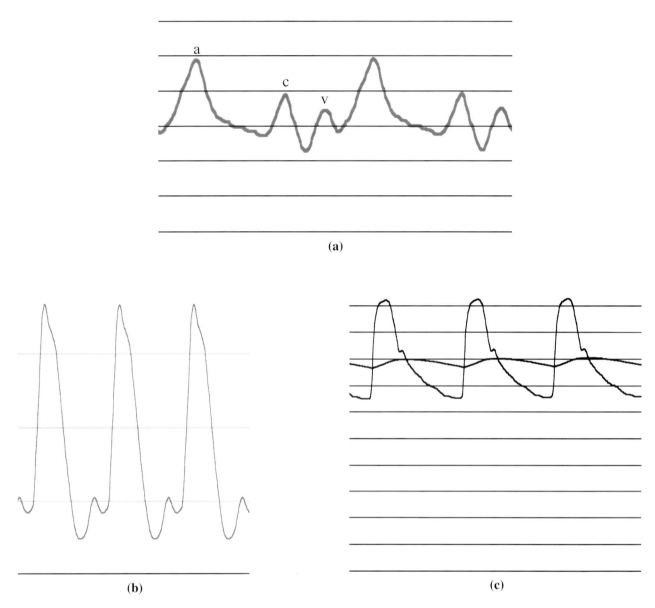

(a)

(b)

(c)

FIGURE 5–3.   Sample pressure tracings. *(a)* Right atrium (with component a, c, and v waves). *(b)* Right ventricle. *(c)* Pulmonary artery. *(d)* Simultaneous pulmonary capillary wedge (approximating left atrium) and left ventricle (with "a wave" approximating the end-diastolic pressure). *(e)* Left ventricle. *(f)* Simultaneous aortic phasic and mean pressures.

The right atrial tracing is composed of three components: the *a* wave, representing atrial contraction, the *c* wave, representing closure of the tricuspid valve, and the *v* wave, caused by atrial filling with a closed tricuspid valve during ventricular systole. The normal mean right atrial pressure is 3 to 5 mm Hg. The right atrial *a* wave is usually

2 to 3 mm Hg higher than the *v* wave, and both are usually <8 to 9 mm Hg.

From the characteristic right ventricular trace, systolic and end-diastolic pressures are obtained. The normal right ventricular systolic pressure is no higher than 30 mm Hg, and the end-diastolic pressure is 5 to 8 mm Hg. During

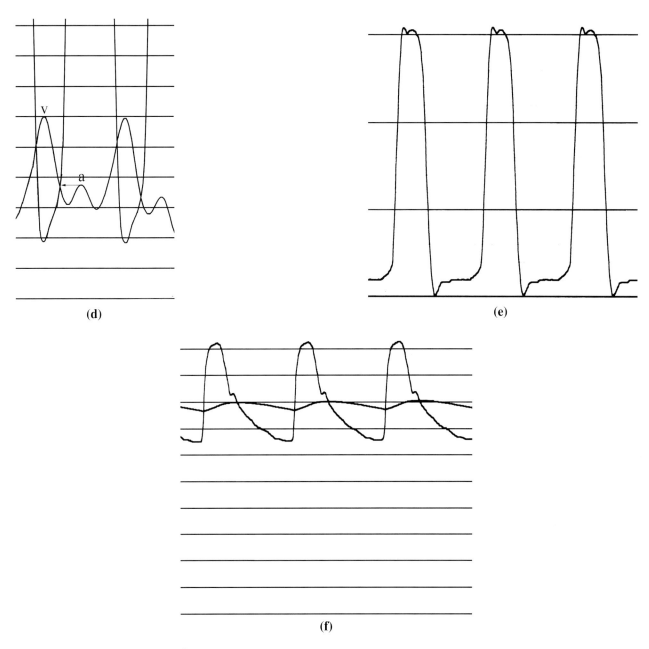

(d)

(e)

(f)

FIGURE 5–3.   (Continued)

diastole, with the tricuspid valve open, the ventricular end-diastolic pressure should equilibrate with the atrial *a* wave. Any process, therefore, that results in ventricular diastolic dysfunction (i.e., poor ventricular compliance) will result in elevated *but equal* right atrial *a* wave and ventricular end-diastolic pressures. An *a* wave that is greater than the end-diastolic pressure indicates obstruction to diastolic flow into the ventricle, which points to tricuspid stenosis. Markedly elevated variable *a* waves suggest atrial arrhythmias causing intermittent atrial contraction when the tricuspid valve is closed. Elevated right ventricular systolic

pressures may be seen with pulmonary hypertension or obstruction to the right ventricular outflow or pulmonary arteries.

Pulmonary artery systolic pressures are normally 15 to 30 mm Hg, and the mean pressures are usually <20 mm Hg. In addition to idiopathic pulmonary hypertension, elevated pulmonary artery pressures may be due to peripheral pulmonary stenosis, pulmonary venous obstruction, mitral stenosis, or left ventricular dysfunction. In the case of a child with a large ventricular septal defect, the right ventricular pressure is equal to the left ventricular pressure.

Without significant obstruction between the right ventricles and the pulmonary arteries, the pulmonary artery pressure will be high as well. Prolonged exposure of the pulmonary arteries to elevated pressure and increased blood flow can lead to irreversible pulmonary vascular disease.

The left atrial trace has similar components to the right atrial trace. Unlike the right atrium, however, the left atrial *v* wave is usually higher than the *a* wave. In addition, the left atrial pressures are usually higher than the corresponding right atrial pressures. This is because the walls of the left ventricle are thicker and less compliant than the right ventricle, causing a higher pressure during diastolic filling. Mean left atrial pressures of 10 to 12 mm Hg are normal. As with the right heart, there should be no gradient between the left atrial *a* wave and the left ventricular end-diastolic pressure, and an increased *a* wave without ventricular end-diastolic elevation usually represents obstruction to left ventricular inflow, as with mitral stenosis or cor triatriatum.

Although it is differently shaped, the left ventricular waveform provides the same information as the right ventricle. Left ventricular systolic pressure varies with age. Premature infants may require only a systolic pressure of 50 mm Hg to maintain adequate cardiac output whereas adolescents need adult-like pressures of 100 to 120 mm Hg. The end-diastolic pressure in the left ventricle is higher than that of the right ventricle, with 12 mm Hg the upper limit of normal. The difference in systolic pressure between the left ventricle and ascending aorta should be no greater than 5 mm Hg in a normal individual. Obstruction to systemic flow at any level will produce left ventricular hypertension, the severity of which will vary with the severity of obstruction. At rest there is no systolic pressure gradient across a normal aortic valve. A sample pressure tracing in a patient with aortic stenosis is shown in Fig. 5–4. The descending aortic systolic pressure is normally 5 to 10 mm Hg higher than the ascending aortic systolic pressure, due to a property of fluid mechanics in large vessels called the standing wave. With minor differences, the sinusoidal pressure tracings in the various portions of the aorta are similar to those commonly seen with peripheral or femoral artery monitoring. Some artificial accentuation of the systolic pressure may occur with peripheral lines due to the position and size of the catheters.

Oxygen Saturations and Shunt Calculations

The measurement of oxygen saturations during catheterization (oximetry) is the most commonly used and easiest method for quantitating blood flows and shunts in patients with congenital heart disease. The current technique of oxygen saturation measurement is done by absorption spectrophotometry, with the absorption of light by blood directly proportional to the oxygen saturation.

Saturation levels are measured in the high and low superior vena cava, right atrium, right ventricle, pulmonary

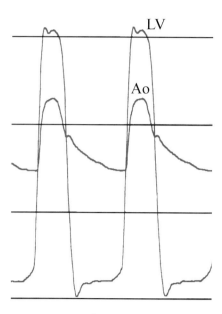

FIGURE 5–4.   Simultaneous pressure tracings from the left ventricle and aorta in a child with valvar aortic stenosis.

arteries, pulmonary veins, left atrium, left ventricle, and aorta. In the absence of intracardiac shunts, normal right heart saturations range from 65% to 75%, and left heart saturations are 95% or higher. On the right side of the heart, increases in saturation from one chamber to the next indicate the addition of oxygenated blood via left-to-right shunting. On the left side of the heart, decreases in the level of saturation indicate a right-to-left shunt. From the oxygen saturation data, oxygen content can be calculated:

$$O_2 \text{ content} = \text{Hgb content} \times 1.36 \times \text{fractional saturation of blood}$$

where 1.36 represents the amount of O_2 in ml that will bind to 1 g of fully saturated hemoglobin. Using the above equation, estimation of blood flow can be calculated using the Fick principle, which states:

$$\text{flow (Q)(L/min)} = \frac{O_2 \text{ consumption (ml/min)}}{\text{arteriovenous } O_2 \text{ difference (ml of oxygen/L of blood)}}$$

Oxygen consumption can either be measured directly or taken from a table of values for children based on sex, age, and heart rate.[3] Oxygen consumption is measured during catheterization by placing a hood over the patient's head to collect and analyze the oxygen content of the patient's expired breaths. To calculate flow for the individual pulmonary and systemic circulations, the appropriate values are substituted in the Fick equation:

$$\text{pulmonary flow }(Q_p) = \frac{O_2 \text{ consumption}}{\text{pulmonary vein } O_2 \text{ content}(PVO_2) - \text{pulmonary artery } O_2 \text{ content}(PAO_2)}$$

$$\text{systemic flow }(Q_s) = \frac{O_2 \text{ consumption}}{\text{systemic artery } O_2 \text{ content}(SAO_2) - \text{mixed venous } O_2 \text{ content}(MVO_2)}$$

These calculations are usually corrected for body surface area, yielding the cardiac index and pulmonary flow index.

To calculate the net left-to-right and right-to-left shunts, the effective pulmonary blood flow must be calculated. The effective pulmonary blood flow (Q_{ep}) is the amount of desaturated systemic venous blood that goes through the pulmonary circulation to become saturated. This excludes saturated blood that is recirculated through the lungs (i.e., left-to-right shunts) and desaturated blood that bypasses the lungs completely (i.e., right-to-left shunts).

$$\text{effective pulmonary flow }(Q_{ep}) = \frac{O_2 \text{ consumption}}{PVO_2 - MVO_2}$$

The amount of shunting can then be calculated as:

$$R \rightarrow L = Q_s - Q_{ep}$$
$$L \rightarrow R = Q_p - Q_{ep}.$$

Another way to express the net left-to-right and right-to-left shunts is by comparing the pulmonary to systemic flow ratio. This ratio ($Q_p{:}Q_s$) can be calculated as follows:

$$Q_p{:}Q_s = \frac{O_2 \text{ consumption}/PVO_2 - PAO_2}{O_2 \text{ consumption}/SAO_2 - MVO_2}$$

Simple mathematics reduces the formula to:

$$Q_p{:}Q_s = \frac{SAO_2 - MVO_2}{PVO_2 - PAO_2}$$

Since O_2 content is proportional to oxygen saturation, the simplified formula is:

$$Q_p{:}Q_s = \frac{SA \text{ sat} - MV \text{ sat}}{PV \text{ sat} - PA \text{ sat}}$$

requiring only measurement of the oxygen saturations in the chambers indicated. For example, in a patient with a ventricular septal defect, a systemic saturation of 95%, a superior vena cava saturation of 75%, and a pulmonary artery saturation of 85%,

$$Q_p{:}Q_s = \frac{95 - 75}{95 - 85} = 2{:}1 \text{ flow ratio}$$

Indicator dilution methods can also be used to quantify intracardiac shunts and measure cardiac output. This method is based on the concept that an indicator injected into the blood can be identified and its concentration measured when blood is sampled from a more distal site in the circulation. With thermodilution measurements, cold saline serves as the indicator, and temperature change of the distal blood is measured. The degree to which the distal, sampled blood cools relative to baseline is proportional to the flow into which the cold fluid is added. Thermodilution measurements are usually performed with the injection in the right atrium and sampling in the pulmonary artery. Significant amounts of pulmonary insufficiency will produce error in the measurement, as will the presence of intracardiac shunts.

Vascular Resistance

Vascular resistance is a measure of the force against which the heart pumps to push blood through the capillary bed in the lungs or body. The calculation of the resistance is analogous to that expressed by Ohm's law for electrical resistance: $V = IR$ where V represents the drop in voltage across the circuit, I is the current through the circuit, and R is the electrical resistance. Substituting for the analogous variables yields $P = QR$ where P represents the pressure drop, Q is the flow across the circuit, and R is the vascular resistance. Rearranging the equation yields: $R = P/Q$. The units of resistance are usually expressed as Wood's units (mm Hg/L/mm) in congenital heart disease. Multiplying the Wood's units by 80 converts them to the more commonly used physiology units of dyn/sec/cm^{-5}.

Calculation of resistances for the pulmonary and systemic circuits requires insertion of the appropriate values into the above equations:

$$PVR = R_p = (PA_p - LA_p)/Q_p$$
$$SVR = R_s = (Ao_p - RA_p)/Q_s.$$

Normal values for pulmonary vascular resistance fall between 1 and 3 Wood units, and the systemic vascular resistance normally is 10 to 30 Wood units. Pulmonary resistances are especially important in surgical planning for congenital heart disease. Abnormally elevated pulmonary vascular resistance increases the risk of procedures requiring passive flow through the pulmonary circuit, as is seen after Glenn or Fontan procedures.

Angiography

Angiography of congenital heart disease is, on the one hand, the easiest part of pediatric cardiac catheterization. Determining which pictures need to be taken (Table 5–2), which projections to use, and how much contrast to inject are to a large degree standard, based on the specific lesion and size of the patient. On the other hand, due to the large variability in complex congenital heart disease, angiography is often the hardest part of catheterization to do well. Nonionic contrast is currently the agent of choice for pediatric angiography because it causes less fluid shifts, reflex tachycardia, and patient discomfort following injection than ionic, high-osmolarity agents. In addition, nonionic agents are better tolerated in children with pulmonary hypertension.

The primary objective of angiography is to delineate the area of interest with the most clarity while avoiding overlapping other areas opacified by the injected contrast. Often movement of the cameras is necessary to achieve this objective in complex congenital heart disease. Biplane fluoroscopy with movable x-ray tubes allows for both rotation around the patient and angulation of the cameras toward the head (cranial) or feet (caudal). Movement of the anteroposterior (AP) camera to the right of the patient yields a right anterior oblique projection. Similarly, movement of the AP camera to the left of the patient, or rotating the lateral camera to less than its baseline 90-degree position, yields a left anterior oblique projection. The interested reader is directed to textbooks devoted entirely to the angiography of congenital heart disease for the evaluation of specific congenital heart lesions.[4]

Special Diagnostic Procedures

Originally the transseptal procedure to access the left heart was developed by adult cardiologists but has become commonplace in the pediatric lab.[5] The most common indication for the transseptal approach in children is the lack of easy and safe arterial access. Common diagnostic indications include direct left atrial pressure measurement for patients with mitral stenosis or direct left ventricular pressure measurement in patients with a prosthetic aortic valve. Common interventional indications include antegrade balloon dilation of mitral or aortic valve stenosis or elctrophysiologic ablation of a left-sided accessory pathway. Using a long sheath and a Brockenbrough needle (a 56- to 71-cm-long stiff needle with a gentle curve at the end), the atrial septum is engaged. The septum is stained using contrast injected through the needle. If the needle is felt to be in the correct position, it is pushed through the septum, into the left atrium. Contrast is then injected to verify position in the left atrium. The long sheath and dilator are then advanced over the needle into the left atrium. Once the sheath is in the left atrium, the needle and dilator are removed. Catheters can then be manipulated through the sheath, and into the left heart as needed. Complications include perforation of either the atrium or aortic root and embolism, either thrombus or air. Obviously the risk increases with decreasing patient age and size, but even in the smallest of infants, the transseptal procedure is extremely safe in experienced hands.

Endomyocardial biopsy is the gold standard for detecting rejection in cardiac transplant patients. Nearly all institutions screen their pediatric transplant patients with cardiac biopsies at regular intervals, although this is less common for neonates. Other, more controversial, indications for biopsy include new-onset cardiomyopathy and suspected myocarditis. In some patients with dilated cardiomyopathy and a very thin intraventricular septum, echocardiography guidance simultaneously with fluoroscopy has proved useful. Although in the past it was thought useful to biopsy both ventricles, data have not supported the additional risk associated with left-sided biopsies. Unless the disease process is limited to the left ventricle, right ventricular biopsy alone is standard practice. Between 4 and 10 samples are obtained, depending on the reason for biopsy and the type of tests required. Samples are obtained from the right ventricular septal surface. Complications associated with this procedure include cardiac perforation, air embolism, and tricuspid valve injury. The risk of perforation is increased in infants due to the smaller heart size and softer consistency of the myocardium. With the development and use of smaller bioptomes and long sheaths to protect the vessels and tricuspid valve, endomyocardial biopsy is a relatively safe procedure.

Complications

Complications during cardiac catheterization include vessel injury or perforation, cardiac perforation, contrast reaction, hemodynamically significant arrhythmias, stroke, and death. The risk of these complications is exceedingly rare, with a combined risk of <1%. Risks have been shown to be higher in newborns and infants, but with careful attention, the procedural risk remains quite low.[6] Minor complications *after* cardiac catheterization are more common and include low-grade fever, hematoma and/or mild discomfort at the site of vascular access, and transient occlusion of the catheterized vessel. In some patients, arterial vasospasm, intimal disruption, or thrombosis may lead to prolonged pulse loss. If the pulse does not return within 4 hours of catheterization, antithrombotic therapy with heparin or with clot-dissolving agents (urokinase or Tissue Plasminogen Activator (TPA)) may be indicated. In a small percentage of patients, pulse loss in the affected leg may be permanent and in rare instances has caused leg length discrepancies.

Interventional procedures carry an increased risk of complications when compared with diagnostic studies. Aortic valvuloplasty may damage the mitral valve or papillary muscles, leading to mitral insufficiency. Coils, stents, and other devices may embolize; if they are not retrieved in the catheterization lab and they are hemodynamically significant, they may require surgical removal. Balloon dilation of pulmonary arteries or aortic coarctation may lead to vascular rupture, which, if uncontrolled, may prove fatal if transcatheter or surgical attempts at control are unsuccessful.[7] In an experienced operator's hands with a properly staffed lab, therapeutic catheterizations have low complication rates.[8]

Interventional/Therapeutic Procedures

Interventional catheterization procedures in children developed in earnest in the early 1980s. Early attempts at interventional catheterization in children were severely limited by technical factors as catheters, sheaths, balloons, and other types of equipment were only available in adult sizes. As technology has improved, younger and smaller patients, even premature neonates, can be safely and effectively treated with transcatheter therapies. In many instances these therapies are definitive cures. Others are palliative, minimizing surgical risk or the need for repeat procedures . The therapeutic procedures performed in pediatric populations can be broadly classified as either dilations or closures. Dilations are performed using balloons alone or in combination with stents, and closures are accomplished using embolization coils or specially designed devices.

Dilations

Balloon Valvuloplasty First reported in 1982, balloon valvuloplasty is now the treatment of choice for valvar pulmonary stenosis in patients of all ages.[9] The subgroup of patients with thickened, dysplastic pulmonary valves, as commonly seen in patients with Noonan's syndrome, has shown a lower success rate.[10] Indications for balloon pulmonary valvuloplasty (BPV) are similar to surgical indications, namely, symptoms or a resting gradient of >50 mm Hg. Patients with mild pulmonic stenosis rarely progress or require intervention.

Although the balloon dilation catheters have improved over time, the technique has not changed significantly since its first description. After a right ventricular angiogram is done to confirm the nature and level of obstruction and to delineate the annulus size, an endhole catheter is placed in the distal pulmonary bed. A stiff, exchange-length wire is placed, and the endhole catheter is exchanged for the valvuloplasty balloon. The diameter of the balloon is chosen to be 100% to 140% (i.e., 1.0 to 1.4 times) the diameter of the pulmonary annulus. Short balloons are used to prevent damage to the right ventricular outflow tract. Using a syringe filled with dilute contrast, the balloon is inflated and deflated quickly to limit the time of outflow obstruction. In patients with a very large pulmonary annulus, the double balloon technique (whereby two balloons are inflated across the valve simultaneously) has proved successful. After dilation, repeat pressure measurements and angiograms are performed. The dilation may be repeated with larger balloons if a significant gradient remains and the anatomy appears amenable to dilation.

Since the initial report, multiple studies have proved the effectiveness and safety of valvuloplasty. Stanger et al.[11]

summarized the results of the Valvuloplasty and Angioplasty of Congenital Anomalies (VACA) Registry for pulmonary stenosis. In 822 patients, right ventricular outflow tract gradients were reduced from 71 ± 33 to 28 ± 21 mm Hg. Major complications, including death, cardiac perforation with tamponade, and tricuspid insufficiency, occurred in 0.6% of cases. That these complications were only seen in neonates and infants confirms the safety of the procedure for older patients and emphasizes the care needed when treating infants. Restenosis after balloon dilation is seen, with 10% to 15% of children requiring repeat dilation.[12,13] Pulmonary insufficiency postdilation is common, occurring in 10% to 40% of patients.[14,15] When compared with surgical valvotomy, however, the incidence and severity of regurgitation was lower in the group treated with valvuloplasty.[15]

Taking the process one step further, multiple techniques have been used to perforate the valve in selected patients with pulmonary atresia. Using the stiff end of a guidewire, transseptal needles, lasers, and, most recently, radiofrequency ablation catheters or wires, the atretic pulmonary valve can be crossed. Complications, specifically perforation of the right ventricular outflow tract, were fairly common early in the experience, but recent reports are encouraging, with higher success rates and lower numbers of complications.[16,17] Once a communication is made between the right ventricle and the pulmonary arteries, a wire can be placed across the valve, and the valve can be dilated in the usual fashion. It is not yet clear which patients with pulmonary atresia and an intact ventricular septum will potentially benefit from this procedure. One group that clearly needs to be excluded are patients with right ventricular–dependent coronary circulation, as they have shown higher mortality rates after surgical decompression.[18] Even with successful valvuloplasty, newborns with hypoplastic right ventricular chambers usually require an additional source of pulmonary blood flow, such as a modified Blalock-Taussig shunt.

The success with balloon dilation for treatment of pulmonary stenosis led to the use of catheter techniques for treatment of congenital aortic stenosis. Balloon aortic valvuloplasty (BAV) is now well established as a therapy for this lesion. Patients with calcific aortic stenosis, moderate to severe aortic insufficiency, or annular hypoplasia, however, are not good candidates for valvuloplasty. Indications for intervention are similar to those for surgical valvotomy including symptoms such as chest pain or syncope, a left ventricular strain pattern on ECG, or a resting peak systolic pressure gradient of 50 to 60 mm Hg. BAV can be performed using either a retrograde (femoral artery) or antegrade (femoral vein, transseptal) approach. Although the femoral artery route is the most commonly used retrograde approach, the umbilical artery or cutdown on the common carotid artery approaches are routinely used in newborns at some institutions.[19,20] Complications associated with the femoral artery retrograde technique include iliofemoral artery damage or thrombosis and aortic valve leaflet perforation. Antegrade BAV significantly reduces these risks but has been complicated by mitral valve and papillary muscle damage, at times severe enough to warrant surgical repair. The choice of which technique is used to cross (and subsequently dilate) the valve is largely operator preference.

BAV is performed in much the same fashion as that described above for the pulmonary valve. After a left ventricular angiogram, the wire is placed across the aortic valve. If the balloon will be delivered retrograde, the wire is coiled in the left ventricle. If the antegrade approach is used, the wire is placed around the arch, in the descending aorta. Balloons measuring 75% to 100% (i.e., 0.75 to 1.0 times) the annulus size are chosen. Longer balloons are helpful in preventing the balloon from being ejected from the ventricle during inflation (Fig. 5–5). After each dilation, pressure measurements are made, and an ascending aortogram is done to assess aortic regurgitation. Expected results include a reduction in the peak-to-peak gradient of 60% to 70% or a final gradient of 25 to 35 mm Hg.

Early results of BAV are comparable with those of surgical valvotomy. In 166 patients ranging in age from 1 day to 39 years, systolic pressure gradients dropped from 71-77 mm Hg to 22-35 mm Hg postdilation. Failure rates defined by a residual gradient >50 mm Hg occurred in up to 10% of patients. An increase in aortic insufficiency of two or more grades was seen in 13% of patients.[21–24] In the neonatal population with severe aortic stenosis, follow-up data to 8 years show survival and freedom from reintervention rates of 88% and 64%, respectively. Reintervention, mostly repeat balloon dilation for recurrent stenosis, was required in 40%, and significant aortic regurgitation was seen in 14%.

Balloon Angioplasty The feasibility of balloon angioplasty in nonatherosclerotic arterial stenoses was first demonstrated experimentally in animals.[25,26] The application of this technique has subsequently applied to both the pulmonary and systemic arteries in the pediatric population, with improving but variable rates of success. Stenosis of the branch pulmonary arteries can be categorized as congenital, acquired, or postsurgical (i.e., at shunt insertion sites, bands, or conduits). Congenital causes of pulmonary artery branch stenosis (PABS) include lesions with pulmonary undercirculation such as tetralogy of Fallot with pulmonary atresia. Additionally, PABS is commonly seen in Williams's syndrome, Alagille's syndrome, and congenital rubella. Stenotic lesions may be single or multiple, proximal or distal, and isolated or diffuse. Successful dilation has been shown to require tearing of the vessel intima and media.[27] Indications for angioplasty include greater than half systemic right ventricular pressure, hypertension in unaffected portions of the vascu-

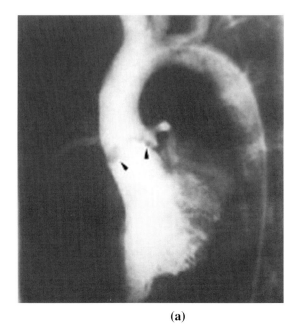

(a)

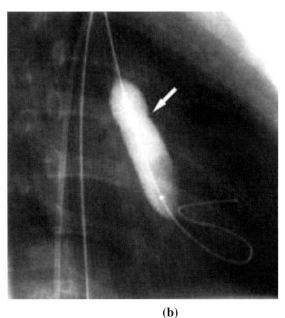

(b)

FIGURE 5–5. *(a)* Long axial oblique angiogram from a patient with valvar aortic stenosis, demonstrating the thickened valve leaflets (arrowheads). *(b)* During valvuloplasty, a waist (arrow) is seen in the balloon during inflation.

lar bed, a marked decrease in flow to an affected portion of the lung, and/or symptoms such as decreased exercise tolerance.

Prior to intervention in patients with suprasystemic right ventricular pressures, the creation of an atrial communication to maintain cardiac output in the event of severe pulmonary vasospasm is indicated to reduce the morbidity and mortality associated with the procedure in this high-risk population. Selective angiograms in the affected lungs or lobes are best to delineate the areas of involvement. The guidewire is positioned in the largest vessel possible to reduce the risk of dilating a small distal vessel and causing aneurysm formation. Using balloons generally three to four times the diameter of the narrowing, the balloon is inflated until the waist disappears or maximal inflation pressure is reached. Postdilation angiography is used to assess the results and evaluate for tears and aneurysms.

Success has been defined as a 50% increase in vessel diameter, a 20% increase in flow in the affected segment, and/or a decrease of >20% in the systolic right ventricle/aorta pressure ratio. Initial success rates using low-pressure balloons was 53% to 58%.[28,29] The more recent use of high-pressure balloons with inflation pressures of up to 22 atm has improved the overall success rate to 72%.[30] Nearly two-thirds of lesions that had failed previous low-pressure attempts were successfully dilated. Lesions not previously addressed had a success rate of 81%. In both groups, dilation of postsurgical stenoses had a higher success rate than that for congenital lesions. Complications were seen in 13% of patients and included two instances of guidewire perforation of a distal pulmonary artery (leading to death in one patient), hypotension in three patients (necessitating CPR in one), and transient complete heart block in one patient.

A combination surgical-transcatheter approach to patients with complex pulmonary artery stenosis has now become more commonplace. Surgical attention to proximal stenoses and associated intracardiac defects with transcatheter therapy of distal pulmonary stenosis and recurrent obstruction now appears to optimize results and survival.[3]

Balloon angioplasty of a recurrent aortic coarctation was first described in 1982.[32] A year later the first report of a successful dilation of a native coarctation was published.[33] Similar to studies done in pulmonary arteries, success depends on tearing the intima and media.[34] Histologic examination several weeks after dilation revealed an intact and normal-appearing intima. Although it is generally agreed that treatment of recurrent coarctation is best done by balloon angioplasty, the decision to chose surgical or transcatheter therapy for native coarctation remains controversial. At this time, most institutions feel that newborn and infant native coarctations are surgical lesions, whereas native coarctation in older children and recoarctations should initially be treated with balloon dilation.

The technique for coarctation angioplasty is, as with other angioplasty procedures, performed over a stiff guidewire. The end of the guidewire is stabilized in either the left ventricle, ascending aorta, or right subclavian artery. A descending aortogram is used to measure the size of the coarctation and the surrounding vessel. Although it is generally agreed that a balloon diameter less than twice the diameter of the coarctation is not likely to achieve success,

there is no consensus for the optimal balloon diameter. In animal studies, a balloon size greater than three times the size of the coarctation was more likely to produce deep and extensive tears.[34] In clinical studies, balloon diameters have been based on either the coarctation diameter, the isthmus diameter, the aorta diameter at the level of the diaphragm, or some combination thereof. It appears prudent to use a balloon no larger than the surrounding native aortic diameter to minimize aneurysm formation. Results from the VACA Registry demonstrated an average balloon-to-coarctation ratio of 3.1 ± 1; however, balloon diameters correlated poorly with procedural success.[35] Postdilation angiography looking for tears, aneurysms, or dissections should be performed after every dilation.

Procedural success for this lesion is defined as a 50% reduction in gradient and a 30% increase in diameter. In 67 patients (ages 2 days to 15 years; mean age 3.6 years) who underwent native coarctation dilation, there was a reduction in peak-to-peak gradient from 47 ± 17 to 11 ± 9 mm Hg.[36] Other cardiac lesions were present in 75% of cases. The procedure was successful in all patients, with one unrelated early death in a neonate, 2 days after dilation. Nearly 20% of patients required blood transfusion, but this was not related to patient age. Late mortality was 4.5% overall and 33% among the neonatal group, all with complex associated heart disease. The overall recoarctation rate was 25%; however, most of these patients were neonates, similar to reports from surgical series. All patients who underwent attempted angioplasty of the recoarctation had successful gradient relief. Three patients (5%) developed an aortic aneurysm, one requiring surgical resection, whereas 14% of patients had partial or complete occlusion of their femoral artery.

In the patients undergoing angioplasty for restenosis of previously repaired coarctations or other aortic obstructions, results have been good, with failures unrelated to the type of previous surgery.[37] The gradient was successfully reduced and the diameter of the stenotic area increased in 83% of patients. The failures occurred in older patients with very mild recoarctations and significantly lower predilation gradients, significantly larger predilation lesion diameters, and significantly older age. Because of the relatively large predilation lesion size, the use of larger, appropriately sized balloons was prohibited due to the risk of injuring the normal surrounding aorta.

Balloon dilation has been used in treating many other uncommon lesions with varying degrees of success. Mitral stenosis has been shown to be amenable to dilation in a subpopulation of patients excluding those with supravalvar mitral rings, parachute mitral valves, and asymmetric papillary muscles.[38] Systemic venous obstructions, specifically those seen after Mustard or Senning repair, are often amenable to balloon dilation; however, as a result of the tremendous elasticity of the venous vessels, these require very large balloons. These lesions are nowadays more often treated with endovascular stents. Pulmonary venous stenosis has been resistant to surgical repair, angioplasty, or endovascular stenting.

Endovascular Stents   Balloon-expandable stents are now used to treat many lesions that are not amenable to balloon dilation alone. Lesions with significant elastic recoil that resist tearing or require overly large balloon-to-vessel ratios can often be treated with endovascular stents. As with balloon angioplasty, stents were initially developed for the treatment of peripheral and coronary artery disease in adults. This technique has now been applied to the treatment of both pre- and postsurgical congenital heart disease patients. The technique of placing a stent in any position requires placement of a long sheath across the lesion to protect the stent during its journey from skin to stenosis. Once the stent is in position, the long sheath is withdrawn, and the balloon is inflated.

The largest experience in pediatrics is with stenting branch pulmonary artery stenosis. Results have shown an increase in vessel diameter, a fall in peak systolic gradient across the obstruction, an increase in flow to the stented lung, and a decrease in right ventricular pressure.[39,40] Restenosis has been seen in approximately one-third of patients, and redilation has been effective.

Similar success has been reported with the use of stents in postoperative systemic venous obstruction, right ventricular to pulmonary artery conduits, and coarctation of the aorta.[41–43] Actuarial freedom from conduit reoperation after placement of endovascular stents in obstructed right ventricle to pulmonary artery conduits was 65% at 30 months postprocedure. The 15% incidence of fractured stents seen in follow-up supports the notion that external compression is probably the cause of conduit obstruction.

Closure Procedures

The idea of leaving foreign material in the vascular space or heart itself has, to some degree, prevented general acceptance of some closure procedures. As time has passed and follow-up has shown the efficacy and safety of these procedures, techniques such as aortopulmonary collateral embolization and patent ductus arteriosus (PDA) coil closure have made their way into routine use. Others, such as device closure of secundum atrial or ventricular septal defects, are limited in their acceptance by lack of general availability, complex implantation techniques, U.S. Food and Drug Administration (FDA) regulations, and lack of long-term follow-up.

Coil Embolization   Aortopulmonary collaterals, arteriovenous malformations, Blalock-Taussig shunts, venous collaterals, coronary artery fistulae, and patent ductus arteriosi have all been successfully occluded using the technique of coil embolization. The embolization coils are composed of a metal wire, either stainless steel or platinum,

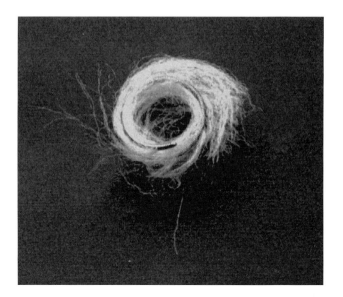

FIGURE 5–6.   Vascular embolization coils composed of a metal wire and Dacron strands. (Reproduced with permission from Cook, Inc.)

with or without Dacron strands; these are available in multiple sizes, lengths, and shapes (Fig. 5–6). Although PDA or coronary artery fistula embolization may obviate the need for surgery, most embolizations serve either to reduce the cardiac workload by decreasing the amount of shunting or to simplify a planned surgical procedure.

The technique for coil closure of collaterals or other communications is straightforward. A catheter is placed in the vessel to be occluded, and a selective angiogram is done to delineate the anatomy and diameter of the vessel to be closed. Coils are chosen that are slightly larger than the diameter of the vessel, as the vessel will distend when the coil is deployed. Using a long "pusher" wire, the coil is advanced through the catheter and deployed in the vessel. Repeat angiography is performed to confirm complete closure. If residual flow remains, additional coils are placed.

PDA coil occlusion has become increasingly popular. Recent reports have demonstrated closure rates of nearly 100% with PDAs measuring 3.5 mm or less and success in PDAs as large as 5.9 mm.[44,45] The ductus can be closed via a retrograde approach from the femoral artery or an antegrade approach from the femoral vein. Unlike occlusion of collateral vessels, when closing a PDA, the coil is not placed entirely inside the PDA. The coil is deployed such that approximately one loop of coil is placed in the pulmonary artery and the remainder is placed in the ductal ampulla (Fig. 5–7). As the ductus is often funnel shaped, this arrangement anchors the coil in the ductus, preventing embolization to either the pulmonary bed or lower body. If, in the case of large PDAs, a single coil does not serve to occlude it completely, multiple coils can be placed until

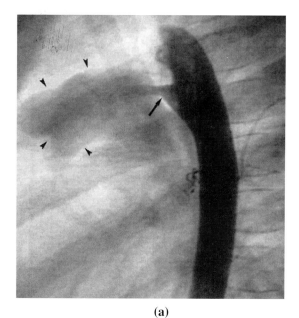

(a)

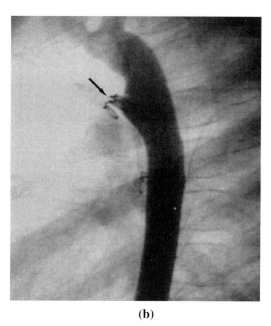

(b)

FIGURE 5–7. *(a)* Lateral angiogram from a patient with a patent ductus arteriosus (PDA). With injection in the aorta, contrast is seen crossing the PDA (arrow) and filling the pulmonary artery (arrowheads). *(b)* After coil occlusion (arrow), no residual flow is seen.

no residual shunting exists.[46] Complications are exceedingly rare and usually consist of coil embolization to the pulmonary artery or pulse loss in small infants. Those coils that embolize to the lungs can be retrieved in the catheterization lab with minimal effort, and using the antegrade

approach in small patients can minimize pulse loss. Rare cases of recanalization, documented by color flow Doppler evidence, have been reported.[47]

Techniques such as the Gianturco-Grifka™ vascular occluder for closing large PDAs or vessels have recently been approved by the FDA and are readily available. This device consists of a nylon sac of varying sizes into which a long, single coil is extruded. The wire and sac are then detached from the catheter and left to occlude the vessel. Animal studies and the limited published results currently available look promising.[48,49] The 8-French delivery system may prevent widespread use in small patients.

Device Closure of Septal Defects　The indications for percutaneous closure of atrial septal defects are similar to those for surgery, including symptoms, right ventricular volume overload, or a defect diameter of >8 mm. However, not all surgical candidates are transcatheter candidates, as device closure is limited to secundum defects that are generally <25 mm in diameter, with an adequate septal rim and geometry to hold the device in place. Currently, the three devices most widely used internationally are the Sideris™ "buttoned" device, the CardioSEAL™ double umbrella, and the AMPLATZER™ Septal Occluder. None of these are currently FDA approved, limiting their use in the United States, but all are currently in phase II clinical trials.

The Sideris™ device has undergone multiple design revisions since its introduction in 1990. Composed of the occluder, a square sheet of polyurethane foam supported by two independent wires in an "X" configuration, and a separate, single wire counter occluder, this device is the simplest from a construction standpoint. The most recent revision addresses the high rate (12%) of device "unbuttoning," separation of the two device components, seen with early devices. In the largest reported experience to date with the newest device, 183 adults underwent attempted closure of an atrial septal defect. Successful implantation was achieved in 98.4% of patients, with the remainder requiring surgical atrial septal defect closure after device unbuttoning. A shunt that was trivial or less was found in 85% of cases with a maximal follow-up of 36 months. Three patients required surgery, and two required an additional device, for significant residual shunt. No thrombus formation or vegetations were noted, and no neurologic sequelae were reported.[50] Intermediate follow-up on a smaller, unrelated subgroup showed an effective closure in 45 of the 46 patients (98%) who had successful implantation during FDA-approved clinical trials. The incidence of residual shunts decreased from 65% at 1 month to 27% at most recent (up to 5.5 years) follow-up. There were no instances of endocarditis or thromboembolism.[51]

The CardioSEAL™ represents the second generation of the original Clamshell device. The trials involving the original device were stopped when a high number of incidental

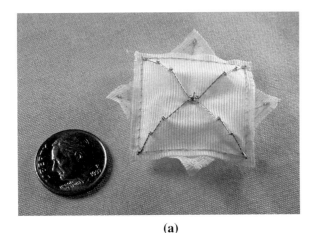

(a)

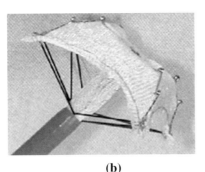

(b)

FIGURE 5–8. *(a)* The CardioSEAL Double Umbrella Device. *(b)* The newest revision will feature the STARFlex Centering System. (Reproduced with permission from Nitinol Medical Technologies, Inc.)

device-arm fractures were noted on routine follow-up. No complications from the fractures have been reported, and no devices required removal as a result. The current device is comprised of two Dacron-covered umbrellas with eight flexible metal arms, four on each umbrella, facing each other and connected by a single post (Fig. 5–8*a*). When implanted, the umbrellas open toward each other and hold the septal tissue between them. The North American Multicenter Atrial Septal Defect Closure Trial using the CardioSEAL™ followed 132 patients ranging in age from 2 to 70 years of age. Short-term results show that procedural success was achieved in 98.5% of patients; the two failures were due to inadequate septal rim tissue. There were no deaths, no blood transfusions were required, and hospital stay was <1 day in 96.2% of patients. At discharge, 93% had at most a small (<2 mm) leak. A balloon stretch diameter >14 mm is correlated with a higher incidence of residual leaks, although none appear to be clinically significant at this time. Four procedural complications were seen: stroke, transient myocardial ischemia, atrial tachycardia, and device embolization requiring surgical retrieval. The only late complication was transient ischemic attack symptoms associated with device thrombi in one patient who then underwent surgical device

removal. The most recent generation CardioSEAL™ features the STARFlex™ Centering System, which makes the device self-centering (Fig. 5–8*b*).

The AMPLATZER™ Septal Occluder, the newest of the three devices, is a self-expandable, double-disc device made from a nitinol (nickel-titanium alloy) wire mesh. The two discs are linked together by a short connecting waist. The device size is chosen such that the waist is slightly larger than the size of the atrial septal defect. To increase its thrombogenicity, the device's discs and waist are filled with polyester patches, which are sewn to the wire frame (Fig. 5–9). Combining the results of the United States and international multicenter trial, 229 patients ranging in age from 9 months to 70 years underwent device closure.[53] Complete closure at 24 hours was documented by color Doppler in 74%; 15% had only a trivial shunt. At 1 month of follow-up, 96% had a trivial or no shunt. Difficulties during the procedure included incorrect deployment of both discs into either the left or right atrium in a few patients. In all cases, the device was retrieved and repositioned correctly. Complications included two cases of device embolization to the right ventricle requiring transcatheter removal, one episode of endocarditis requiring device removal, and one patient with transient ischemic attack.

Other Device Uses Each of the devices described above, or modifications thereof, have been used to close other communications. Limited studies have reported varying degrees of success in closing post–myocardial infarction or muscular ventricular septal defects, PDAs, Fontan fenestrations, and perivalvar leaks. Several new experimental devices specifically designed for ventricular septal defect closure are currently being tested.

Conclusions

Noninvasive modalities for initial assessment, preoperative evaluation, and long-term follow-up of patients with congenital heart disease are now standards of care. However, for hemodynamic and angiographic data unavailable by noninvasive means, cardiac catheterization remains the gold standard and is critical for surgical planning and optimizing outcomes for many congenital lesions.

Much in the same fashion that echocardiography has affected cardiac catheterization, so has catheterization altered surgical practices, that is, although interventional catheterization has reduced the surgical caseload for some lesions, overall surgical volumes have not been similarly reduced. Simple lesions such as uncomplicated valvar pulmonary stenosis or PDA are easily and effectively dealt with in the catheterization lab, and complex, previously fatal lesions are now able to undergo surgical palliation or repair. Interventional catheterization often plays a major role in the success of these complex patients as well. For example, coiling unwanted aortopulmonary collaterals or

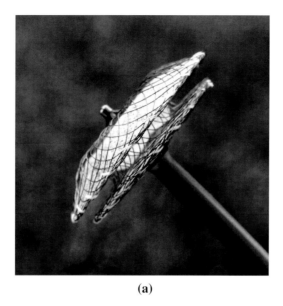

(a)

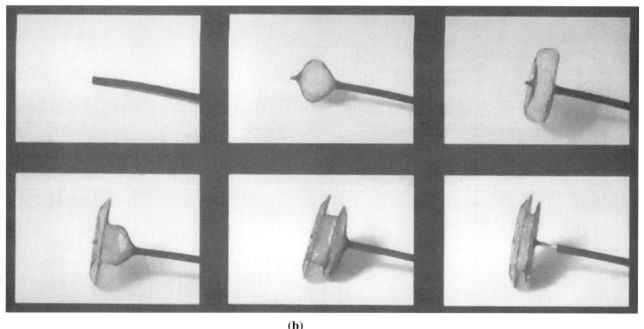

(b)

FIGURE 5–9. *(a)* The AMPLATZER Septal Occluder shown deployed while still attached to the introducer sheath and delivery cable. At this stage, the device can be retrieved into the sheath if necessary. *(b)* The deployment sequence. (Reproduced with permission from AGA Medical Corporation.)

dilating stenotic pulmonary arteries prior to the Fontan procedure can minimize the complexity of surgery and improve outcome.

Cardiac catheterization is, and will remain, a crucial component in the evaluation and treatment of patients with congenital heart disease. Close collaboration between surgeons and catheterizers has already led to tremendous advances in the care of these patients. Continued partnership will no doubt make the seemingly impossible quite ordinary in years to come.

References

1. SHIM D, LLOYD TR, CHO KI, et al. Transhepatic cardiac catheterization in children. Evaluation of efficacy and safety. *Circulation* 1995;92:1526–1530.

2. BRIDGES ND, FREED MD. Cardiac catheterization. In: Emmanouilides GC, et al., eds. *Heart Disease in Infants, Children, and Adolescents.* Williams & Wilkins, Philadelphia 1995:312–314.

3. LAFARGE CG, MIETTINEN OS. The estimation of oxygen consumption. *Cardiovasc Res* 1970;4:23–30.

4. FREEDOM RM, MAWON JB, YOO SJ, et al., eds. *Congenital Heart Disease Textbook of Angiocardiography.* Armonk, NY: Futura Publishing; 1997.

5. DUFF DF, MULLINS CE. Transseptal left heart catheterization in infants and children. *Cathet Cardiovasc Diagn* 1978;4:213–223.

6. COHN HE, FREED MD, HELLENBRAND WE, et al. Complications and mortality associated with cardiac catheterization in infants under one year. *Pediatr Cardiol* 1985;6:123–131.

7. BAKER CM, MCGOWAN FX, LOCK JE, et al. Management of pulmonary artery trauma due to balloon dilation. *J Am Coll Cardiol* 1998;31:2(57A).

8. VITIELLO R, MCCRINDLE BW, NYKANEN D, et al. Complications associated with pediatric cardiac catheterization. *J Am Coll Cardiol* 1998;32:1433–1440.

9. KAN JS, WHITE RI JR, MITCHELL SE, et al. Percutaneous balloon valvuloplasty: a new method for treating congenital pulmonary valve stenosis. *N Engl J Med* 1982;307:540–542.

10. BALLERINI L, MULLINS CE, CIFARELLI A, et al. Percutaneous balloon valvuloplasty of pulmonary valve stenosis, dysplasia, and residual stenosis after surgical valvotomy for pulmonary atresia with intact ventricular septum: long-term results. *Cathet Cardiovasc Diagn* 1990;19:165–169.

11. STANGER P, CASSIDY SC, GIROD DA, et al. Balloon pulmonary valvuloplasty: results of the Valvuloplasty and Angioplasty of Congenital Anomalies Registry. *Am J Cardiol* 1990;65:775–783.

12. MCCRINDLE BW. Independent predictors of long-term results after balloon pulmonary valvuloplasty. *Circulation* 1994;89:175l–1759.

13. WITSENBURG M, TALSMA M, ROHMER J, et al. Balloon valvuloplasty for valvular pulmonary stenosis in children over 6 months of age: initial results and long-term follow-up. *Eur Heart J* 1993;14:1657–1660.

14. MASURA J, BURCH M, DEANFIELD JE, et al. Five-year follow-up after balloon pulmonary valvuloplasty. *J Am Coll Cardiol* 1993;2:132–136.

15. O'CONNOR BK, BEEKMAN RH, LINDAUER A, et al. Intermediate-term outcome after pulmonary balloon valvuloplasty: comparison with a matched surgical control group. *J Am Coll Cardiol* 1992;20:169–173.

16. JUSTO RN, NYKANEN DG, WILLIAMS WG, et al. Transcatheter perforation of the right ventricular outflow tract as initial therapy for pulmonary valve atresia and intact ventricular septum in the newborn. *Cathet Cardiovasc Diagn* 1997;40:408–413.

17. GIBBS JL, BLACKBURN ME, UZUN O, et al. Laser valvotomy with balloon valvuloplasty for pulmonary atresia with intact ventricular septum: five years' experience. *Heart* 1997;77:225–228.

18. ROME JJ, MAYER JE, CASTANEDA AR, et al. Tetralogy of Fallot with pulmonary atresia. Rehabilitation of diminutive pulmonary arteries. *Circulation* 1993;88:1691–1698.

19. BEEKMAN RH, ROCCHINI AP, ANDES A. Balloon valvuloplasty for critical aortic stenosis in the newborn: influence of new catheter technology. *J Am Coll Cardiol* 1991;17:1172–1176.

20. FISCHER DR, ETTEDGUI JA, PARK SC, et al. Carotid artery approach for balloon dilation of aortic valve stenosis in the neonate: a preliminary report. *J Am Coll Cardiol* 1990;15: 1633–1636.

21. SHOLLER GF, KEANE JF, PERRY SB, et al. Balloon dilation of congenital aortic valve stenosis. Results and influence of technical and morphological features on outcome. *Circulation* 1988;78:351–360.

22. SHADDY RE, BOUCEK MM, STURTEVANT JE, et al. Gradient reduction, aortic valve regurgitation and prolapse after balloon aortic valvuloplasty in 32 consecutive patients with congenital aortic stenosis. *J Am Coll Cardiol* 1990;16:451–456.

23. O'CONNOR BK, BEEKIHAN RH, ROCCHINI AP, et al. Intermediate-term effectiveness of balloon valvuloplasty for congenital aortic stenosis. A prospective follow-up study. *Circulation* 1991;84:732–738.

24. WITSENBURG M, CROMME-DUKHUIS AH, FROHN-MULDER IM, et al. Short- and midterm results of balloon valvuloplasty for valvular aortic stenosis in children. *Am J Cardiol* 1992;69:945–950.

25. CASTENEDA-ZUNIGA WR, FORMANEK A, TADAVARTHY M, et al. The mechanism of balloon angioplasty. *Radiology* 1980;135:565–571.

26. LOCK JE, NIEMI T, EINZIG S, et al. Transvenous angioplasty of experimental branch pulmonary artery stenosis in newborn lambs. *Circulation* 1981;64:886–893.

27. EDWARDS BS, LUCAS RV, LOCK JE, et al. Morphologic changes in the pulmonary arteries after percutaneous balloon angioplasty for pulmonary artery stenosis. *Circulation* 1985;71:195–201.

28. HOSKING MC, THOMAIDIS C, HAMILTON R, et al. Clinical impact of balloon angioplasty for branch pulmonary artery stenosis. *Am J Cardiol* 1992;69:1467–1470.

29. ROTHMAN A, PERRY SB, KEANE JF, et al. Early results and follow-up of balloon angioplasty for branch pulmonary artery stenosis. *J Am Coll Cardiol* 1990;15:1109–1117.

30. GENTLES TL, LOCK JE, PERRY SB. High pressure balloon angioplasty for branch pulmonary artery stenosis: early experience. *J Am Coll Cardiol* 1993;22:867–872.

31. ROME JJ, MAYER, JE, CASTANEDA AR, et al. Tetralogy of Fallot with pulmonary atresia. Rehabilitation of diminutive pulmonary arteries. *Circulation* 1993;88:1691–1698.

32. SINGER MI, ROWEN M, DORSEY TJ. Transluminal aortic balloon angioplasty for coarctation of the aorta in the newborn. *Am Heart J* 1982;103:131–132.

33. LABABIDI Z. Neonatal transluminal balloon coarctation angioplasty. *Am Heart J* 1983;106:752–753.

34. LOCK JE, CASTANEDA-ZUNIGA WR, BASS JL, et al. Balloon dilatation of excised aortic coarctations. *Radiology* 1982;143:689–691.

35. TYNAN M, FINLEY JP, FINTES V, et al. Balloon angioplasty for the treatment of native coarctation: results of Valvuloplasty and Angioplasty of Congenital Anomalies registry. *Am J Cardiol* 1990;65:790–792.

36. RAO PS, GALAL O, SMITH P, et al. Five- to nine-year follow up results of balloon angioplasty of native aortic coarctation in infants and children. *J Am Coll Cardiol* 1996;27:462–470.

37. PERRY SB, ZEEVI B, KEANE JF, et al. Interventional catheterization in left heart lesions, including aortic and mitral valve stenosis and coarctation of the aorta. *Cardiol Clin* 1989;7:341.

38. MOORE P, ADATIA I, SPEVAK PJ, et al. Severe congenital mitral stenosis in infants. *Circulation* 1994;89: 2099–2106.

39. FOGELMAN R, NYKANEN D, SMALLHORN JF, et al. Endovascular stents in the pulmonary circulation: clinical impact on the management and medium term follow-up. *Circulation* 1995;92:881–885.

40. O'LAUGHLIN MP, SLACK MC, GRIFKA RG, et al. Immediate and intermediate-term follow-up of stents in congenital heart disease. *Circulation* 1993;88:605–614.

41. BU'LOCK FA, TOMETZKI AJ, KITCHINER DJ, et al. Balloon expandable stents for systemic venous pathway stenosis late after Mustard's operation. *Heart* 1998;79:225–229.

42. POWELL AJ, LOCK JE, KEANE JF, et al. Prolongation of RV-PA conduit life span by percutaneous stent implantation: intermediate-term results. *Circulation* 1995;92:3282–3288.

43. EBEID MR, PRIETO LR, LATSON LA. Use of balloon-expandable stents for coarctation of the aorta: initial results and intermediate-term follow-up. *J Am Coll Cardiol* 1997;30:1847–1852.

44. ROTHMAN A, LUCAS VW, SKLANSKY MS, et al. Percutaneous coil occlusion of patent ductus arteriosus. *J Pediatr* 1997;130:447–454.

45. OWADA CY, TEITEL DF, MOORE P. Evaluation of Gianturco coils for closure of large (> or = 3.5 mm) patent ductus arteriosus. *J Am Coll Cardiol* 1997;30:1856–1862.

46. HIJAZI ZM, GEGGEL RL. Transcatheter closure of large patent ductus arteriosus (> or = 4 mm) with multiple Gianturco coils: immediate and mid-term results. *Heart* 1996;76:536–540.

47. DANIELS CJ, CASSIDY SC, TESKE DW, Reopening after successful coil occlusion for patent ductus arteriosus. *J Am Coll Cardiol* 1998;31:444–450.

48. GRIFKA RG, MULLINS CE, GIANTURCO G, et al. New Gianturco-Grifka vascular occlusion device. Initial studies in a canine model. *Circulation* 1995;91:1840–1846.

49. GRIFKA RG, VINCENT JA, NIHILL MR, et al. Transcatheter patent ductus arteriosus closure in an infant using the Gianturco-Grifka vascular occlusion device. *Am J Cardiol* 1996;78:721–723.

50. RAO PS, BERGER F, SCHRADER R, et al. Transvenous occlusion of atrial septal defects in adults with the fourth generation buttoned device. *J Am Coll Cardiol* 1998;31:171–176.

51. ZAMORA R, RAO PS, LLOYD TR, et al. Intermediate-term results of phase I Food and Drug Administration trials of buttoned device occlusions of secundum atrial septal defects. *J Am Coll Cardiol* 1998;31:674–676.

52. MOORE P, BENSON LN, et al. CardioSEAL device closure of secundum ASDs: how effective is it? *Circulation* 1998;98:17.

53. MASURA J, WILKINSON JL, KRAMER HH, et al. US/international multicenter trial of atrial septal catheter closure using the Amplatzer septal occluder: initial results. *J Am Coll Cardiol* 1998;31:2 (56A).

54. MULLINS CE, MAYOR DC, eds. *Congenital Heart Disease: A Diagrammatic Atlas.* New York: John Wiley & Sons; 1994.

CHAPTER 6

Pediatric Cardiac Anesthesia

Laureen L. Hill, MD, Cathy R. Lammers, MD, and M. Gail Boltz, MD, FAAP

Introduction

The pediatric patient with congenital heart disease presents the anesthesiologist with unique challenges. A thorough understanding of the anatomic defects and subsequent alterations in normal circulatory flow patterns, the physiologic disturbances related to changes in pulmonary and systemic perfusion, and the impact of anesthetic agents and techniques on cardiopulmonary performance is essential to the safe and successful perioperative care of these patients. In this chapter, we discuss the classification and pathophysiology of congenital cardiac malformations, review interpretation of cardiac catheterization data, and consider the anesthetic management of patients presenting for corrective or palliative repair.

Normal Fetal and Neonatal Circulation

For a better understanding of the pathophysiology associated with congenital cardiac disease, it is necessary to review normal fetal and neonatal circulation. In utero, pulmonary and systemic circulations exist in parallel. The presence of both the patent foramen ovale (PFO) and patent ductus arteriosus (PDA) allows for mixing between the two circulations. The increased pulmonary vascular resistance causes much of the blood flow to be directed away from the lungs, (i.e., from the right atrium), through the PFO into the left atrium, or from the main pulmonary artery through the PDA into the descending aorta. Following delivery, a number of changes take place in which a series circulation pattern evolves. With spontaneous ventilation, pulmonary vascular resistance decreases, pulmonary blood flow increases, and the PDA begins to close in response to increased PO_2.[1] The increased delivery of pulmonary venous blood to the left atrium increases left atrial pressure (LAP) above right atrial pressure (RAP) causing functional closure of the PFO. The loss of the low-resistance placental circulation increases

systemic vascular resistance and reverses PDA blood flow (Fig. 6–1).

Classification

Congenital cardiac malformations are generally classified by the direction of central cardiac shunting and by the presence or absence of obstructive lesions (Table 6–1). Simple shunts are not associated with obstructive defects, so the magnitude and direction of shunting are determined by the size of the shunt orifice (restrictive versus nonrestrictive) and the relative differences in vascular resistance in pulmonary and systemic circulations. In general, simple shunts that produce blood flow from *left to right* increase pulmonary blood flow (PBF) and create a significant volume load for the right heart. Depending on the magnitude of shunting, the increased PBF can produce pulmonary edema and ultimately lead to fixed pulmonary vascular obstructive changes, pulmonary hypertension, and a condition known as *Eisenmenger's syndrome* in which the direction of the shunting is reversed, (i.e., right-to-left).

Anatomic defects that produce *right-to-left* shunting are associated with increased venous admixture, arterial desaturation, and cyanosis. The compensatory response to hypoxemia is polycythemia, with hematocrits in excess of 70% in some cyanotic patients. Polycythemia increases blood viscosity and may actually compromise tissue perfusion due to increased resistance to flow and a greater workload on the heart.

Certain cardiac malformations, referred to as *mixing lesions,* are characterized by mixing of pulmonary and systemic circulations. The resultant physiologic effects depend on the relative differences in pulmonary and systemic vascular resistances and the net blood flow through each of the parallel circulations. Factors that alter vascular tone in both the pulmonary and systemic vascular beds can be manipulated to affect the direction of blood flow and control oxygen saturation and systemic perfusion.

TABLE 6–1. Common Congenital Cardiac Defects Classification

Characteristics	Defect

Left-to-right shunts
  Lesions with increased
  pulmonary blood
  flow (failure)
	Atrial septal defect
	Ventricular septal defect
	Patent ductus arteriosus
	Endocardial cushion
	  defect
	Aortopulmonary window

Right-to-left shunts
  Lesions with decreased
  pulmonary blood
  flow (cyanotic)
	Tetralogy of Fallot
	Pulmonary atresia
	Tricuspid atresia
	Ebstein's anomaly

Complex shunts
  Mixing of pulmonary and
  systemic circulation
	Truncus arteriosus
	Transposition of the great
	  vessels
	Total anomalous
	  pulmonary venous
	  return
	Double-outlet right
	  ventricle
	Hypoplastic left heart
	  syndrome

Obstructive lesions	Aortic stenosis Mitral stenosis Pulmonic stenosis Coarctation of the aorta Cor triatriatum Interrupted aortic arch

Source: From Bell C, Kain ZN, eds: *The Pediatric Anesthesia Handbook*, 2nd ed. St. Louis: Mosby; 1997:140, with permission.

Complex malformations are those lesions characterized by both shunting and obstructive defects. The direction and magnitude of shunting is determined by the size of the shunt orifice and the outflow resistance. When there is complete obstruction to flow, as in tricuspid or pulmonary atresia, the degree and direction of shunting is fixed. This type of complete shunting can only occur in the presence of another shunt in the distal circulation, allowing mixing of pulmonary and systemic blood.

Determination of Shunt Direction and Magnitude

Cardiac catheterization provides useful information regarding both the anatomic features and the physiologic sequelae of congenital cardiac disease. Using catheters directed into the affected chamber(s) or vessel(s), pressure measurements can be obtained and gradients can be calculated. Similarly, oxygen saturations can be measured in each cardiac chamber and great vessel to determine the location and direction of intracardiac shunts. For example, there is normally a slight decrease in oxygen saturation between the right atrium and right ventricle due to drainage from the coronary sinus; therefore, an increase in oxygen saturation between the right atrium and right ventricle would indicate the presence of a left-to-right shunt at the ventricular level. A decrease in left atrial saturation may be due to right-to-left shunting at the atrial level, whereas low pulmonary venous saturations would suggest a pulmonary etiology for hypoxemia, i.e., pneumonia, atelectasis, pulmonary edema.

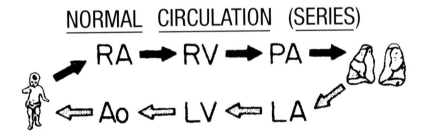

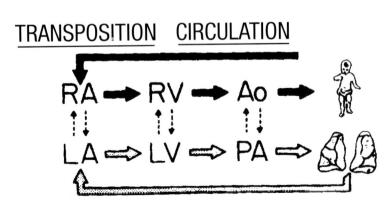

FIGURE 6–1.

TABLE 6–2. Correlation Between Q_p/Q_s Ratios and Congenital Cardiac Lesions

Q_p/Q_s	Shunt Direction	Clinical Manifestations	Examples
<1	R → L	Cyanosis	Tetralogy of Fallot
1–2	L → R	Often asymptomatic	Atrial septal defect
2–3	L → R	±Pulmonary edema Murmur	Ventricular septal defect
>3	L → R	Congestive heart failure Murmur Cardiomegaly	Atrioventricular canal

The amount of pulmonary blood flow (Q_p) and systemic blood flow (Q_s) can be calculated using oxygen content data derived from blood samples collected from cardiac catheterization. The oxygen consumption ($\dot{V}o_2$) can be measured but is often estimated from tables based on age, sex, and heart rate:

$$Q_p(L/min) = \dot{V}o_2/Cpvo_2 - Cpao_2 \qquad (1)$$

$$Q_s(L/min) = \dot{V}o_2/Cao_2 - Cmvo_2 \qquad (2)$$

$$Q_p/Q_s = Sao_2 - Smvo_2/Spvo_2 - Spao_2 \qquad (3)$$

where, $Cpvo_2$ = pulmonary venous oxygen content (mL/L), $Cpao_2$ = pulmonary arterial oxygen content (mL/L), Cao_2 = arterial oxygen content (mL/L), $Cmvo_2$ = mixed venous oxygen content (mL/L), Sao_2 = arterial oxygen saturation, $Smvo_2$ = mixed venous oxygen saturation, $Spvo_2$ = pulmonary venous oxygen saturation, and $Spao_2$ = pulmonary arterial oxygen saturation.

The Q_p/Q_s is useful in predicting the clinical manifestations and degree of compromise expected in patients with cardiac malformations (Table 6–2).

Effective pulmonary blood flow (Q_{ep}) is defined as the amount of desaturated venous blood that reaches the lungs (Fig. 6–2) and can be calculated using the following equation:

$$Q_{ep} (L/min) = \dot{V}o_2/Cao_2 - Cpao_2 \qquad (4)$$

By using the total pulmonary and systemic blood flow calculations and subtracting the effective pulmonary blood flow, one can calculate the amount and direction of

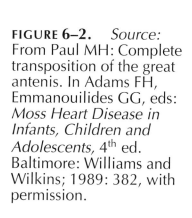

FIGURE 6–2. *Source:* From Paul MH: Complete transposition of the great antenis. In Adams FH, Emmanouilides GG, eds: *Moss Heart Disease in Infants, Children and Adolescents,* 4th ed. Baltimore: Williams and Wilkins; 1989: 382, with permission.

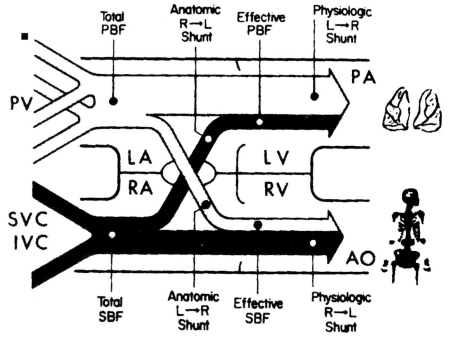

shunting present:

$$left\text{-}to\text{-}right\ shunt = Q_p - Q_{ep} \tag{5}$$

$$right\text{-}to\text{-}left\ shunt = Q_s - Q_{ep} \tag{6}$$

Perioperative Monitoring of the Pediatric Cardiac Patient

Placement and interpretation of both invasive and noninvasive monitors are an essential part of anesthetic care (Table 6–3). Commonly used noninvasive monitors for pediatric patients are similar to those used in adults: (1) electrocardiography with multiple lead capabilities; (2) oscillometric blood pressure measurement; (3) precordial and esophageal stethoscopes; (4) pulse oximetry; (5) temperature (usually two separate sites, reflecting both core and cerebral temperatures); and (6) transesophageal echocardiography (TEE). In pediatric patients, invasive monitors are usually placed after the induction of general anesthesia, endotracheal intubation, and the establishment of peripheral venous access. It is imperative to be vigilant at all times for sources of emboli, particularly air. In patients with septal defects, there is always the potential for *paradoxical emboli* to the cerebral circulation.[1]

Arterial catheterization is usually performed by percutaneously cannulating the radial artery. In infants and small children, a 22-gauge catheter is placed and in children over 5 years of age or weighing >25 kg, a 20-gauge catheter is used. Arterial cannulation is associated with little morbidity, although thrombosis, bleeding, and hematoma formation are known complications. The transducer and the flushing devices of the system must be carefully examined for evidence of air bubbles and/or entrainment, as these can be a source of air emboli, a substantial concern in patients

with intracardiac shunts.[1] In infants, infusion pumps primed with heparinized saline administer a continuous flush to the transducer to prevent volume overload. Additionally, a continuous flush attenuates the problem of paradoxical emboli that are associated with the high-velocity jet of intermittent flush devices. If it is not possible to cannulate the radial artery, other sites can be used; the femoral, dorsalis pedis, axillary or brachial arteries, and (in newborn infants) the umbilical artery are all acceptable sites for arterial monitors. If percutaneous placement of an arterial catheter is difficult, a surgical cutdown of the vessel can be performed.

Central Venous Catheters

Central venous catheter placement is not essential for anesthesia, surgery, or cardiopulmonary bypass (CPB), as transthoracic intracardiac lines may be placed by the surgeon. Percutaneous placement of a central venous line prior to initiation of the operative procedure facilitates the rapid administration of vasoactive drugs or fluid and provides information regarding ventricular preload. The preferred site of percutaneous placement is the internal jugular vein. Other sites that have been utilized are the external jugular, femoral, and subclavian veins. In the newborn, the umbilical vein is commonly threaded into the intrathoracic inferior vena cava by the pediatrician in the nursery.

Ultrasound guidance is an increasingly popular technique to aid placement of the central venous catheter in the internal jugular vein. Transcutaneous ultrasound of the neck structures permits identification of the vessels and visualization of vessel depth from the skin. This approach decreases the incidence of inadvertent carotid puncture and hematoma formation. It also increases the likelihood of successful catheter placement in small infants.[2]

Pulmonary Artery Catheters

Although frequently used for monitoring in the adult population, pulmonary artery catheters (PACs) are infrequently placed in the pediatric population. The use of PACs in children is limited because of the difficulty in placing a balloon-tipped catheter in a very small patient with an intracardiac lesion and because the catheter is proportionally larger in infants than adults and may require fluoroscopy for placement. If measurement of pulmonary artery pressures is required, the surgeon can place a transthoracic pressure line directly into the main pulmonary artery. Other transthoracic lines that are routinely placed by the surgeon include right atrial and left atrial catheters. Transthoracic lines have minimal morbidity associated with their use.

Transesophageal Echocardiography

Pediatric TEE has become a rapidly evolving field in the past decade since the development of the miniature

TABLE 6–3. Monitoring Techniques for Pediatric Cardiac Surgery

Noninvasive
  Precordial and esophageal stethoscope
  Pulse oximeter
  Electrocardiogram
  Blood pressure
  End-tidal CO_2
  Temperature (multiple sites)
  Electroencephalogram
Invasive
  Blood pressure
  Bladder catheter
  Central venous pressure
  Right atrial pressure
  Left atrial pressure
  Pulmonary artery pressure
  Optional

multiplane probe. Intraoperative TEE is routinely performed in children as small as 3 kg, although there have been reports of TEE used in children as small as 2.4 kg. Stevenson et al.[3] demonstrated that TEE offers substantial utility in detection of residual problems requiring reoperation. Although there have been no large outcome studies, data have demonstrated that patients with acceptable surgical results substantiated by echocardiography had a >90% likelihood of a long-term acceptable outcome. At many pediatric cardiac centers, TEE has become a standard of care for the intraoperative assessment of most congenital heart repairs prior to chest closure. TEE is a valuable tool for intraoperative anesthetic and surgical management.[4] Diagnoses can be confirmed preoperatively and the operative plan revised accordingly. The interpretation of intraoperative TEE images requires collaboration among the anesthesiologists, cardiologists, and the surgeon.

Pulse Oximeters

Pulse oximetry combines pulse plethesmography and calculates the ratio of reduced hemoglobin to oxyhemoglobin. The reliability of the pulse oximeter is affected by tissue hypoperfusion, hypothermia, ambient light, electrocautery, patient motion, and some intravenous dyes. Importantly, fetal hemoglobin has no effect on pulse oximeter function. A common practice in pediatric cardiac cases is the use of multiple sites for placement of the probes, usually preductal and postductal.

Temperature

Body temperature is monitored routinely in all pediatric cases. In cardiac surgery, temperature is monitored at two separate sites to correlate the brain (nasopharynx, tympanic membrane) and core temperatures for both the cooling and rewarming phases of CPB. The locations commonly monitored are the nasopharynx, rectum, bladder, esophagus, and tympanic membrane.

Urine Output

Bladder catheterization and indwelling Foley placement is indicated for all procedures requiring CPB and generally for all cardiothoracic procedures. Urine output is a reflection of renal perfusion and is affected by changes in temperature, blood pressure, and blood glucose and administration of diuretics. Urine output should be evaluated every 30 minutes while the patient is on CPB and should be in the range of 0.5 to 1.0 cc/kg/hr.

Blood Gases

Arterial blood gases are sampled at critical points during the operation and every 15 to 20 minutes while the patient is on CPB. Under current debate is the issue of temperature correction during hypothermic CPB (alpha stat versus pH stat).

Both strategies may be appropriate at specific perioperative intervals.

Anticoagulation

Management of hemostasis in the pediatric cardiac patient is very similar to that in the adult. The commonly used monitors are the *activated clotting time* (ACT) using an automated method, such as the Hemochron™ or one of the Hepcon™ systems. The ACT measures the effects of heparin on the coagulation cascade. Normal ACT values range between 120 and 140 seconds. A common approach to heparin dosing is based on the patient weight in U/kg. An initial dose of heparin is 3 to 4 mg/kg (300 to 400 U/kg) prior to the initiation of CPB with a resultant ACT in excess of 450 seconds. This level is adequate to prevent complications of fibrinolysis and disseminated intravascular coagulation while the patient is on CPB. A more accurate method may be to base the dose on the patient's blood volume and the circuit priming volume, since the activity of the drug is based partly on its concentration. Direct measurement of heparin levels has not been widely adopted, as heparin concentrations inhibiting fibrinolysis have not been defined. The ACT is measured frequently during CPB, as it may be affected by changes in temperature and hemodilution while the patient is on CPB. The effect of heparin is reversed with protamine. The initial dose of protamine is empirically based on the dose of heparin administered (1.5 mg protamine/1.0 mg heparin). However, subsequent doses are administered based on the ACT, the heparin concentration, and visual inspection of the operative field for excessive bleeding. For pediatric patients who undergo procedures requiring bypass, the surface exposure of the cardiopulmonary bypass circuit is proportionally greater than that of adults, perhaps increasing the inflammatory response to CPB and also increasing the risk of significant fibrinolysis. There is interest in the development of techniques to reduce the inflammatory response to CPB, including heparin-coated circuits and the intraoperative use of antifibrinolytics.[5]

Left-to-Right Shunts

All the lesions in this category are characterized by anatomic defects that allow unidirectional shunting of oxygenated blood from the left heart or systemic circulation, where the pressures are normally greater, to the right heart or pulmonary artery. This left-to-right shunting results in excessive PBF, which clinically manifests as pulmonary congestion, edema, and recurrent pulmonary infections. The shunt volume increases the volume load on the right and left heart; if such volume is significant or long-standing, cardiomegaly and heart failure may result. The left-to-right shunt lesions include atrial septal defect (ASD), ventricular septal defect (VSD), atrioventricular (AV) septal defect, and patent ductus arteriosus (PDA).

Atrial Septal Defect

ASD is characterized by a defect within the interatrial septum, allowing communication between the left and right atria. ASDs are classified according to the specific anatomic location of the defect, as follows: (1) ostium secundum, (2) ostium primum, (3) patent foramen ovale, and (4) sinus venosus. *Ostium secundum* lesions are the most common, may be quite large in size, and are typically located in the center of the septum. *Ostium primum* defects occur within the lower portion of the septum and, if associated with mitral valve abnormalities, may be termed *partial atrioventricular canal.* A *patent foramen ovale* has been shown to occur in as many as 50% of children aged 1 to 5 years and up to 35% of adults; however, small patent foramen ovale defects are usually hemodynamically inconsequential. *Sinus venosus* defects occur high in the atrial septum above the fossa ovalis, near the junction of the superior vena cava and right atrium. These ASDs are relatively uncommon and are usually associated with anomalous pulmonary venous return. Small, restrictive defects are associated with limited shunt flow and minimal symptoms, whereas larger defects may allow considerable left-to-right shunting and produce significant symptoms of pulmonary congestion and heart failure. Rarely, patients with large defects, if left uncorrected for several decades, may develop pulmonary vascular occlusive disease (PVOD) with reversal of the shunt, cyanosis, and right heart failure (i.e., Eisenmenger's syndrome).

Ventricular Septal Defect

VSDs are characterized by defects within the interventricular septum and, like ASDs, are classified according to their specific anatomic locations. *Perimembranous VSDs* are the most common and are located in the membranous septum below the crista supraventricularis. *Supracristal VSDs* lie above the crista supraventricularis just below the aortic annulus. This superior location allows blood to shunt from the left ventricle directly into the pulmonary artery and may create a prolapse of the aortic valve cusp into the defect with concomitant aortic insufficiency. *Muscular VSDs* occur within the muscular septum and may be multiple in number (i.e., "swiss cheese" defects). Blood flows from left to right through these defects, with the degree of shunting determined by the size of the lesion and the differences in right and left ventricular pressures. If the right ventricular pressure remains less than the left ventricular pressure, the defect is termed *restrictive.* When equalization of ventricular pressures occurs, the defect is termed *nonrestrictive.* Small, restrictive defects may have minimal effects on the right ventricle and pulmonary circulation, whereas large defects lead to pulmonary overcirculation, biventricular enlargement, and congestive heart failure. Patients may develop PVOD within the first few years of life due to excessive pulmonary blood flow at systemic pressures.

Atrioventricular Septal Defect

Two types of AV canal defects exist: *partial* and *complete.* A *partial AV canal* is synonymous with an ostium primum ASD. No interventricular communication exists because the AV valves are fused to the ventricular septum. The more common *complete AV canal* lesion is characterized by a single common AV valve and communication between all four chambers through both atrial and ventricular septal defects. Blood flows left to right through the multiple defects with the amount of shunting determined by the relationship between pulmonary and systemic vascular resistances, the degree of atrioventricular valve incompetence, and the presence of left ventricular outflow tract obstruction. Patients with complete AV canal usually present in the first 2 years of life with pulmonary congestion, biventricular enlargement, frequent respiratory infections, and failure to thrive. Early correction is necessary to prevent the development of PVOD.

Patent Ductus Arteriosus

Failure of the ductus arteriosus to close following birth in response to the increase in the partial pressure of oxygen (PO_2) results in a PDA. Premature infants have poor development of the ductal muscular layers that contract in response to the increase in PO_2 and therefore have an increased incidence of PDA. Other factors common to premature infants including anemia, hypoxemia, and positive pressure ventilation contribute to maintained patency of the ductus.[6,7]

As pulmonary vascular resistance falls and the systemic vascular resistance increases after birth, blood preferentially shunts left to right from the descending thoracic aorta to the pulmonary artery via the patent ductus. Clinical signs and symptoms are dependent on the degree of shunting and the ability of the left ventricle to accommodate the increased volume load. Patients may be asymptomatic or may develop cough, dyspnea, tachypnea, and/or tachycardia secondary to pulmonary vascular congestion.

Anesthetic Considerations

Management decisions will be guided by the degree of shunting and presence of signs and symptoms related to pulmonary overcirculation. Infants and children with good cardiopulmonary function and no evidence of congestive failure will tolerate inhalational induction and maintenance and may be considered appropriate candidates for early extubation, employing low-dose opiate or regional anesthesia techniques. Left-to-right shunts theoretically decrease inhalation induction time, particularly for soluble agents, but this is rarely clinically significant.

Patients with evidence of pulmonary congestion, particularly neonates with mechanical ventilator dependence secondary to a large PDA and infants with large VSDs or AV canal lesions may not tolerate the depressant and hypotensive effects of inhalational anesthetics and should be managed with intravenous opiates, muscle relaxants, and benzodiazepines to preserve hemodynamic performance. Infants in significant congestive failure are likely to be hospitalized for optimization prior to surgery and will therefore have established intravenous access. Intramuscular ketamine (4 to 8 mg/kg) may be used to establish intravenous access in patients with cardiopulmonary compromise. Although these lesions are characterized by left-to-right shunting, meticulous attention must be paid to all drugs and fluids administered to prevent paradoxical embolism during transient right-to-left shunting resulting from increases in right heart pressures.

Ventilation management should be directed toward avoiding further decreases in the pulmonary-to-systemic vascular resistance (PVR/SVR) ratio to ensure adequate systemic and coronary blood flow, particularly in patients with large, nonrestrictive defects. Although a number of factors contribute to changes in pulmonary vascular tone (including patient age, anatomic defects that alter PBF, endogenous catecholamines, and vasoactive drugs), alterations in inspired oxygen concentration and blood pH have the greatest impact on PVR.[8] Hypoxia and hypoxemia increase pulmonary arteriolar vasoconstriction, especially as the PO_2 falls below 50 mm Hg, and this response is exaggerated in the presence of metabolic or respiratory acidosis. These two variables can be intentionally altered to influence pulmonary vascular tone and PBF. Following surgical repair, maneuvers to decrease PVR are appropriate to minimize right ventricular afterload without compromising systemic perfusion. Potent opiate agents such as fentanyl and sufentanil are useful in blunting pulmonary vascular reactivity in patients at risk for developing pulmonary hypertension and right ventricular failure. Inotropes may be required after CPB to improve myocardial performance and to support cardiac output.

Right-to-Left Shunts

All defects in this category comprise a communication between the pulmonary and systemic circulations and an obstruction to PBF via the outflow tract, the pulmonary vessels, or the pulmonary vascular bed. This results in an incresed venous admixture, arterial desaturation, and cyanosis. It is important to note that not all infants who are cyanotic at birth have congenital heart disease. The differential diagnosis for cyanosis must include polycythemia of the newborn, pulmonary lesions such as hypoplasia, atelectasis, and lobar emphysema, neurologic or metabolic disturbances, sepsis, and other congenital malformations. The right-to-left shunt lesions include tetralogy of Fallot, tricuspid atresia, pulmonary atresia with intact ventricular septum, and Ebstein's anomaly.

One of the principle guidelines for the operative correction of right-to-left shunt lesions is the degree of arterial

desaturation of the patient. Frequently, palliative shunts are used to improve pulmonary blood flow and relieve hypoxemia. Increased PBF acts to stimulate growth in the pulmonary artery in anticipation of future surgery if the patient is not a candidate for total repair at birth. The type of shunt used is based on patient size, diagnosis, and anatomy of the lesion.

Tetralogy of Fallot

Tetralogy of Fallot is the most common cyanotic cardiac defect in children. It occurs in approximately 10% to 15% of children with congenital heart disease. This condition is applied to a tetrad of anatomic malformations that include (1) right ventricular outflow tract obstruction (i.e., infundibular stenosis, pulmonic stenosis, or supravalvular stenosis); (2) VSD, usually in the subaortic position, (3) the aortic origin overriding the right ventricle; and (4) right ventricular hypertrophy. There is wide anatomic variation of this condition and as a result, varying clinical presentation. The critical factor is the degree of right ventricular outflow obstruction, determining the amount of right-to-left shunting across the VSD. This is a somewhat dynamic process, as the degree of obstruction can be related to infundibular spasm and changes in pH, PaO_2, and $PaCO_2$.

Hypercyanotic episodes, or "tet spells," initially present at 2 to 3 months of age and are characterized by acute cyanosis and hyperventilation. These episodes are associated with irritability, crying, feeding, or defecation. Left untreated, this condition can progress to seizures and a semicomatose state. The etiology of tet spells is unclear, but they are probably related to infundibular hypercontractility or spasm. The recommended treatment for hypercyanotic episodes is given in Table 6–4.

Tricuspid Atresia

Absence of the tricuspid valve, hypoplasia of the right ventricle, and lack of communication between the right atrium and ventricle characterize this malformation. Survival is dependent on the presence of an interatrial communication via a patent foramen ovale or secundum ASD to permit right atrial outflow. Unless the interatrial defect is restrictive, there are no features of congestive heart failure.

Cyanosis is the predominant feature in patients with tricuspid atresia. All patients with tricuspid atresia experience some degree of hypoxia because all systemic venous blood must mix with oxygenated blood in the left atrium. The degree of hypoxia is dependent on the ratio of systemic to pulmonary blood flow (Q_p/Q_s) and total PBF. About 70% of patients with tricuspid atresia have reduced PBF secondary to a small VSD and concomitant right ventricular outflow tract obstruction. Patients with tricuspid atresia may experience hypercyanotic spells similar to those seen in tetralogy of Fallot due to VSD closure or infundibular narrowing that further reduces PBF. Such patients usually require early

TABLE 6–4.   Treatment of Hypercyanotic "tet" Spells

Treatment	Effect
High FIO$_2$, (0.50–1.0)	Pulmonary vasodilator, decreases pulmonary vascular resistance
Volume administration	Opens right ventricular outflow tract
Morphine	Sedation, decreases sympathetic stimulation
Ketamine	Sedation, analgesia, maintains systemic vascular resistance, may improve pulmonary blood flow
Phenylephrine	Increases systemic vascular resistance
Beta-blockers (esmolol)	Decreases heart rate, negative inotrope, decreases infundibular spasm
Halothane	Negative inotrope in dose-dependent fashion, not indicated in severe ventricular failure
Abdominal compression	Increases systemic vascular resistance and systemic venous return
Knee-chest position	Increases systemic vascular resistance and systemic venous return

surgical intervention with a palliative shunt to increase PBF. The remaining 30% of patients without right ventricular outflow tract obstruction will be hypoxic but with increased PBF and features of congestive heart failure. This condition exists because there is no obstruction to PBF, and the VSD accentuates the volume load on the left ventricle. These patients may undergo pulmonary artery banding to relieve the symptoms of congestive heart failure.

Pulmonary Atresia with Intact Ventricular Septum

Pulmonary atresia with intact ventricular septum (PA/IVS) is defined by complete obstruction of the right ventricular outflow tract, an intact ventricular septum, and variable hypoplasia of the right ventricle and tricuspid valve. This is a highly lethal and complex anomaly associated with abnormalities in right ventricular myocardial architecture and coronary circulation. Because of the diminutive size of the right ventricle, suprasystemic pressures develop in the right ventricle during fetal life. The myocardium becomes hypertrophied and may also have fistulous connections between the endocardium and the coronary arteries. These vascular channels, referred to as *sinusoids*, result in retrograde perfusion of the coronary circulation, placing the myocardium at extreme risk for ischemia and infarction.

Infants with PA/IVS present immediately after birth with cyanosis and tachypnea. PBF is derived from a PDA. Preoperative management considerations include the correction of hypoxia and acidosis by optimizing ductal blood flow with the use intravenous prostaglandins. Since the right ventricular outflow tract is obstructed, systemic venous return to the right atrium is decompressed through an interatrial defect (i.e., patent foramen ovale or ASD). If the defect is small and restrictive, enlarging the communication with *balloon septostomy* is often performed.

Surgical correction of PA/IVS is performed in two stages. The first stage is palliative and attempts to establish adequate PBF. This is accomplished by pulmonary valvotomy, a systemic-to-pulmonary artery shunt, or both. The second stage depends on the size of the right ventricular cavity. If the right ventricle is of adequate size, a definitive *biventricular repair* is performed. Univentricular correction (i.e., Fontan procedure) is performed if the right ventricle is underdeveloped or in the presence of a right ventricle-dependent coronary circulation.

Ebstein's Anomaly

This deformity of the tricuspid valve is characterized by downward displacement of the posterior and septal leaflets in a spiral fashion below the true annulus. The leaflets are dysplastic, thickened, and often adherent to the right ventricular septum. This displacement leaves a portion of the right ventricle above the valve as a part of the right atrium, referred to as the "atrialized ventricle." The distal right ventricular chamber is variable in size but the right atrium is usually enlarged, sometimes massively. There is virtually always a patent foramen ovale or an ASD present. This is a rare anomaly, comprising 0.3% to 0.6% of all congenital heart defects.

Hemodynamic alterations seen with Ebstein's anomaly correspond to a broad spectrum of pathologic changes associated with this defect. Symptoms are generally related to the degree of tricuspid valve regurgitation, the presence of an ASD, the degree of right ventricular dysfunction, and the presence of other cardiac malformations. During the early postnatal period, the degree of tricuspid regurgitation is accentuated by the initially elevated PVR, leading to increased right-to-left shunting and marked cyanosis. These neonates may also develop severe congestive heart failure. If the neonate survives this period, the degree of cyanosis diminishes as the PVR decreases. In older patients, the predominant symptoms include fatigue, dyspnea on exertion, cyanosis, and dysrhythmias.

In the neonate, treatment is determined by the degree of cyanosis and right ventricular dysfunction. Infusion of prostaglandins may maintain ductal patency, increase pulmonary blood flow, and decrease right-to-left shunting. Generally, surgery is reserved for patients with severe symptoms. Both valvoplasty and replacement of the tricuspid valve have been performed with success.

Anesthetic Considerations

Anesthetic management is predicated on whether pulmonary blood flow is restricted or excessive because the systemic and pulmonary vascular resistances can be manipulated to favor an increase in PBF if it is restricted. It is important to avoid conditions that increase PVR or exacerbate right ventricular outflow tract obstruction. Other management goals include maintaining or increasing SVR and preserving adequate cardiac output.

Altered pharmacokinetics should be expected. Inhalation induction may be prolonged due to the reduced PBF. Intravenous induction agents should have a more rapid onset of action since they could enter the systemic circulation faster, but this is rarely observed clinically. The continuous infusion of prostaglandin to maintain ductal patency preoperatively is very important since adequate PBF must be maintained. Conditions that favor ductal closure must be avoided until surgical palliation or correction is performed. In hemodynamically stable patients, adequate premedication is recommended to prevent agitation and anxiety, which would otherwise increase PVR and exacerbate right-to-left shunting and hypoxia.

In some cases (e.g., tricuspid atresia, VSD, and unobstructed right ventricular outflow tract) excessive PBF leads to congestive heart failure. These patients require normal to high PVRs; therefore, conditions that decrease PVR should be avoided. Furthermore, agents that depress myocardial function should be avoided. Infants may require inotropic support prior to cardiopulmonary bypass to maintain coronary perfusion and an adequate cardiac output.

The method of anesthetic induction for a particular patient is generally dictated by the cardiac anomaly and the degree of hemodynamic compromise. If the patient is stable, either an intravenous or inhalation induction may be accomplished. In unstable patients with poor ventricular function, intravenous narcotics and muscle relaxants have been shown to be safe and effective. The patient with dynamic outflow tract obstruction is generally a better candidate for an inhalational induction. Adequate hydration is important as this maintains adequate right-sided filling pressures, which, in turn, minimizes right ventricular outflow tract obstruction. If needed, ketamine can be used either intramuscularly or intravenously for its sedative and analgesic properties. Once the induction is accomplished, an intravenous line is placed and potent narcotics (i.e., fentanyl or sufentanil) may be administered.

Complex Mixing Lesions

This group of defects is characterized by complete mixing of the arterial and venous circulations, resulting in systemic desaturation. The relative pulmonary and systemic blood flows are determined by the relative pulmonary and systemic vascular resistances and the presence or absence of obstruction to flow. The complex mixing shunts include transposition of the great arteries (TGA), truncus arteriosus, double-outlet right ventricle (DORV), total anomalous pulmonary venous connections (TAPVC), and hypoplastic left heart syndrome (HLHS).

Transposition of the Great Arteries

This lesion is characterized by discordance of the ventriculoarterial connections. The aorta arises from the right ventricle, and the pulmonary artery arises from the left ventricle. The prefix *D-* or *L-* refers to the anatomic relationship between the two great vessels: specifically, whether the aorta lies to the right or left of the pulmonary artery. The term *congenitally corrected* TGV is used when there is atrioventricular discordance in addition to the ventriculoarterial discordance.

In TGA, the pulmonary and systemic circulations flow in parallel. Deoxygenated blood returns to the right heart and is ejected through the aorta to the systemic circulation without circulating through the lungs for gas exchange. Oxygenated blood simply recirculates through the left heart and pulmonary vasculature. Therefore, survival is dependent on mixing of pulmonary and systemic blood at some level (i.e., ASD, VSD, PDA). An atrial septostomy may be performed preoperatively in the catheterization laboratory to promote mixing.

Patients with congenitally corrected TGV have normal circulatory patterns. Deoxygenated blood returns to the right atrium, empties into the left ventricle, and is ejected through the pulmonary artery into the pulmonary circulation for gas exchange. Pulmonary venous return flows into the left atrium, which empties into the right ventricle and is ejected via the aorta into the systemic circulation.

Truncus Arteriosus

This lesion is characterized by one large vessel, or *truncus,* arising from both right and left ventricles, a single semilunar valve, and a large VSD. The truncus may subsequently divide into the pulmonary artery and aorta, or the pulmonary arteries may arise from the lateral or posterior surfaces of the truncus. The absence of the normal separation between pulmonary artery and aorta produces extensive mixing of the pulmonary and systemic circulations. The normal decrease in pulmonary vascular resistance after birth creates excessive PBF, congestive failure, and the rapid development of pulmonary vascular occlusive disease. Systemic blood flow may be severely compromised at the expense of excessive pulmonary blood flow, leading to metabolic acidosis and inadequate coronary artery perfusion.

Double-Outlet Right Ventricle

In DORV, both great vessels arise from the right ventricle, and there is a large, nonrestrictive VSD. Depending on the position of the VSD (i.e., subaortic, subpulmonic) and the presence of other anatomic abnormalities such as pulmonic or aortic stenosis, the pathophysiology varies widely. The balance between pulmonary and systemic circulations is dependent on the relative pulmonary and systemic vascular resistances and coexisting anatomic obstructions to flow.

In *DORV with a subaortic VSD*, oxygenated left ventricular blood is directed to the aorta, and deoxygenated systemic venous return from the right ventricle is directed to the pulmonary artery, resulting in minimal to no cyanosis. Left-to-right shunting across the VSD results in pulmonary overcirculation, pulmonary hypertension, and congestive heart failure. When coupled with pulmonic stenosis, the aorta receives a greater proportion of deoxygenated venous return, leading to cyanosis; this pathophysiology resembles that found in tetralogy of Fallot.

In *DORV with a subpulmonic VSD*, oxygenated left ventricular blood is directed to the pulmonary artery, and deoxygenated systemic venous return from the right ventricle is directed to the aorta, leading to pulmonary overcirculation and cyanosis. In the absence of pulmonic stenosis, this pathophysiology resembles that of TGA with a VSD.

Total Anomalous Pulmonary Venous Connection

In TAPVC, the entire pulmonary venous return drains into the right atrium, usually via a common pulmonary venous confluence. The anomalous drainage patterns are classified as supracardiac, cardiac, or infracardiac. In *supracardiac* TAPVC, the common pulmonary vein confluence drains into the right atrium via an ascending vertical vein leading into the left innominate vein or the superior vena cava. In the *cardiac* configuration, the common pulmonary vein drains into the coronary sinus or directly into the right atrium. In the *infracardiac* pattern, the common pulmonary vein drains through the diaphragm into the hepatic/portal venous system. Pulmonary venous return to the right atrium is subject to stenosis or obstruction, leading to pulmonary congestion and hypertension. Furthermore, the excess volume load placed on the right heart contributes to early right heart failure.

A right-to-left shunt (i.e., PFO, ASD) permits intercirculatory mixing and is essential for survival in TAPVC. The magnitude and direction of shunting across a large, unrestrictive defect is determined by the relative pulmonary and systemic vascular resistances. The degree of systemic arterial desaturation is determined by the degree of intercirculatory mixing.

Hypoplastic Left Heart Syndrome

HLHS is characterized by variable degrees of left heart structure hypoplasia (i.e., left ventricle, aorta, mitral and aortic valves). There is a single functional right ventricle that supplies both pulmonary and systemic blood flow. Oxygenated pulmonary venous blood must cross an ASD and mix with systemic venous return before being ejected by the right ventricle through a PDA into the systemic circulation.

Cyanosis, congestive heart failure, and systemic hypoperfusion result as PVR decreases and PBF increases at the expense of systemic perfusion.

Anesthetic Considerations

The anesthetic goals for patients with complex mixing lesions depend on the specific anatomic and physiologic disturbances present. Management decisions are often driven by the amount of PBF present and the desire to achieve a balance between pulmonary and systemic circulations. In general, patients with increased PBF and extensive intercirculatory mixing will not benefit from efforts to decrease PVR; in fact, such efforts may adversely affect systemic and coronary perfusion, leading to poor myocardial performance, metabolic acidosis, and hepatic and renal hypoperfusion. Patients with diminished PBF, limited mixing, or pulmonary hypertension may benefit from interventions to reduce PVR, promote PBF, and improve arterial oxygen saturation. A complete review of ventilatory management in the neonatal intensive care unit and meticulous adjustments of ventilatory parameters to maintain the desired balance between pulmonary and systemic blood flow is essential in the care of infants with complex mixing lesions. Hypoxic gas mixtures (i.e., <21% oxygen) may be required to prevent pulmonary overcirculation. The appropriate gas mixtures, usually blends of oxygen and nitrogen, must be available in the operating room and transport unit.

Endogenous catecholamine levels will increase pulmonary vascular tone and may lead to the detrimental effects of pulmonary hypertension. Opiate-based anesthetic techniques will decrease pulmonary vasoreactivity and blunt catecholamine-mediated responses. Infants possess a highly reactive pulmonary vasculature and may benefit from high-dose opiate therapy for a number of days perioperatively to prevent pulmonary hypertensive crises. Therapy with systemic vasoactive drugs to decrease pulmonary artery pressures may be limited by systemic hypotension. Inhaled nitric oxide (iNO) can selectively decrease pulmonary artery pressures by promoting pulmonary vascular smooth muscle relaxation. Any iNO that reaches the circulation is bound to hemoglobin and rapidly inactivated, producing no systemic effects. Delivered iNO concentrations must be monitored, and methemoglobin levels must be checked to prevent toxicity in infants who have reduced levels of methemoglobin reductase.

Polycythemia, resulting from persistent hypoxia, may decrease flow through important vascular beds due to hyperviscosity. This phenomenon is particularly prevalent when the hematocrit exceeds 65%. Maintenance of intravascular volume is essential to prevent sludging and end-organ ischemia. Following surgical repair, maintaining hematocrits of 30% is appropriate to provide adequate oxygen-carrying capacity in patients with normal pulmonary and systemic circulations. If patients continue to have mixing of venous and arterial blood, systemic oxygen saturation will be decreased, and therefore the hematocrit should be maintained at a higher level (i.e., 40% to 45%) to improve oxygen delivery.

Compromised cardiac performance due to pressure and volume overloads may require anesthetic techniques and drugs that augment cardiac contractility. Inotropes are used following bypass to improve myocardial function and to support cardiac output. Dobutamine, isoproterenol, and milrinone are commonly used inotropic agents that do not significantly increase PVR; dopamine and epinephrine increase cardiac output at the expense of increasing pulmonary vascular tone.

Obstructive Lesions

Lesions in this category obstruct flow in the form of valvular stenosis or vascular bands. Obstruction causes pressure overload and ventricular hypertrophy, which, in turn compromise ventricular perfusion. Long-standing obstruction in utero leads to significant cardiac dysfunction and failure. Defects included in this category include coarctation of the aorta, interrupted aortic arch, aortic stenosis, mitral stenosis, and cor triatriatum.

Coarctation of the Aorta

Aortic coarctation is a discrete narrowing of the aorta. It is described in relationship to the ductus arteriosus. *Preductal* lesions are proximal to the ductus and present in infancy with ductal closure. Presentation of the infant is characterized by congestive heart failure secondary to left ventricular outflow tract obstruction, hypoperfusion of the lower body, and, in severe cases, cardiovascular collapse. Prostaglandin infusion is used to maintain ductal patency and to stabilize perfusion. *Postductal* and juxtaductal coarctation present at a later age. Postductal coarctation is usually characterized by hypertension, decreased or absent femoral pulses, and the development of extensive collateral blood flow from the subclavian and intercostal arteries. Surgery is indicated if the pressure gradient across the coarctation exceeds 40 mm Hg or if the systolic blood pressure exceeds 180 mm Hg.

Blood pressure monitoring is critical in patients with aortic coarctation. Ideally, both preductal (i.e., right radial artery) and postductal intraarterial blood pressure and pulse oximetry are monitored to guide both proximal and distal blood pressure management. The preductal blood pressure is the most critical, as this indicates upper body and brain perfusion pressure. If the patient does not require central venous access for monitoring or infusion of vasoactive drugs, peripheral venous access is sufficient. Hypertension during aortic cross-clamping can be treated with either inhalational agents or intravenous vasodilators in the stable patient. In infants, volatile agents may not be well tolerated.

Paraplegia is a rare (0.5% to 1.5%) but devastating complication of coarctation repair. Paraplegia is generally believed to result from diminished spinal cord perfusion during aortic cross-clamping. Measures that have been used for cord preservation include intravascular shunting, partial CPB, mild hypothermia (33°C), low-dose anticoagulation, and evoked potential monitoring.

Postoperatively, systemic hypertension is common and requires both vasodilator and beta-blocker therapy. Regional anesthesia is sometimes used to reduce intraoperative anesthetic requirements and for perioperative pain control.

Interrupted Aortic Arch

In interrupted aortic arch, there is a lumenal interruption between the ascending and descending aorta. Systemic arterial perfusion is dependent on a PDA. There are three different types of interrupted aortic arch (types A, B, and C), corresponding to the level of interruption. Associated anomalies include VSD, truncus arteriosus, DORV, and DiGeorge syndrome. The pathophysiology and the anesthetic management of patients with this lesion are similar to those of preductal aortic coarctation.

Aortic Stenosis

There are three types of congenital aortic stenosis: valvular, subvalvular, and supravalvular. All are characterized by ventricular hypertrophy and elevated ventricular filling pressures leading to a decrease in coronary perfusion pressure. These physiologic manifestations have important implications for the anesthetic management of patients with aortic stenosis. Avoiding excessive increases in preload while maintaining adequate systemic diastolic pressures and normal heart rates is necessary to maintain a favorable balance of myocardial oxygen supply and demand.

Infants with valvular aortic stenosis have an increased incidence of associated cardiac malformations and endocardial fibroelastosis. These infants typically present in congestive heart failure and have a significantly higher mortality. Patients with subvalvular stenosis present with a dynamic left ventricular outflow tract obstruction requiring a different management approach. Reducing inotropy and heart rate and maintaining preload and afterload minimizes left ventricular outflow tract obstruction and improves forward flow.

Mitral Stenosis

This is a relatively rare congenital lesion that may occur in isolation as a result of leaflet fusion, annular malformation, or deranged chordae and papillary muscle structures. Mitral stenosis may also occur as part of *Shone's complex,* which includes a supravalvular ring, "parachute" mitral valve, subaortic stenosis, and coarctation of the aorta. Mitral stenosis results in diminished cardiac output secondary to restricted flow across the mitral valve and elevated left atrial pressures leading to pulmonary hypertension and right heart failure.

Anesthetic management of patients with mitral stenosis can be quite challenging. It is essential to control the heart rate to allow adequate time for left ventricular filling. Preload should be maintained for adequate ventricular filling while avoiding volume overload and pulmonary edema. Careful attention to acid-base balance and ventilatory management is crucial to avoid further increases in PVR.

Cor Triatriatum

Cor triatriatum is characterized by a web-like membrane within the left atrium, dividing it into superior and inferior chambers. Pulmonary venous drainage has restricted access to the mitral valve orifice, producing functional mitral stenosis. Management issues are as described above for mitral stenosis.

References

1. MORRAY J. A hazard of continuous flush systems for vascular pressure monitoring in infants. *Anesthesiology* 1983;58:187–189.

2. VERGESE ST, PATEL RI, SELL JE, et al. Ultrasound-guided internal jugular venous cannulation in infants: a prospective comparison with the traditional palpation method. *Anesthesiology* 1999;91:71–77.

3. STEVENSON SG, HARTMAN D, et al. Transesophageal echocardiography during repair of congenital heart defects: identification of residual problems necessitating reoperation. *J Am Soc Echocardiologr* 1993;6:356–365.

4. MUHIUDEEN RUSEELL IA, SILVERMAN NH. Intraoperative transesophageal echocaridography for pediatirc patients with congenital heart disease. *Anesth Analg* 1988;87:1058–1076.

5. DESPOTIS GJ, FIBS K, LEVY J. Anticoagulation monitoring during cardiac surgery. *Anesthesiology* 1999;91:1122–1151.

6. KNIGHT D. Patent ductus arteriosus: how important to which babies? *Early Hum Development* 1992;29:287–292.

7. OBERHANSLI-WEISS I, RUDOLPH AM, MELMON KL. The pattern and mechanism of response to oxygen by the ductus arteriosus and umbilical artery. *Pediatr Res* 1972;6:693–700.

8. RUDOLPH AM. Response of the pulmonary vasculature to hypoxia and H+ ion concentration changes. *J Clin Invest* 1966;45:399–411.

PART 2

Congenital Cardiac Defects: Pathophysiology and Correction

CHAPTER 7

Obstructive Lesions

David D. Yuh, MD, and Bruce A. Reitz, MD

Introduction

This group of congential cardiac defects comprises obstructive lesions which **impede ventricular outflow.** Left untreated, the resultant increase in ventricular afterload generally leads to ventricular hypertrophy, which in turn predisposes to the development of arrhythmias and myocardial ischemia or infarction. Surgical correction generally consists of resecting the anatomic obstruction to flow.

7.1 Pulmonary Stenosis with Intact Ventricular Septum (Fig. 7–1)

Incidence: 8% to 10% of all congenital heart defects; 1:1 male:female

Pathophysiology: Usually involves a stenotic pulmonary valve that obstructs right ventricular emptying and pulmonary blood flow, producing right ventricular hypertrophy and cyanosis. Subvalvar (infundibular) and supravalvar (pulmonary artery) stenoses are other forms of this defect.

Clinical Features: Most patients are usually asymptomatic, with symptoms of dyspnea and fatigue developing as the lesion progresses. Critically ill neonates with severe pulmonary stenosis are dyspneic and cyanotic, with significant right-to-left shunting across a patent foramen ovale or atrial septal defect. A systolic ejection murmur and ejection click at the left upper sternal border is often present. Two-dimensional echocardiography is diagnostic, with the identification of a stenotic pulmonary valve.

Concepts of Corrections: To open the stenotic pulmonary valve with a valvotomy or the hypertrophied right ventricular outflow tract with infundibular resection

Corrective Operation(s):

- Balloon or open pulmonary valvotomy
- Transannular patch (hypoplastic pulmonary valve annulus)
- Infundibular resection with patch-widening of right ventricular outflow tract (subvalvar stenosis)

General Considerations

Pulmonary stenosis is usually at the level of the pulmonary valve, with a wide spectrum of pulmonary **valvar** morphologies, but it may also be **subvalvar** (infundibular) or **supravalvar** (pulmonary artery stenosis). In most cases of isolated valvar pulmonary stenosis (70%), the valve is tricuspid with fused commissures, producing a dome-like structure with a central opening of varying diameter. Thirty percent to 40% of patients with pulmonary valvar stenosis have a patent foramen ovale or small atrial septal defect, producing an atrial level right-to-left shunt. After the neonatal period, poststenotic pulmonary artery dilation and varying degrees of right ventricular hypertrophy are observed, depending on the degree of stenosis. The severity of stenosis varies considerably and is most simply defined by determining the systolic pressure gradient between the right ventricle and the pulmonary artery. Significant pulmonary stenosis, indicating operative correction, is associated with a peak systolic pressure gradient ≥ 50 mm Hg. Critically ill neonates with severe pulmonary stenosis often require resuscitation (i.e., inotropic and/or ventilatory support) and prostaglandin E_1 to maintain ductal patency and pulmonary blood flow.

Diagnostic Keys

Most patients diagnosed with pulmonary stenosis beyond the neonatal period are minimally symptomatic on initial presentation. With moderate stenosis, the right ventricle gradually hypertrophies, resulting in dyspnea and easy fatigability due to inadequate pulmonary blood flow, particularly with physical exertion. Critically ill neonates with severe pulmonary stenosis present within the first week of life, with severe cyanosis and tachypnea due to atrial right-to-left shunting. Cardiac auscultation reveals a systolic ejection murmur at the upper left sternal border in association with an ejection click. Hepatomegaly secondary to tricuspid regurgitation may also be seen. Chest radiography reveals a

95

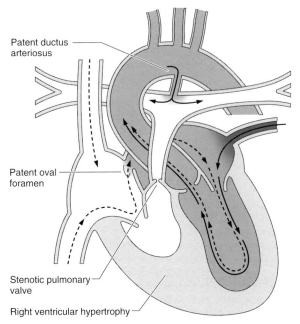

Patent ductus arteriosus

Patent oval foramen

Stenotic pulmonary valve

Right ventricular hypertrophy

Pulmonary valvar stenosis

FIGURE 7–1. Schematic drawing of pulmonary stenosis with intact ventricular septum. (■)——→, Oxygenated; (□)---→, Deoxygenated; (▨)==→, mixed.

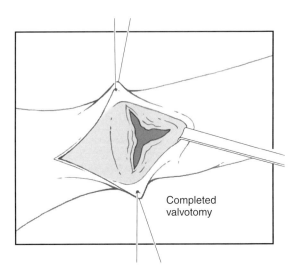

Completed valvotomy

FIGURE 7–1.1. Open pulmonary valvotomy. After cardiopulmonary bypass and cardioplegic arrest has been established, the stenosed pulmonary valve is accessed via a longitudinal arteriotomy. The fused commissures are incised completely with a #11 or #15 scalpel blade. The pulmonary arteriotomy is closed with a running 6-0 Prolene™ suture.

normal to moderately enlarged cardiac silhouette, a prominent main pulmonary artery segment with poststenotic dilation, and diminished pulmonary vascularity in severe cases. Electrocardiography may reveal right atrial dilation and right ventricular hypertrophy in moderate to severe cases of pulmonary stenosis. Two-dimensional echocardiography is usually diagnostic, with identification of a stenotic, thickened, and often hypoplastic pulmonary valve; estimation of pulmonary valve gradients and right ventricular pressures may be obtained with Doppler measurements.

Operative Correction

Balloon pulmonary valvotomy is the procedure of choice for significant pulmonary valvar stenosis in all phases of life. Performed during cardiac catheterization, sequentially graduated balloons are inflated across the stenotic pulmonary valve until a residual transvalvar gradient of <30 mm Hg is achieved.

Open pulmonary valvotomy under cardiopulmonary bypass with cardioplegic arrest is indicated when balloon valvotomy is either unavailable or unsuccessful. Once cardiopulmonary bypass with mild hypothermia has been established, cardioplegic arrest is instituted. The ductus arteriosus is temporarily closed with a snare. The stenotic pulmonary valve is approached through a longitudinal pulmonary arteriotomy, and the fused commisures are opened

with a #11 scalpel blade (Fig. 7–1.1). The valve is then gently dilated with a mosquito clamp, the annular diameter is appropriately calibrated with Hegar dilators (based on body surface area), and the arteriotomy is closed. Adequate opening of the valve is of paramount importance; portions of the valve may need to be excised in a severely dysplastic valve. In most cases, the patent foramen ovale or atrial septal defect is closed via a right atriotomy, and the patient is weaned from cardiopulmonary bypass.

Intraoperative epicardial two-dimensional echocardiography with Doppler is performed immediately after the repair to measure the residual gradient across the right ventricular outflow tract, the residual tricuspid regurgitation, and atrial level shunt. The heretofore snared ductus arteriosus is permanently ligated if the arterial PO$_2$ is ≥35 mmHg; if the arterial PO$_2$ is <35 mmHg, the snare is released and PGE$_1$ infusion is continued to maintain ductal patency. In the setting of inadequate early right ventricular function (e.g., arterial PO$_2$ < 35 mm Hg despite a patent ductus arteriosus), the patent foramen ovale is left open, and a temporary Blalock-Taussig systemic-pulmonary artery shunt is constructed. After the right ventricle develops properly and its function improves, these shunts are closed.

In rare cases when the pulmonary valve annulus is hypoplastic (<10%; Z score <−3) and the right ventricular cavity is small, the annular diameter can be augmented by placing a patch of autologous pericardium across it. When **transannular patching** is indicated, the pulmonary

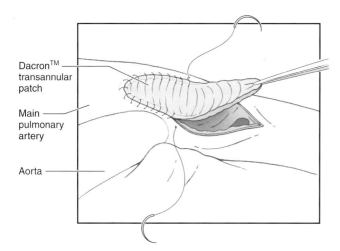

FIGURE 7–1.2. Transannular patch augmentation of hypoplastic pulmonary valve annulus. A vertical pulmonary arteriotomy is carried onto the infundibulum. The extent of annular widening is determined by passing an appropriately sized Hegar dilator across the pulmonary valve annulus into the right ventricular outflow tract. An autologous pericardial patch is placed with a continuous 5-0 Prolene™ suture.

arteriotomy is carried proximally across the annulus onto the infundibular free wall. An appropriately sized Hegar dilator is then used to calibrate the size and placement of the pericardial patch (Fig. 7–1.2).

In cases of subvalvar stenosis, **infundibular resection** with patch widening of the right ventricular outflow tract may be indicated. A vertical ventriculotomy is made in the infundibulum, and varying amounts of hypertrophied muscular trabeculae are resected. The ventriculotomy is then closed with an autologous pericardial patch.

Closed transventricular pulmonary valvotomy does not require cardiopulmonary bypass and can be performed rapidly compared with the open procedure; it is useful in critically ill neonates with severe pulmonary stenosis. In this technique, sequentially graduated Hegar dilators are passed across the right ventricular outflow tract and pulmonary valve via an incision made in the right ventricular infundibulum. Disadvantages of this technique include a higher perioperative mortality rate (10% to 20%) and more frequently required reinterventions. The perioperative mortality for patients undergoing balloon or open valvotomy for noncritical pulmonary valvar stenosis is 1% to 3%. Hanley and associates report 30-day and 4-year survival rates of 89% and 81%, respectively, among a multiinstitutional series of patients who underwent interventional treatment (all modes) for critical pulmonary stenosis.[1] Right ventricular size approaches normal in 90% of successfully

treated patients. Complications of pulmonary valvotomy include residual or recurrent valvar stenosis, persistent postoperative hypoxemia, and pulmonary valvar incompetence.

7.2 Pulmonary Atresia with Intact Ventricular Septum (Fig. 7–2)

Incidence: 1% to 1.5% of all congenital heart defects

Pathophysiology: Atretic pulmonary valve combined with varying degrees of tricuspid valve and right ventricular hypoplasia, leading to inadequate pulmonary blood flow (supported by patent ductus arteriosus) and hypoxia. Right ventricular-to-coronary artery fistulae are seen in 50% to 60% of patients, resulting in a right ventricular-dependent coronary circulation in 10% to 20%.

Clinical Features: Majority (90%) present in the first 3 days of life with generalized cyanosis, worsening as the patent ductus arteriosus constricts. Chest radiography may reveal a "boot-shaped" heart from a flat/concave pulmonary artery segment. Echocardiography is used to evaluate right ventricular cavity and outflow tract, tricuspid insufficiency, ductal flow, and coronary artery fistulae.

Concepts of Correction: Initial goals of correction are to improve pulmonary blood flow with a systemic-to-pulmonary artery shunt and to promote right ventricular development by relieving right ventricular outflow tract obstruction (RVOTO).

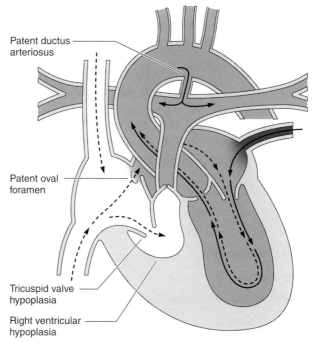

Pulmonary valvar atresia

FIGURE 7–2. Schematic drawing of pulmonary atresia with intact ventricular septum. (■)——➤, Oxygenated; (□)---➤, Deoxygenated; (▨)----➤, mixed.

Satisfactory right ventricular development leads to a "normal" biventricular system. Otherwise, a Fontan operation or cardiac transplantation is indicated.

Corrective Operation(s):

- Modified Blalock-Taussig shunt and transannular patch
- Bidirectional Glenn shunt ("one-and-a-half ventricle" repair)
- Bidirectional Glenn shunt and Fontan procedure
- Cardiac transplantation

General Considerations

Pulmonary atresia with intact ventricular septum (PA-IVS) is composed of an atretic pulmonary valve resulting in severe RVOTO. The malformed valve resembles a diaphragm formed by fusion of three commissures. Associated maldevelopment of the right ventricle, tricuspid valve, and coronary circulation are generally felt to be induced by the hemodynamic perturbations of severe RVOTO in utero. The right ventricle is usually hypoplastic, with marked wall hypertrophy, although the ventricular size is infrequently normal or supranormal. Similarly, the tricuspid valve annulus is usually hypoplastic. An interatrial communication, in the form of a secundum atrial septal defect or patent foramen ovale, is almost always present. About 50% of patients with PA-IVS display coronary sinusoids with **right ventricular-to-coronary artery fistulae,** particularly patients with markedly hypoplastic right ventricles and tricuspid valves, and 20% possess a right ventricular-dependent coronary circulation. Significant coronary artery stenoses may occur proximal or distal to these fistulae. Cumulatively, these malformations markedly compromise pulmonary blood flow, resulting in cyanosis. In PA-IVS, pulmonary blood flow is dependent on a patent ductus arteriosus, often necessitating the use of prostaglandin E_1 to maintain ductal patency after birth. PA-IVS entails a high early mortality, with 2-week and 6-month survival rates of 50% and 15%, respectively. Death results from severe hypoxia and metabolic acidosis stemming from spontaneous ductal closure.

Diagnostic Keys

Moderate cyanosis and a systolic murmur of ductal flow are usually evident within the first several days of life, with cyanosis becoming more severe as the ductus arteriosus closes. Electrocardiography often reflects right atrial enlargement (i.e., prominent P wave) stemming from tricuspid regurgitation. Chest radiography classically reveals a "boot-shaped" heart resulting from the atretic pulmonary artery segment. Echocardiography is diagnostic and is used to evaluate the right ventricular outflow tract and cavity, tricuspid valve, atrial septum, ductal flow, and right ventricular-to-coronary artery fistulae. Cardiac catheterization and angiography are essential to define the coronary anatomy precisely, identify fistulae, and determine the presence of a right ventricular-dependent coronary circulation.

Operative Correction

Immediate operative intervention is indicated in all cases of PA-IVS. The optimal operative result in patients with PA-IVS is a "normal" biventricular circulation, with a right ventricle capable of delivering adequate pulmonary blood flow at normal filling pressures. Since the choice of procedures to accomplish this goal has been controversial, a consensus approach based on a prospective multicenter study initiated by the Congenital Heart Surgeon's Society (CHSS) has been formulated (Fig. 7–2.1).[2]

The initial operation is directed toward (1) establishing satisfactory ductal-independent pulmonary blood flow with a systemic-to-pulmonary artery shunt (i.e., modified Blalock-Taussig shunt); and (2) promoting normal right ventricular development by relieving RVOTO and decompressing the right ventricle with a transannular patch (or, rarely, a pulmonary valvotomy). The atrial septal defect is usually not closed at the initial operation to prevent systemic venous hypertension.

In PA-IVS patients with a normal tricuspid valve diameter and a normal right ventricular cavity, relief of RVOTO with a transannular patch is performed. In patients with mild-to-moderate tricuspid valve annular hypoplasia, a transannular patch and concomitant systemic-to-pulmonary artery shunt is indicated. Patients with severe right ventricular and tricuspid annular hypoplasia should initially receive a systemic-to-pulmonary artery shunt alone since the prospect of a biventricular repair is unlikely.

There are two recognized contraindications to relieving RVOTO in PA-IVS: (1) PA-IVS patients with a right ventricle–dependent coronary circulation should not undergo right ventricular decompression, since abrupt reduction in right ventricular systolic pressures could result in irreversible myocardial ischemia; and (2) PA-IVS patients with severe tricuspid insufficiency should not undergo transannular patching of the pulmonary valve since the potential pulmonary insufficiency combined with the existing tricuspid regurgitation may result in severe congestive right heart failure. Therefore, PA-IVS patients with a right ventricle–dependent coronary circulation or severe tricuspid regurgitation should only receive a Blalock-Taussig shunt. Exceptions to this rule are patients with severe tricuspid regurgitation who undergo tricuspid valve annuloplasty to reduce regurgitation.

Patients who undergo right ventricular outflow tract reconstruction should undergo follow-up echocardiography and catheterization at 3 to 6 months of age to assess right ventricular and tricuspid valvar development. If these are deemed adequate to support a biventricular circulation, trial occlusion of the shunt and atrial septal defect is performed in the catheterization laboratory. If an adequate systemic oxygen saturation is maintained with temporary shunt occlusion, it may be closed permanently. Furthermore, if temporary balloon occlusion of the atrial septal defect does

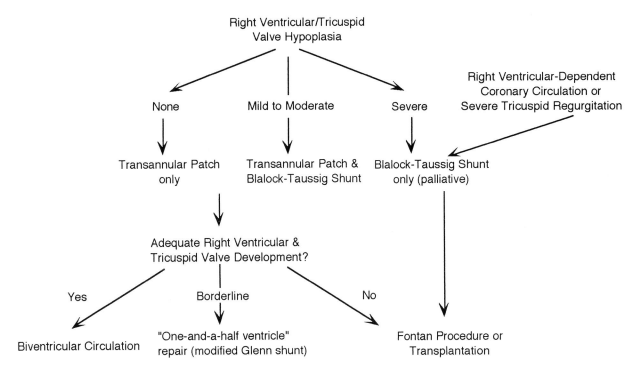

FIGURE 7–2.1. Congenital Heart Surgeon's Society (CHSS) consensus approach to pulmonary atresia with intact ventricular septum.

not result in a marked increase in right atrial pressures and/or decreases in systemic arterial pressures and mixed venous oxygen saturations, this too can be closed permanently at this time or within 6 months. Patients in whom minimal to no right ventricular development is appreciated at follow-up should be tracked to a **Fontan procedure or cardiac transplantation.** The Fontan operation and its variants serves to direct systemic venous return to the pulmonary artery, by-passing the right ventricle (see Tricuspid Atresia section in Chapter 9). Cases of borderline interval right ventricular development at the initial follow-up evaluation may continue to be followed at 6-month intervals, with the hope of further development permitting a biventricular repair. A small subset of patients in this borderline category may undergo a definitive **"one-and-a-half ventricle repair"** in which a superior vena cava-to-pulmonary artery bidirectional connection (**modified Glenn shunt**) is performed, the interatrial communication is closed, and the systemic-to-pulmonary artery shunt is taken down. In this configuration, pulmonary blood flow supplied by the underdeveloped right ventricle is supplemented by the modified Glenn shunt.

Patients who cannot undergo right ventricular outflow tract reconstruction due to marked right ventricular and tricuspid annular hypoplasia, right ventricle–dependent coronary circulation, or severe tricuspid regurgitation should be immediately tracked toward a Fontan procedure or cardiac

transplantation. These patients should undergo follow-up catheterization at 3 to 6 months of age to plan for a bidirectional Glenn shunt (i.e., bidirectional superior cavopulmonary shunt) between 3 and 12 months of age followed by a completion Fontan operation between 1 and 4 years of age.

Modified Blalock-Taussig Shunt Through a right thoracotomy or median sternotomy, the pericardium is opened, and the innominate and right subclavian arteries are dissected. A side-biting clamp is placed across the subclavian artery, an arteriotomy is made, and an end-to-side anastomosis is performed between this artery and a 4- or 5-mm GoreTex™ tube graft using a running 6-0 or 7-0 Prolene™ suture (Fig. 7–2.2). The distal anastomosis is similarly constructed between the graft and right pulmonary artery. After the occluding clamps are removed, the ductus arteriosus is temporarily occluded; it may be permanently ligated if arterial saturations are >80%.

Transannular Patch and Modified Blalock-Taussig Shunt Through a median sternotomy, the heart is cannulated, and cardiopulmonary bypass with mild hypothermia (30° to 34°C) is established. A longitudinal pulmonary arteriotomy is created and extended across the pulmonary valve annulus and onto the infundibulum. A pericardial patch is secured across the arteriotomy with a continuous

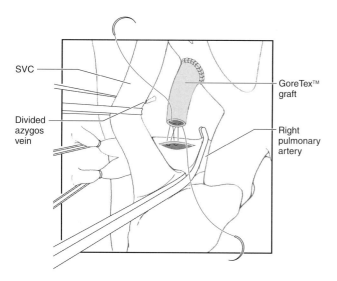

FIGURE 7–2.2. Modified Blalock-Taussig systemic-to-pulmonary artery shunt. A side-biting clamp is placed across the right subclavian artery, a longitudinal arteriotomy is made, and an end-to-side anastomosis is performed between this artery and a 4- or 5-mm GoreTex™ tube graft using a running 6-0 or 7-0 Prolene™ suture. The distal anastomosis between the graft and the right pulmonary artery is similarly performed. SVC = superior vena cava.

5-0 Prolene™ suture (Fig. 7–2.3). The size and shape of the patch are calibrated using an appropriately sized Hegar dilator placed across the pulmonary valve and the right ventricular outflow tract. A Blalock-Taussig shunt is then constructed as described above, and rewarming is started. A right atrial pressure line is inserted, and the patient is weaned from cardiopulmonary bypass.

The most common early complication following right ventricular outflow tract reconstruction and a systemic-to-pulmonary artery shunt is low cardiac output manifested by hypoperfusion and metabolic acidosis. This is most commonly due to coronary hypoperfusion caused by a right ventricular–dependent coronary circulation. Excessive shunt flow may also result in low cardiac output.

A CHSS multiinstitutional series of 171 PA-IVS patients have achieved 1-month and 4-year survival rates of 77% and 58%, respectively, with the best results obtained from transannular patching or valvulotomy with systemic-to-pulmonary artery shunting.

Modified Glenn Shunt and Fontan Procedure For a discussion of this procedure, see the Tricuspid Atresia section in Chapter 9.

Cardiac Transplantation For discussion, see the Hypoplastic Left Ventricle section in Chapter 10.

7.3 Left Ventricular Outflow Tract Obstruction (Fig. 7–3)

Incidence: Comprises 5% of congenital heart defects, with a 4:1 male:female predominance

Pathophysiology: Left ventricular tract obstruction (LVOTO) leads to left ventricular hypertrophy, ischemia, and dysfunction. The obstruction is at the valvar, subvalvar, or supravalvar level.

Clinical Features: Most children beyond infancy with mild-to-moderate aortic stenosis are asymptomatic. Angina, dyspnea, and syncope are associated with severe aortic stenosis. Physical examination reveals a harsh systolic ejection murmur (URSB). Echocardiography with Doppler is diagnostic,

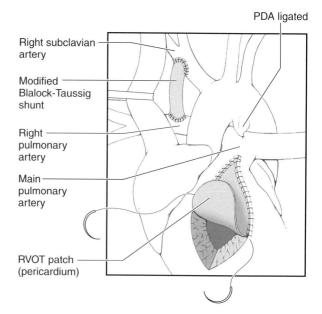

FIGURE 7–2.3. Transannular patch and modified Blalock-Taussig shunt. Once cardiopulmonary bypass is instituted, a longitudinal pulmonary arteriotomy is extended across the atretic pulmonary valve annulus and onto the infundibulum. The patent ductus arteriosus is also snared. A right-sided modified Blalock-Taussig shunt is constructed with a 4-mm GoreTex™ tube graft placed between the right subclavian/innominate and pulmonary arteries. A pericardial transannular patch is secured across the infundibular incision to enlarge the right ventricular outflow tract (RVOT). The patent ductus arteriosus is permanently ligated; the atrial septal defect is usually left open at the initial procedure.

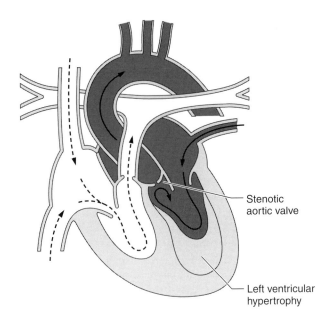

FIGURE 7–3. Schematic drawing of left ventricular outflow tract obstruction. (■)——▶, Oxygenated; (□)----▶, Deoxygenated; (▨)----▶, mixed.

revealing structural lesions of the LVOT, left ventricular hypertrophy, and left ventricular dysfunction. Neonates with critical aortic stenosis are dependent on ductal patency for systemic perfusion; they may present in shock upon spontaneous ductal closure.

Concepts of Correction: Valvar stenosis is relieved with open valvotomy or percutaneous balloon valvuloplasty, often followed by aortic valve replacement. Valve replacement in infants may require an aortoventriculoplasty to enlarge the aortic annulus for accommodation of a prosthetic valve or pulmonary autograft. Subvalvar stenosis is treated by resection of a discrete subvalvar membrane or idiopathic hypertrophic subaortic stenosis (IHSS). Valve replacement is required for tunnel-type LVOTO with aortic valve hypoplasia. Supravalvar stenosis is relieved patch widening of the narrowed aorta.

Corrective Operation(s):

- Surgical aortic valvotomy versus percutaneous balloon valvuloplasty
- Resection of subvalvar membrane or hypertrophied septal muscle
- Konno aortoventriculoplasty with prosthetic valve replacement
- Ross or Ross-Konno procedure

General Considerations

Congenital aortic stenosis represents a group of malformations that obstruct blood flow from the left ventricle to the aorta. Also identified as LVOTO, these malformations

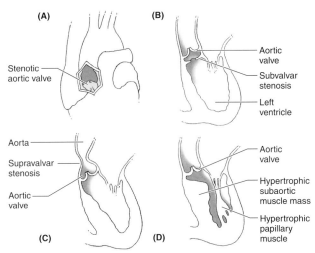

FIGURE 7–3.1. Types of left ventricular outflow tract obstruction. *(A)* Valvar aortic stenosis. *(B)* Discrete subvalvar aortic stenosis. *(C)* Supravalvar aortic stenosis. *(D)* Diffuse subvalvar aortic stenosis (IHSS). *(Source: From Verrier.[3])*

are broadly classified as **valvar, subvalvar,** and **supravalvar** (Fig. 7–3.1A–C). Approximately 25% of patients diagnosed with congenital aortic stenosis have other cardiovascular defects including coarctation of the aorta, patent ductus arteriosus, ventricular septal defect, and pulmonary stenosis.

Valvar aortic stenosis is the most common type of aortic stenosis and is comprised of varying degrees of valve leaflet thickening and incomplete commissural separation. A **bicuspid aortic valve** is the most common form (70%). Poststenotic dilation of the ascending aorta commonly develops over time.

Subvalvar aortic stenosis may take the form of a *discrete fibromuscular membrane, diffuse septal muscle hypertrophy* causing dynamic narrowing of the left ventricular outflow tract, or a rigid, *fibromuscular tunnel-like narrowing.* The discrete fibromuscular type of obstruction is the most common form of subvalvar aortic stenosis, occurring in 75% to 85% of these patients. The diffuse septal hypertrophic form of subvalvar stenosis (Fig. 7–3.1–D) is a manifestation of the cardiomyopathy known as IHSS. Tunnel-type subvalvar stenosis is commonly associated with a severely hypoplastic aortic valve. Aortic regurgitation usually develops in 30% to 50% of patients with subvalvar aortic stenosis. Associated cardiac malformations are particularly common with subvalvar aortic stenosis, occurring in 50% to 65% of patients. These include ventricular septal defect, coarctation of the aorta, patent ductus arteriosus, and left superior vena cava. Consequently, left and right cardiac catheterization is recommended in the workup of subvalvar aortic stenosis to identify these concomitant lesions.

Supravalvar aortic stenosis is composed of three forms: an *hourglass*-shaped deformity (50% to 75%), *diffuse* narrowing of the ascending aorta (25%), or a *discrete membranous* obstruction above the aortic valve. Concomitant abnormalities of the aortic arch vessel orifices and the aortic valve itself are commonly seen. Accelerated coronary artery occlusive changes are identified in patients with supravalvar aortic stenosis, presumably due to prolonged exposure of the coronary arteries to supranormal pressures. Supravalvar aortic stenosis is often associated with Williams's syndrome, a genetic disorder consisting of mental retardation, "elfin facies," and multiple peripheral pulmonary artery stenoses.

In congenital aortic stenosis, the left ventricle experiences an increase in pressure and wall tension generally leading to concentric left ventricular hypertrophy and reduced capacity. An associated increase in the systolic ejection period necessitates a diminished diastolic interval during the cardiac cycle and hence a reduction in coronary perfusion. **Endocardial fibroelastosis** may also be present in affected infants, presumably due to subendocardial ischemia. Therefore, the combined effects of left ventricular hypertrophy and diminished coronary perfusion lead to left ventricular ischemia and dysfunction; sudden death is frequently observed in untreated patients with severe left ventricular outflow tract obstruction.

Diagnostic Keys

Most children (95%) beyond infancy with mild-to-moderate valvar aortic stenosis are asymptomatic, experiencing normal growth and development. Severe aortic stenosis in children, however, can be associated with angina pectoris, exertional dyspnea, syncope, and even sudden death (1% to 2%). Physical examination classically reveals a harsh systolic ejection murmur at the upper right sternal border. An ejection click may be heard with valvar aortic stenosis, and a diastolic decrescendo murmur may present in patients with a bicuspid aortic valve or discrete subvalvar stenosis. A narrow pulse pressure is associated with severe aortic stenosis. Electrocardiography and chest radiography are usually normal in mild cases; however, severe cases may be associated with left ventricular hypertrophy, ascending aortic poststenotic dilation, and signs of congestive heart failure (e.g., cardiomegaly, pulmonary congestion). Two-dimensional echocardiography is diagnostic, revealing structural abnormalities of the left ventricular outflow tract (e.g., aortic valve) as well as left ventricular hypertrophy and diminished contractility. Doppler flow velocity measurements can identify abnormal flow patterns and estimate transvalvar pressure gradients. Mild to moderate transvalvar gradients range from 40 to 50 mm Hg; peak systolic gradients >50 to 75 mm Hg or a valve area <0.5 cm²/m² constitute severe aortic stenosis. Intervention to relieve the LVOTO is indicated when the transvalvar gradient exceeds 50 mm Hg and/or symptoms attributable to aortic stenosis are present (e.g., syncope, angina). Cardiac catheterization is useful for pinpointing and characterizing the site of LVOTO in equivocal cases and for identifying coexistent cardiac defects.

Neonates with *critical aortic stenosis* may develop signs of congestive heart failure (i.e., tachypnea, feeding problems, failure to thrive) within the first few days, weeks, or months of life. Systemic perfusion is heavily dependent on ductal patency in these patients, and ductal closure often results in hypotensive shock and cyanosis. Physical findings include a soft ejection murmur, poor peripheral pulses, and precordial lift. Chest radiography typically reveals cardiomegaly, sometimes associated with pulmonary congestion. As in older children, two-dimensional echocardiography is usually diagnostic and, additionally, provides crucial assessment of left ventricular size and function as well as the presence of endocardial fibroelastosis, which may directly affect the surgical approach and outcome. Acute deterioration in these newborns may require inotropic and ventilatory support as well as prostaglandin E₁ to maintain ductal patency and systemic perfusion.

Operative Correction

Neonates in congestive heart failure from critical valvar aortic stenosis require immediate intervention. Careful echocardiographic examination of left ventricular size and function is of particular importance in evaluating these critically ill neonates. In cases of severe left ventricular hypoplasia or endocardial fibroelastosis, the **Norwood procedure** or **cardiac transplantation** are indicated. A Rashkind balloon atrial septostomy is often required as a temporizing move in these cases, to reduce pulmonary venous hypertension.

In neonates with satisfactory left ventricular function, critical valvar aortic stenosis is usually treated with **surgical valvotomy** (Fig. 7–3.2) or **percutaneous balloon valvuloplasty**. Open aortic valvotomy is performed through a median sternotomy using cardiopulmonary bypass or inflow occlusion. The aortic valve is exposed through a transverse ascending aortotomy directed toward the noncoronary cusp. The fused valve commissures are then sharply separated just enough with a #11 or #15 scalpel blade to relieve the stenosis without creating aortic insufficiency. Unfortunately, this procedure is associated with a 25% to 50% operative mortality rate in critically ill neonates and, among survivors, a high rate of recurrent aortic stenosis and/or aortic regurgitation. The percutaneous technique does not require cardiopulmonary bypass. A balloon dilation catheter is passed retrograde across the aortic valve over a percutaneously placed guidewire. The aortic valve is then dilated with a series of balloon inflations, with special care taken to avoid excessive valve dilation and resultant aortic insufficiency.

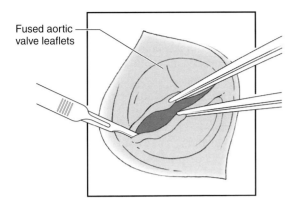

FIGURE 7–3.2. Open surgical aortic valvotomy. The aortic valve is exposed through a transverse aortotomy just above the level of the valve cusps and extending to the noncoronary sinus of Valsalva. The fused commissure(s) are incised to within 1 to 2 mm of the annulus. Care must be taken to avoid overextending the commissural incision, as aortic valvar incompetence may result.

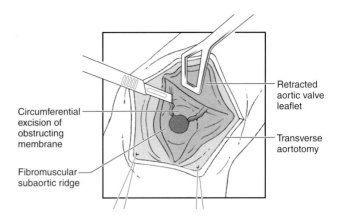

FIGURE 7–3.3. Resection of subaortic membrane in discrete subvalvar stenosis. Through a transverse aortotomy, the right coronary cusp is retracted, exposing the obstructing subvalvar fibromuscular ring. A radial incision into septal portion of the ring is performed. Wedge resection of the septum may be required for complete relief of the obstruction; however, care must be taken to avoid creating a ventricular septal defect or damaging the bundle of His. The obstructing subvalvar fibromuscular membrane is then circumferentially resected. Care must be taken to avoid incising the bases of the mitral valve anterior leaflet or aortic valve leaflets, as this would result in valvar insufficiency.

Hospital mortality rates are generally lower with this closed procedure compared with its open counterpart, with comparable success rates at some centers. Open and closed aortic valvotomies are largely palliative procedures, with aortic valve replacement often required later in life.

In older children with valvar aortic stenosis, intervention is indicated for severe disease indicated by a high transvalvar pressure gradient (i.e., 50 to 75 mm Hg) and/or symptoms. Standard treatment is with open aortic valvotomy or percutaneous balloon valvuloplasty. Aortic valve replacement constitutes another therapeutic option.

The surgical correction of significant subvalvar aortic stenosis varies according to the form of obstruction; all are performed through a median sternotomy and require cardiopulmonary bypass with cardioplegic arrest. Discrete subvalvar stenosis is treated with **resection of the obstructing subvalvar membrane** (Fig. 7–3.3). A transverse aortotomy is created just above the aortic valve commissures. The fibrous subaortic membrane or ridge extending from beneath the aortic valve right coronary leaflet to the border of the anterior mitral leaflet is visualized by retracting the aortic valve leaflets and is circumferentially resected. Special care must be taken to avoid injury to the membranous ventricular septum (containing the bundle of His) or mitral and aortic valve leaflets.

In the diffuse form of subaortic stenosis, **ventricular septoplasty** (Fig. 7–3.4) is the treatment of choice. The ventricular septum is exposed through an oblique subpulmonic infundibular incision extending to the level of the aortic annulus. The septum is incised longitudinally and

extended along the subaortic left ventricular outflow tract. Any hypertrophied septal muscle along the left ventricular outflow tract is then excised, avoiding injury to the bundle of His. The resultant defect is then closed with an autologous pericardial or Dacron patch. The infundibular incision is then closed (or patched in the case of RVOTO), and cardiopulmonary bypass is discontinued.

Tunnel subvalvar stenosis has traditionally been treated by enlarging the left ventricular outflow tract with the **Konno-Rastan aortoventriculoplasty** (Fig. 7–3.5). This procedure is designed to enlarge a severely hypoplastic aortic annulus anteriorly to accommodate a prosthetic aortic valve that is large enough to accomodate growth. The procedure can provide a substantial increase (up to 50%) in the diameter of the aortic annulus, but it is technically challenging and subject to complications including hemorrhage, septal patch dehiscence, conduction system injury, and diminished left ventricular function. Furthermore, a mechanical prosthetic valve entails lifelong anticoagulation. Once cardiopulmonary bypass with cardioplegic arrest has been established, a vertical aortotomy is created on the anterior surface of the ascending aorta and extended inferiorly

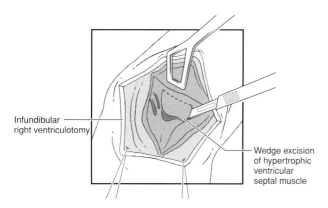

Infundibular right ventriculotomy

Wedge excision of hypertrophic ventricular septal muscle

FIGURE 7–3.4. Ventricular septoplasty for diffuse subvalvar stenosis. A subpulmonic infundibular right ventriculotomy is extended to the level of the aortic annulus to expose the interventricular septum. A septal incision is extended along the subvalvar left ventricular outflow tract. Obstructive, hypertrophic septal muscle is then resected. The resultant septal defect is closed with autologous pericardium or Dacron.™ The right ventriculotomy is closed primarily or patched in the setting of RVOTO.

through the aortic annulus (to the left of the right coronary ostium) and into the right ventricular outflow tract. The interventricular septum is also incised from the level of the aortic annulus, extending inferiorly along the same line as the aortotomy. Together, these two incisions significantly widen the left ventricular outflow tract, including the aortic valve annulus. The native aortic valve cusps are excised. The left ventricular outflow tract is then reconstructed by securing a diamond-shaped Dacron™ patch across the septal incision with a running 3-0 or 4-0 Prolene™ suture. An appropriately sized prosthetic aortic valve is then secured to the aortic annulus and this patch using interrupted pledgeted mattress sutures. Finally, a second triangular Dacron™ patch is used to close the right ventriculotomy, thereby widening the right ventricular outflow tract.

Aortic valve replacement by translocation of a pulmonary autograft and replacement of the pulmonary artery root with a cryopreserved homograft, the **Ross procedure** (Fig. 7–3.6), is an attractive alternative to mechanical valve replacement in children because anticoagulation is not required and there is the potential for autograft growth. The rationale of this procedure lies in the placement of an autogenous tissue valve in the high-pressure aortic position, and a homograft tissue valve in the low-pressure pulmonary position, where the development of valve incompetence would be better tolerated. Once cardiopulmonary bypass is established, the aortic root is explored through a transverse

aortotomy. The aortic root, including the aortic valve, is then excised from the ventriculoarterial junction to the midascending aorta except for two coronary ostial "buttons"; this is similar to coronary ostial mobilization in arterial switch operations. The pulmonary artery is dissected away from the aorta to the level of its bifurcation where it is divided. The main pulmonary trunk, containing the pulmonary valve, is then separated from the right ventricular outflow tract above the infundibulum. The resultant pulmonary autograft is sutured to the aortic annulus with interrupted 3-0 Prolene™ sutures and hence placed in continuity with the left ventricular outflow tract. The coronary artery ostia are implanted into the pulmonary autograft with continuous 5-0 Prolene™ sutures, and the distal end-to-end anastomosis to the aorta is performed with a running 3-0 Prolene™ suture line. Finally, a cryopreserved pulmonary homograft is anastomosed between the pulmonary artery bifurcation and the right ventricular outflow tract with continuous 3-0 Prolene™ sutures. The **modified Ross-Konno** procedure accomplishes augmentation of the left ventricular outflow tract and uses a pulmonary autograft for the aortic valve replacement.

Supravalvar aortic stenosis is treated with **aortoplasty** (Fig. 7–3.7), namely, widening of the aorta just superior to the aortic annulus with a Dacron™ or an autologous pericardial patch. An inverted "Y" aortotomy is made along the narrowed ascending aortic segment, extending into the non- and right coronary sinuses. This aortotomy is then patch-widened with a bifurcated Dacron™ patch. Any discrete obstructing ridges of intraluminal tissue are concomitantly excised. When the supravalvar aortic stenosis is severe due to multiple levels of obstruction or a deformed aortic valve, a replacement of the ascending aorta or aortic root may be necessary.

7.4 Coarctation of the Aorta (Fig. 7–4)

Incidence: Comprises approximately 5% to 8% of congenital heart defects.

Pathophysiology: Narrowed aorta produces increased left ventricular afterload and wall stress, left ventricular hypertrophy, and congestive heart failure. Systemic perfusion is dependent on ductal flow and collateralization in severe coarctation.

Clinical Features: Classically presents with upper extremity hypertension, absent/diminished lower extremity pulses, and systolic ejection murmur. Infants with severe coarctation are dependent on ductal and collateral flow for systemic perfusion and may present in congestive heart failure upon ductal closure. Older children usually present with lower extremity weakness and dyspnea. Electrocardiography may reveal left ventricular hypertrophy. Chest radiograph may produce the classic "3" sign (hourglass morphology) of coarctation. Echocardiography with Doppler is diagnostic.

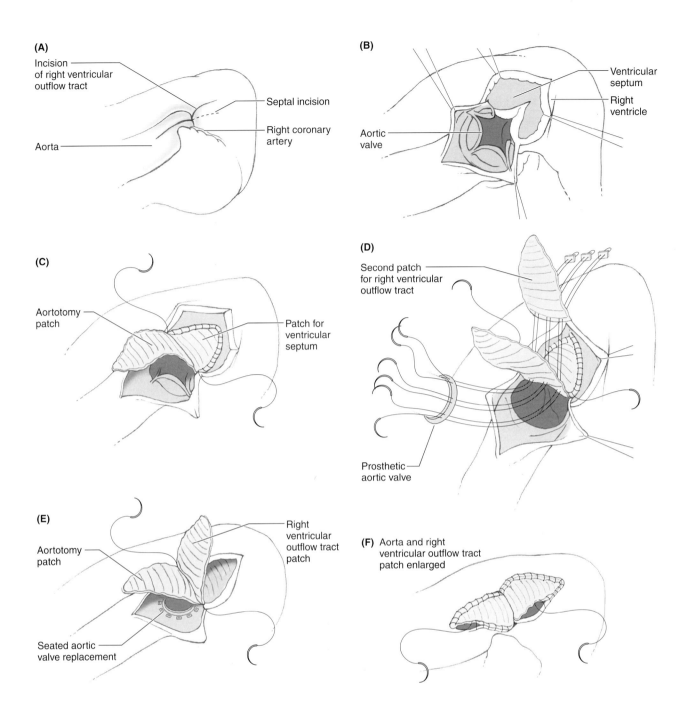

(A)
Incision of right ventricular outflow tract

Septal incision

Right coronary artery

Aorta

(B)
Ventricular septum

Right ventricle

Aortic valve

(C)
Aortotomy patch

Patch for ventricular septum

(D)
Second patch for right ventricular outflow tract

Prosthetic aortic valve

(E)
Aortotomy patch

Right ventricular outflow tract patch

Seated aortic valve replacement

(F) Aorta and right ventricular outflow tract patch enlarged

FIGURE 7–3.5.   Konno-Rastan aortoventriculoplasty and aortic valve replacement for tunnel subvalvar stenosis: *(A)* A vertical aortotomy is extended across the aortic valve annulus to the left of the right coronary artery and onto the right ventricle. The interventricular septum is then incised beginning at the aortic annulus and carried downward and to the left of the bundle of His. These two incisions greatly widen the left ventricular outflow tract and facilitate excision of the native aortic valve. *(B, C)* The left ventricular outflow tract is enlarged by placing a diamond-shaped Dacron™ patch across the septal incision and aortotomy in conjunction with a prosthetic aortic valve replacement; the patch is also secured to the anterior aspect of the valve sewing ring. The base of a second triangle-shaped Dacron™ patch is attached to the midpoint of the diamond-shaped patch. *(D, E)* This second patch is used to close the right ventriculotomy, thereby widening the right ventricular outflow tract. The free end of the diamond-shaped patch is used to close the aortotomy. These are secured with continuous 4-0 or 5-0 Prolene™ sutures.

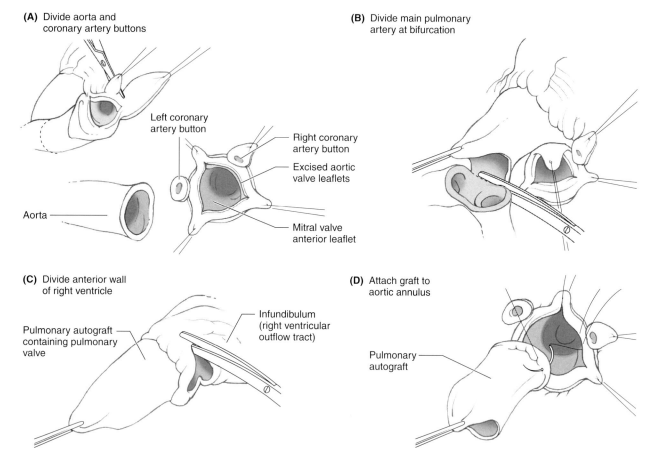

FIGURE 7–3.6. Ross procedure (pulmonary autograft) for tunnel subvalvar stenosis. *(A)* The ascending aorta is transected just above the aortic root. The sinus aorta including the valve is excised except for two "buttons" containing the right and left coronary ostia. *(B)* The pulmonary trunk is dissected away from the aorta from the infundibulum up to the level of the bifurcation, where it is transected. *(C)* The pulmonary trunk, containing the pulmonic valve, is then separated from the right ventricular outflow tract above the infundibular septum, creating the pulmonary autograft. Care must be taken to avoid injury to the first septal branch of the anterior descending coronary artery. *(D)* The proximal end of the pulmonary autograft is secured to the aortic annulus of the left ventricular outflow tract using interrupted 3-0 Prolene™ sutures. *(E)* The left and right coronary ostia are anastomosed to the autograft using continuous 5-0 Prolene™ sutures. *(F)* The distal end of the autograft is anastomosed end to end to the aorta using continuous 4-0 Prolene™ sutures. *(G, H)* A pulmonary homograft is interposed end to end between the pulmonary artery bifurcation and the right ventricular outflow tract using continuous 4-0 and interrupted 3-0 Prolene™ sutures at the respective anastomoses. *(I)* The completed repair.

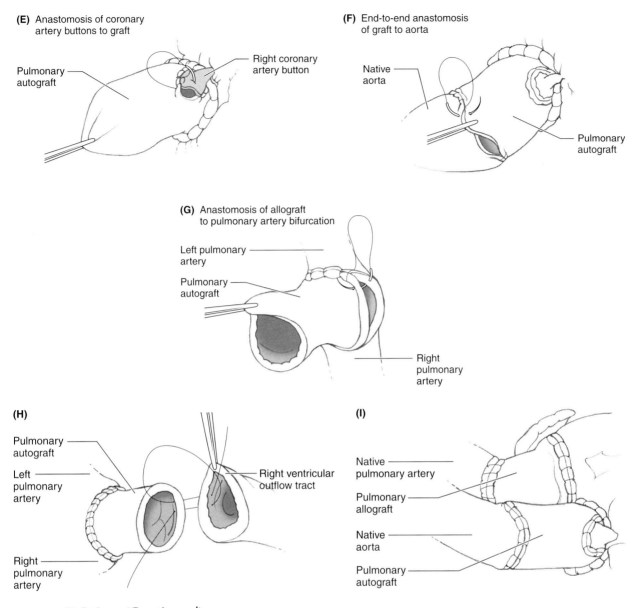

(E) Anastomosis of coronary artery buttons to graft

Pulmonary autograft

Right coronary artery button

(F) End-to-end anastomosis of graft to aorta

Native aorta

Pulmonary autograft

(G) Anastomosis of allograft to pulmonary artery bifurcation

Left pulmonary artery

Pulmonary autograft

Right pulmonary artery

(H)

Pulmonary autograft

Left pulmonary artery

Right pulmonary artery

Right ventricular outflow tract

(I)

Native pulmonary artery

Pulmonary allograft

Native aorta

Pulmonary autograft

FIGURE 7-3.6. (Continued)

- **Concepts of Correction:** To repair the aortic coarctation, relieve the obstruction to left ventricular outflow, and establish adequate systemic perfusion.
- **Corrective Operation(s):**
- Resection with end-to-end anastomosis
- Subclavian flap aortoplasty
- Patch aortoplasty
- Percutaneous balloon dilatation

General Considerations

Coarctation of the aorta is a congenital narrowing of the upper descending thoracic aorta and comprises approximately 5% to 8% of all congenital defects. There are two general morphologic forms of this defect: (1) an isolated discrete aortic narrowing adjacent to the ductus arteriosus and (2) a diffuse tubular hypoplasia of the distal aortic arch and isthmus with a large patent ductus arteriosus. Aortic coarctation is frequently associated with other significant cardiac anomalies including ventricular septal defect, bicuspid aortic valve, hypoplastic aortic arch, and hypoplastic left ventricle syndrome; it is also associated with Turner's syndrome and von Recklinghausen's disease. The etiology of coarctation is not clear, but the prevalent theories have associated the localized narrowing with closure of the ductus arteriosus and disruption of normal fetal blood flow patterns. A pressure gradient exists across the length of aortic narrowing that can be quite severe. The lumenal cross-sectional area must be reduced by more than 50% before a hemodynamically significant gradient exists, although longer coarctations may

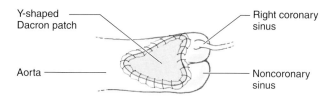

FIGURE 7-3.7.   Aortoplasty for supravalvar stenosis. An ascending aortotomy in an inverted Y pattern is created along the length of stenotic aorta, extending into the noncoronary and right coronary sinuses of Valsalva, incising the sinus ridges at these two points. A bifurcated Dacron™ patch is then fashioned to reconstruct the aorta, with the bifurcated ends used to close the sinus incisions.

result in significant gradients with lesser narrowing. Severe coarctation presents a large afterload to the left ventricle, which, if left untreated, eventually leads to left ventricular failure, mitral insufficiency, left-to-right intracardiac shunting (e.g., atrial septal defect, patent foramen ovale), and pulmonary congestion. Neonates with severe coarctation are dependent on ductal flow for lower body systemic perfusion; spontaneous ductal closure results in visceral and lower extremity hypoperfusion and metabolic acidosis. In older patients with mild-to-moderate coarctation, collateral circulation develops over time (which partially circumvents the narrowed aortic segment) and is composed of enlarged internal mammary, intercostal, subscapular, and other arteries.

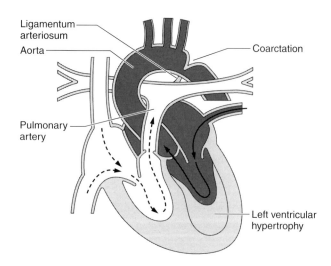

FIGURE 7–4.   Schematic drawing of coarctation of the aorta. (■)——▶, Oxygenated; (□)----▶, Deoxygenated; (▨)----▶, mixed.

These vessels become dilated and sometimes aneurysmal and may be a significant source of hemorrhage if not respected during surgical repair.

In 5% to 10% of infants with coarctation of the aorta, left ventricular failure may be severe and even fatal during the first month of life without correction. After the first year of life, congestive heart failure rarely occurs before the age of 20 years. Without treatment, the average life expectancy among these patients is between 30 and 40 years. The most common causes of death include aortic rupture, cardiac failure, intracranial hemorrhage, and bacterial endocarditis.

Diagnostic Keys

Classically, the combination of upper extremity hypertension with absent or diminished lower extremity pulses suggests aortic coarctation. A systolic murmur is usually audible over the left hemithorax. Infants with severe coarctation are dependent on ductal and collateral flow for systemic perfusion. At the time of ductal closure, these infants often present in severe congestive heart failure including pulmonary edema, renal failure, and acidosis. These signs are often accompanied by marked cardiomegaly and pulmonary congestion on chest radiography. Electrocardiography reveals signs of right ventricular hypertrophy as the result of right ventricular–dependent lower body perfusion.

Older children and adolescents with coarctation usually present with more subtle findings, complaining of headaches, lower extremity weakness, dyspnea on exertion, and fatigue. Electrocardiography and chest films typically reveal signs of left ventricular hypertrophy from long-standing hypertension. Chest films also may display signs of rib notching and the classic "3" sign produced by the hourglass configuration of the aorta in the region of coarctation.

Echocardiography is usually diagnostic, with anatomic definition of the coarctation associated with accelerated pulse Doppler flow. A ventricular septal defect, bicuspid aortic valve, and left ventricular hypertrophy may be observed. Careful assessment of the transverse aortic arch should be performed. Hypoplasia of the arch requiring arch reconstruction should be considered in neonates if the arch measures (in millimeters) <1 plus the infant's weight (in kilograms). Cardiac catheterization should be reserved for equivocal echocardiographic findings.

Operative Correction

Severe congestive heart failure in neonates with coarctation warrants immediate operative correction. However, every effort should be made to stabilize the patient with prostaglandin E_1 (to maintain ductal patency), inotropes, mechanical ventilation, and/or diuretics prior to surgery.

Generally accepted techniques of repair include **resection with end-to-end anastomosis** of the descending aorta to the distal aortic arch, **subclavian flap aortoplasty,** and

(A) Excise coarctated segment

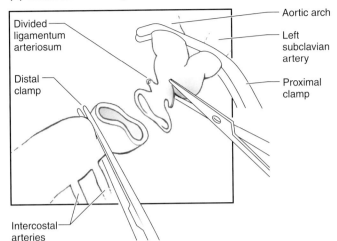

Divided
ligamentum
arteriosum

Distal
clamp

Intercostal
arteries

Aortic arch

Left
subclavian
artery

Proximal
clamp

(B) End-to-end aortic anastomosis

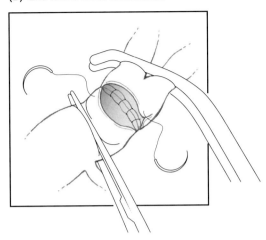

FIGURE 7–4.1. Resection of discrete aortic coarctation with end-to-end anastomosis. *(A)* Through a left posterolateral thoracotomy, the distal aortic arch, left subclavian artery, isthmus, descending aorta, and ductus arteriosus are dissected and mobilized. Care is taken to identify and preserve the phrenic and vagus nerves. The ductus arteriosus is ligated and divided. The aorta is crossclamped proximal and distal to the coarctation, which is resected along with all ductal tissue. *(B)* An end-to-end anastomosis is performed using a continuous 5-0 to 7-0 Prolene™ suture, completing the repair.

patch aortoplasty. All three techniques may be performed through a left posterolateral thoracotomy through the third or fourth intercostal space. Exposure is obtained by retracting the left upper lobe of the lung anteriorly and inferiorly, identifying the vagus and phrenic nerves, and incising the pleura overlying the distal aortic arch, isthmus, and ductus arteriosus. Special care must be taken to avoid injury to the nearby thoracic duct. Patients with aortic coarctation associated with other significant cardiac anomalies (e.g., large ventricular septal defect) or a hypoplastic aortic arch should undergo repair via a median sternotomy with the addition of circulatory arrest for aortic reconstruction.

Resection with end-to-end anastomosis (Fig. 7–4.1) is the preferred technique for repair of discrete aortic coarctation since it entails complete removal of all ductal tissue at the site of coarctation and can be readily extended to treat tubular hypoplasia of the distal aortic arch. After adequately dissecting and mobilizing the distal aortic arch, left subclavian artery, isthmus, ductus arteriosus, and descending aorta, the coarctation is isolated by crossclamping the distal aortic arch (proximally) and descending aorta (distally). After ligating and dividing the ductus arteriosus, the coarctation is segmentally resected, removing all ductal tissue. An end-to-end anastomosis is performed with the remain-

ing ends of the aorta using a running 5-0 to 7-0 Prolene™ suture, taking care to avoid excessive tension narrowing at the suture line. If the distal aortic arch is hypoplastic, this technique can be modified by applying the proximal crossclamp to the arch just distal to the innominate artery, preserving cerebral circulation (Fig. 7–4.2). The descending aorta is crossclamped below the coarctation and point of ductus insertion. An axial incision is then made along the undersurface of the hypoplastic arch, and an end-to-side anastomosis between the descending aorta and undersurface of the arch can be performed after excising the intervening coarctation.

Subclavian flap aortoplasty (Fig. 7–4.3) requires less aortic dissection and mobilization than resection with end-to-end anastomosis and hence may be the preferred technique when previous aortic surgery has been performed (including prior coarctation resection) and substantial scar periaortic adhesions are present. Also, since this technique does not require ductal ligation and division, it may be used when continued ductal flow is desired. After the left subclavian artery is ligated distally, the distal aortic arch between the left carotid and left subclavian artery origins is crossclamped; the distal crossclamp is placed below the coarctation. The left subclavian artery is then divided distally and

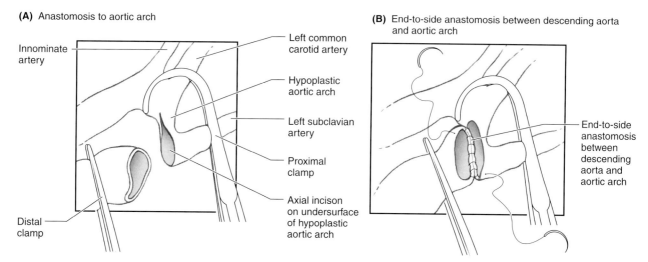

(A) Anastomosis to aortic arch

Innominate artery

Distal clamp

Left common carotid artery

Hypoplastic aortic arch

Left subclavian artery

Proximal clamp

Axial incison on undersurface of hypoplastic aortic arch

(B) End-to-side anastomosis between descending aorta and aortic arch

End-to-side anastomosis between descending aorta and aortic arch

FIGURE 7–4.2. Repair of aortic coarctation in the setting of tubular hypoplasia of the aortic arch. *(A)* Through a left posterolateral thoracotomy, the proximal crossclamp is applied to the arch just distal to the innominate artery, preserving cerebral circulation. The descending aorta is crossclamped below the coarctation and point of ductus insertion. The ductus arteriosus is ligated and divided. An axial incision is then made along the undersurface of the hypoplastic arch. The coarctation is resected between the clamps, and the isthmus is ligated with a transfixing ligature. *(B)* An end-to-side anastomosis is then performed between the descending aorta and undersurface of the arch.

incised longitudinally along its posterior surface, extending this incision distally along the distal aortic arch, isthmus, and descending aorta, completely traversing the coarctation. The resultant "flap" of subclavian artery is then brought down to augment the coarctation with a running 5-0 to 7-0 Prolene™ suture line.

Patch aortoplasty (Fig. 7–4.4) can be performed fairly rapidly with minimal preparative dissection and therefore may be indicated in the rare instances of critically ill neonates in whom ductal flow cannot be reestablished or discrete recoarctation is not amenable to balloon dilation. After mobilizing the aortic isthmus and ligating the ductus arteriosus, a single side-biting crossclamp can be applied across the entire coarctation, extending from the base of the left subclavian artery to the descending aorta beyond the coarctation. A longitudinal aortotomy is made along the coarctation, and an oval Dacron™ patch is applied across the aortotomy with a continuous 5-0 to 7-0 Prolene™ suture, thereby augmenting the narrowed aortic segment.

Some centers have experience with **percutaneous balloon dilation** of native coarctation, but presently, percutaneous procedures are generally limited to the treatment of postoperative recurrence of the coarctation, which is usually related to scarring of residual ductal tissue left at the anas-

tomotic site. A multicenter review of native coarctations treated initially with balloon dilation cites an aneurysm formation rate of 12%.

Several considerations with respect to intraoperative hemodynamics should be mentioned. Intraoperative arterial pressure monitoring should comprise a right radial arterial line and a lower extremity sphygmomanometer. Aortic crossclamping may result in an acute rise in left ventricular wall tension and decompensation requiring temporary inotropic support. This condition is ameliorated in the setting of a significant ventricular septal defect allowing for left ventricular decompression (i.e., left-to-right shunt); however, in this setting, pulmonary overcirculation at the expense of systemic hypoperfusion may result. Measures directed toward elevating pulmonary vascular resistance, thereby reducing the shunt volume, include utilizing low levels of the fraction of inspired oxygen (FIO_2) and avoiding hyperventilation. Finally, the arterial pressure gradient across the repair should be measured using an intraluminal catheter; a resting gradient of ≤ 20 mm Hg is generally acceptable.

Perioperative mortality from repair of isolated coarctation of the aorta ranges from 5% to 15%. Paradoxical systemic hypertension in the early postoperative period is a well-recognized phenomenon after coarctation repair and

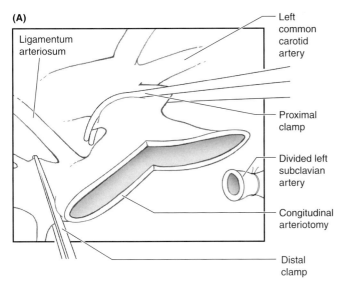

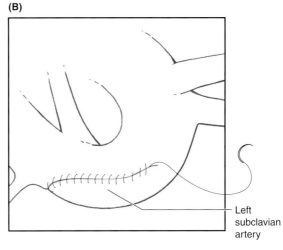

FIGURE 7–4.3. Subclavian flap aortoplasty. *(A)* Through a left posterolateral thoracotomy, the distal aortic arch, left subclavian artery, and descending aorta below the ductus arteriosus is dissected. After the left subclavian artery is ligated distally, the distal aortic arch between the left carotid and left subclavian artery origins is crossclamped; the distal aortic crossclamp is placed below the coarctation. The left subclavian artery is then divided distally and incised longitudinally along its posterior surface, extending this incision distally along the distal aortic arch, isthmus, and descending aorta, completely traversing the coarctation. *(B)* The resultant "flap" of subclavian artery is then brought down to augment the coarctation with a running 5-0 to 7-0 Prolene™ suture line.

is generally felt to be due to perturbations in baroreceptor activity, the renin-angiotensin axis, and sympathetic discharge. Rare complications associated with coarctation repair include paraplegia from aortic crossclamping, intestinal ischemia due to splanchnic vasospasm, chylothorax from thoracic duct injury, and recoarctation.

Interrupted Aortic Arch (Fig. 7–5)

Incidence: Comprises <1% of all congenital heart defects.

Pathophysiology: Lumenal interruption between the ascending and descending aorta is found, and distal blood flow is dependent on a patent ductus arteriosus. Spontaneous ductal closure results in systemic hypoperfusion, metabolic acidosis, and end-organ failure. Associated cardiac anomalies are common, particularly a nonrestrictive ventricular septal defect.

Clinical Features: Most neonates with interrupted aortic arch become critically ill at the time of ductal closure, with signs and symptoms of circulatory shock and congestive heart failure. Physical exam classically reveals abnormal extremity pulse patterns depending on the type of interruption. Two-dimensional echocardiography with Doppler and/or angiography are diagnostic, revealing a narrow ascending aorta, ab-

sent arch, and descending aorta in continuity with the ductus arteriosus.

Concepts of Correction: To reestablish continuity between the ascending and descending aorta with a multi- or single-staged procedure.

Corrective Operation(s):

• Multistage repair: (first) GoreTex™ interposition graft between the ascending and descending aorta with pulmonary artery banding, (second) ventricular septal defect repair and pulmonary artery band removal, and (third) graft revision.

• Single-stage repair—primary anastomosis between the ascending and descending aorta with ventricular septal defect closure.

General Considerations

Interrupted aortic arch is a rare congenital cardiac anomaly in which there is an interruption of lumenal continuity between the ascending and descending aorta. Three types of interrupted aortic arch have been anatomically defined (Fig. 7–5.1) and correlate with the different embryologic derivations of the aortic arch. **Type A interruption** (25%

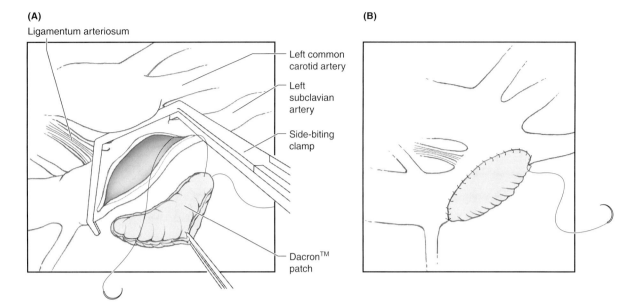

(A)
Ligamentum arteriosum
Left common carotid artery
Left subclavian artery
Side-biting clamp
Dacron™ patch

(B)

FIGURE 7–4.4. Patch aortoplasty. *(A)* Through a left posterolateral thoracotomy, the aortic isthmus is mobilized, and the ductus arteriosus is ligated. A single side-biting crossclamp can then be applied across the entire coarctation, extending from the base of the left subclavian artery to the descending aorta beyond the coarctation. A longitudinal aortotomy is made along the coarctation. *(B)* An oval Dacron™ patch is then applied across the aortotomy with a continuous 5-0 to 7-0 Prolene™ suture, thereby augmenting the narrowed aortic segment.

to 35%) occurs at the level of the aortic isthmus distal to the left subclavian artery. The innominate, left carotid, and left subclavian arteries originate from the ascending aorta, whereas the descending aorta derives its blood flow from a

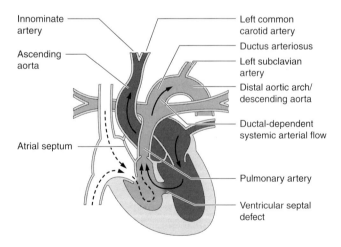

Innominate artery
Ascending aorta
Atrial septum
Left common carotid artery
Ductus arteriosus
Left subclavian artery
Distal aortic arch/ descending aorta
Ductal-dependent systemic arterial flow
Pulmonary artery
Ventricular septal defect

FIGURE 7–5. Schematic drawing of interrupted aortic arch. (■)——▶, Oxygenated; (□)----▶, Deoxygenated; (▦)--–-▶, mixed.

patent ductus arteriosus. *Type B interruption,* the most common form of this anomaly (60% to 70%), occurs between the left common carotid and left subclavian arteries. This form is frequently associated with an aberrant origin of the right subclavian artery from the descending aorta and left ventricular outflow tract obstruction secondary to subaortic stenosis. *Type C interruption* is the rarest form (<5%), occurring between the innominate and left common carotid arteries. A patent ductus arteriosus is the sole provider of blood flow to the descending aorta and is, therefore, essential for survival in virtually all patients with interrupted aortic arch. Interrupted aortic arch is rarely an isolated defect, and most cases are associated with other cardiac anomalies. The condition is most commonly associated with a patent ductus arteriosus and a large, nonrestrictive ventricular septal defect (70% to 90%). Other associated defects include bicuspid aortic valve (60%), subaortic stenosis (20%), and truncus arteriosus (10%). *DiGeorge's syndrome,* characterized by an absent thymus, hypocalcemia, and immunodeficiency, is observed in 15% to 30% of patients with interrupted aortic arch.

Since systemic blood flow is dependent on ductal patency in cases of interrupted aortic arch, most cases present during the first few days of life at the time of spontaneous ductal closure. As end-organ perfusion is reduced

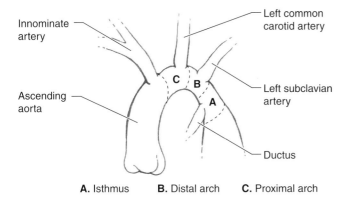

FIGURE 7–5.1. Celoria and Patton[3] classification of interrupted aortic arch. Type A: Interruption at the aortic isthmus. Type B: Interruption between the left common carotid and left subclavian arteries. Type C: Interruption between the innominate and left common carotid arteries.

during ductal closure, metabolic acidosis, acute renal failure, necrotizing enterocolitis, hepatic ischemia, and severe congestive heart failure ensues. Prompt, aggressive medical resuscitation includes the use of prostaglandin E_1, mechanical ventilation, inotropes, and sodium bicarbonate. Prostaglandin E_1 is essential to maintain ductal patency. Maximizing pulmonary vascular resistance to maintain right-to-left flow across the ductus is facilitated by mechanical ventilation paralysis; the FIO_2 and ventilation can be accurately regulated.

Diagnostic Keys

Most neonates with interrupted aortic arch become critically ill at the time of spontaneous ductal closure, presenting with signs and symptoms of circulatory shock and congestive heart failure including cyanosis, tachypnea, tachycardia, and acidosis. Abnormal peripheral pulse patterns depend on the type of interruption. In type B interruption, only the right radial pulse is palpable, with the left radial and both femoral pulses being absent; an exception to this is in the case of an aberrant right subclavian artery origin, in which there may be no palpable extremity pulses. Type A interruption is associated with palpable radial pulses bilaterally and absent femoral pulses. Cardiomegaly and pulmonary vascular congestion are often evident on chest radiography. Electrocardiography may indicate right ventricular hypertrophy. Two-dimensional echocardiography with Doppler and/or angiography are diagnostic, revealing a narrow ascending aorta, an absent arch, and descending aorta in continuity with the ductus arteriosus.

Operative Correction

Surgical correction is indicated in all cases of interrupted aortic arch and is accomplished with a **staged correction** or a **single-stage complete repair**. The best modality remains controversial, although the staged approach may be preferable in cases of complex associated defects. Complete medical resuscitation, with optimization of acid-base, cardiopulmonary, renal, and hepatic parameters, must be established prior to surgery. Preoperative placement of right radial, umbilical, and lower extremity arterial pressure monitors is essential to monitor upper and lower body perfusion during cardiopulmonary bypass and to assess the adequacy of the repair.

The staged approach is based on an initial procedure to establish continuity between the ascending and descending aorta with a synthetic conduit and to limit left-to-right shunting across the ventricular septal defect. The ventricular septal defect is then closed at a later date. The first stage is generally performed through a left posterolateral thoracotomy. The patent ductus arteriosus is ligated and divided and an 8- or 10-mm GoreTex™ graft is anastomosed between the ascending and descending aorta to restore distal blood flow. A pulmonary artery band is also placed. In the second stage, performed 2 to 3 months later through a median sternotomy and using cardiopulmonary bypass, the ventricular septal defect is patched, and the pulmonary artery band is removed. In most cases, a third operation to replace the polytetrafluoroethylene graft with a larger graft is required at 8 to 12 years.

The single-stage complete repair (Fig. 7–5.2) entails direct anastomosis of interrupted arch and closure of the ventricular septal defect during the neonatal period. Through a median sternotomy, circulatory arrest is established followed by mobilization of the ascending and descending aorta, arch vessels, and ductus arteriosus. In some cases of type B interruption, ligation and division of the left subclavian artery may facilitate aortic mobilization and minimize tension at the ensuing aortic anastomosis. The ductus arteriosus is ligated and divided, and the ascending and descending aorta are anastomosed in an end-to-side fashion with a 6-0 Prolene™ continuous suture. The ventricular septal defect is then closed through a pulmonary arteriotomy or right atriotomy. Rewarming is commenced after completion of these repairs, and separation from bypass is initiated with concomitant assessment of the gradient across the aortic anastomosis.

Early postoperative mortality rates for interrupted aortic arch range from about 25% for the staged approach to <10% for the single-stage complete repair. Recognized complications include anastomotic hemorrhage (single-stage repair), often due to excessive anastomotic tension, and late development of a pressure gradient across the synthetic conduit (staged repair) or the direct anastomosis (single stage repair). Anastomotic strictures across the

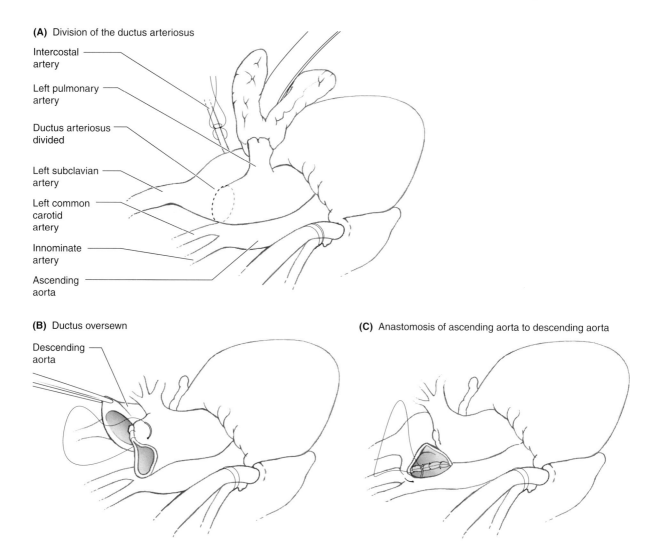

(A) Division of the ductus arteriosus

- Intercostal artery
- Left pulmonary artery
- Ductus arteriosus divided
- Left subclavian artery
- Left common carotid artery
- Innominate artery
- Ascending aorta

(B) Ductus oversewn

- Descending aorta

(C) Anastomosis of ascending aorta to descending aorta

FIGURE 7–5.2. Single-stage complete repair for type B interrupted aortic arch. *(A)* The ascending and descending aorta, arch vessels, and ductus arteriosus are fully mobilized. Division of the left subclavian artery may be necessary to obtain adequate mobilization of the distal arch. *(B)* The ductus arteriosus is oversewn. *(C)* Using circulatory arrest, end-to-side anastomosis is performed between the ascending and descending aorta. Care must be taken to avoid excessive tension on the anastomosis.

direct aortic anastomosis can often be successfully treated with balloon dilation; however, conduit replacement is usually necessary for those undergoing the staged repair.

References

1. HANLEY FL, SADE RM, FREEDOM RM, et al. Outcomes in critically ill neonates with pulmonary stenosis and intact ventricular septum: A multiinstitutional study. *J Am Coll Cardiol* 1993;22:183–192.

2. HANLEY FL, SADE RM, BLACKSTONE EH, et al. Outcomes in neonatal pulmonary atresia with intact ventricular septum. A multiinstitutional study. *J. Thorac Cardiovasc Surg.* 1993;105:406–423.

3. CELORIA GC, PATTON RB. Congenital absence of the aortic arch. *Am Heart J.* 1959;58:407.

CHAPTER 8

Left-to-Right Shunt Defects

David D. Yuh, MD, and Bruce A. Reitz, MD

Introduction

This category of congenital cardiac defects comprises lesions which permit shunting of systemic arterial blood into the pulmonary circulation. The compliance of the thick-walled left ventricle is greater than that of the thin-walled right ventricle, and the resistance of the systemic vascular bed is greater than that of the pulmonary bed; therefore, the pressures in the left heart chambers and systemic arteries are greater than those found in the right heart and pulmonary arteries. In the setting of these differential pressures, anatomic communications between the left- and right-sided systems permit oxygenated blood to recirculate through the pulmonary capillary bed. The resultant pulmonary overcirculation, if severe enough, can lead to pulmonary vascular congestion manifested clinically as pulmonary edema and frequent respiratory infections. If this condition is left untreated, pulmonary vascular occlusive disease due to intimal and medial hyperplasia may develop, leading to irreversible pulmonary hypertension and, ultimately, right heart failure. Furthermore, left-to-right shunting causes diastolic volume overload of one or both ventricles, leading to ventricular dilatation, elevated end-diastolic pressures, and ventricular failure.

Surgical correction generally consists of two strategies: pulmonary artery banding and closure of the anatomic defect. Banding of the main pulmonary artery restricts pulmonary arterial flow, reducing pulmonary overcirculation. This modality is generally considered palliative and is reserved for neonates or infants in whom definitive repair is considered too risky. Surgical closure of the anatomic shunt is definitive therapy.

8.1 Atrial Septal Defect (Ostium Secundum) (Fig. 8–1)

Incidence: 10% to 15% of congenital heart defects.

Pathophysiology: Secundum atrial defects (ASDs) permit left-to-right shunting, increasing pulmonary blood flow. Over time, increased pulmonary overcirculation leads to pulmonary vascular occlusive disease, pulmonary hypertension, right ventricular failure, and atrial arrhythmias.

Clinical Features: Secundum defects are usually asymptomatic in infancy and early childhood. Symptoms are those of congestive heart failure stemming from pulmonary hypertension. Atrial arrhythmias present after the third decade. Physical examination characteristically reveals a soft midsystolic pulmonary flow murmur, a widely split and fixed S2, and a diastolic tricuspid flow murmur. Electrocardiography reveals right atrial enlargement and right ventricular hypertrophy. Chest radiograph reveals an enlarged right ventricle and atrium, increased pulmonary vascularity, and a prominent main pulmonary artery. Two-dimensional echocardiography is diagnostic and demonstrates right atrial, right ventricular, and pulmonary artery enlargement along with the secundum defect. Sinus venosus defects are more readily visualized with transesophageal echocardiography or with cardiac catheterization.

Concepts of Correction: Secundum ASDs that fail to spontaneously close should be repaired in early childhood to avoid long-term complications (e.g., congestive heart failure, endocarditis, paradoxical emboli). Adults with significant left-to-right shunts ($Q_p/Q_s > 1.5{:}1$) should undergo ASD closure.

Corrective Operation(s): Direct suture or patch closure.

General Considerations

Atrial septal defects (ASDs) are among the most common congenital cardiac defects, constituting 10% to 15% of congenital heart defects. ASDs vary widely in size and location and are broadly classified as ostium secundum, ostium primum, sinus venosus, and coronary sinus types (Fig. 8–1.1). Ostium secundum defects, the most common type of ASD (80%), result from a failure of the septum secundum to develop completely and cover the foramen ovale; these defects are usually located in the midportion of the interatrial septum, contained within the fossa ovalis. A secundum

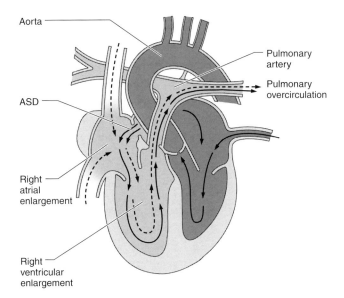

FIGURE 8–1. Schematic drawing of ASD (ostium secundum). (■)———▶, Oxygenated; (□)---▶, Deoxygenated; (▨)---▶, mixed.

defect in which the limbus and septum primum are intact is also known as a **patent foramen ovale.** Sinus venosus defects (5% to 10%) can occur in any position along the remnant of the right horn of the sinus venosus, which extends between the superior and inferior vena cava orifices; these defects are most commonly located at the junction of the superior vena cava and the right atrium. Sinus venosus defects are frequently (>90% of cases) associated with partial anomalous connections of the right upper and middle lobe pulmonary veins to the superior vena cava or right atrium. Low or inferior vena cava defects are sinus venosus

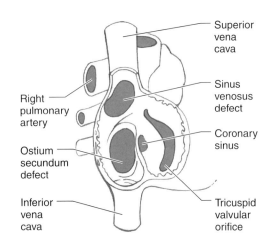

FIGURE 8–1.1. Typical anatomic locations of ostium secundum and sinus venosus ASDs as viewed through a right atriotomy.

defects located between the entrance of the inferior vena cava and the inferior limbic septum. Coronary sinus septal defects (<5%), also known as *unroofed coronary sinus*, consist of varying communications between the coronary sinus tube and left atrium. This rare entity is usually associated with a persistent left superior vena cava. **Ostium primum ASDs** are classified as endocardial cushion or atrioventricular (AV) canal defects and are discussed in the following section.

Most ostium secundum ASDs present as an isolated defect; however, they are frequently associated with other congenital cardiac anomalies. The initial physiologic effect of an ASD is a left-to-right shunting of blood across the interatrial septum. The degree of shunting, represented as the ratio of pulmonary and systemic blood flow (Q_p/Q_s) derived from cardiac catheterization measurements, is a function of the defect size and relative compliances of the left and right ventricles during diastole. During the newborn period, left and right ventricular compliances are similar, with minimal shunting across the ASD. However, as the pulmonary vascular resistance decreases, right ventricular pressures decrease and right ventricular compliance increases, leading to an increase in left-to-right shunting. This shunting, in turn, leads to right ventricular volume overload and an augmentation of pulmonary blood flow that may reach two to four times systemic flow in unrestrictive ASDs. Most infants are asymptomatic despite this shunt due to the high compliance and capacity of the pulmonary vascular bed to accommodate this increased blood flow. However, over time, the increased pulmonary blood flow leads to pulmonary vascular disease and pulmonary hypertension. These chronic changes promote a decrease in right ventricular compliance and a consequent reversal of the shunt (i.e., right-to-left), cyanosis, and right ventricular failure by the third or fourth decades of life; this phenomenon is known as **Eisenmenger's syndrome.**

Diagnostic Keys

Isolated ASDs rarely produce symptoms in infancy or early childhood. Symptoms of congestive heart failure, including dyspnea on exertion, tachypnea, and frequent respiratory infections, occur as a result of pulmonary overcirculation. Approximately 1% of patients with large ASDs are symptomatic during the first year of life. Atrial arrhythmias including paroxysmal atrial tachycardia and atrial fibrillation usually present after the age of 30; paradoxical embolization through an ASD may lead to a cerebrovascular accident. Physical examination characteristically reveals a soft midsystolic pulmonary flow murmur at the upper left sternal border, a widely split and fixed S2, and a diastolic tricuspid flow murmur. Electrocardiography demonstrates right atrial enlargement and right ventricular hypertrophy. Chest radiography often reveals an enlarged right ventricle and right atrium, increased pulmonary vascular markings, and a prominent main pulmonary artery. Two-dimensional echocardiography is diagnostic and will demonstrate right atrial, right ventricular, and pulmonary artery enlargement in association with secundum defects. Sinus venosus defects and any anomalous pulmonary venous drainage patterns are more readily visualized with transesophageal echocardiography or with cardiac catheterization. Although not routinely used in the workup of this defect, cardiac catheterization may be helpful in measuring pulmonary artery pressures and pulmonary vascular resistances as well as Q_p/Q_s ratios in older patients prior to intervention.

Operative Correction

The rate of spontaneous ASD closures during the first 4 years of life is approximately 40%; higher rates are noted with small defects. Spontaneous closure is extremely rare after the age of 2 years. In general, children found to have significant ASDs should undergo elective closure, ideally between the ages of 3 and 5 years. Since most children are diagnosed by history and physical examination in conjunction with echocardiography, the magnitude of the shunt is not generally calculated preoperatively. Adults with significant left-to-right shunts ($Q_p/Q_s > 1.5:1$) should undergo ASD closure. Adult patients with severe pulmonary vascular disease (pulmonary vascular resistance >10 Wood units

or two-thirds systemic vascular resistance) or left-sided cardiac failure may not be candidates for closure, since elective repair will not improve or may even worsen cardiopulmonary function.

Repairs of ostium secundum defects are usually performed through a median sternotomy on cardiopulmonary bypass with bicaval cannulation (Fig. 8–1.2). A right anterolateral thoracotomy through the fourth intercostal space is also satisfactory and provides female patients with a superior cosmesis. The ASD is accessed through a right atriotomy extending obliquely from the right atrial appendage toward the inferior vena cava, staying well anterior to the sinoatrial node. The entire ASD, all systemic and pulmonary vein orifices, and the coronary sinus should be identified. Secundum defects can usually be closed directly with sutures; however, if the defect is large, a patch made of autologous pericardium or GoreTex™ is used to avoid excess tension on the suture line. The left atrium should be evacuated of air by filling it with cold saline just prior to completing the ASD closure. After completing the suture line, the right atriotomy is closed, and separation from cardiopulmonary bypass is commenced.

Sinus venosus defects are repaired through a median sternotomy under cardiopulmonary bypass. The upper venous cannula is inserted high in the superior vena cava or the innominate vein to facilitate exposure the defect and

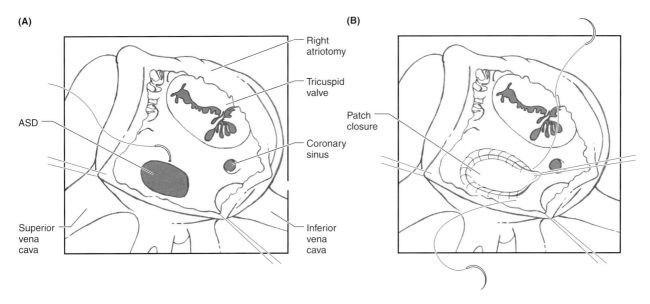

(A)

- Right atriotomy
- Tricuspid valve
- ASD
- Coronary sinus
- Superior vena cava
- Inferior vena cava

(B)

- Patch closure

FIGURE 8–1.2. Primary *(A)* and patch *(B)* repair of ostium ASDs. After cardiopulmonary bypass has been established, the ASD is accessed through an oblique right atriotomy. Small defects may be closed primarily with a running Prolene™ suture beginning at the inferior rim of the defect. Care must be taken to avoid injury to the nearby coronary sinus or AV node. Larger defects may require patch closure to avoid excessive suture line tension.

any anomalous pulmonary venous connections to the right atrium or superior vena cava. If the sinus venous defect is large and the pulmonary venous drainage is normal or at the sinoatrial junction, adequate exposure can be obtained through an incision made in the right atrial appendage. The defect is repaired with an autologous pericardial patch in such a way as to allow any anomalous pulmonary venous drainage to be directed through the defect into the left atrium. For sinus venous defects associated with anomalous pulmonary venous drainage into the superior vena cava above the sinoatrial junction, a longitudinal incision is made along the posterolateral surface of the superior vena cava extending across the sinoatrial junction, staying posterior to the sinoatrial node. These defects usually require an autologous pericardial patch placed within the superior vena cava and the right atrium to baffle the anomalous pulmonary venous flow through the defect into the left atrium (Fig. 8–1.3). A second, external patch may be used to close the caval incision, to prevent caval obstruction after the baffle has been sutured in place. Isolated coronary sinus septal defects are usually exposed through a right atriotomy and closed with a simple autologous pericardial patch.

Repair of isolated ASDs are associated with a hospital mortality well below 1%. The prognosis is generally excellent. Damage to the conduction system, particularly the sinoatrial node, is an infrequent, but recognized complication of ASD repair.

8.2 Atrioventricular Septal Defect (Ostium Primum and Complete Atrioventricular Canal) (Fig. 8–2)

Incidence: 5% of congenital cardiac defects

Pathophysiology: Partial AV canal defects result from the failure of the endocardial cushions to meet the septum primum, producing a low-lying (ostium primum) defect in the atrial septum; a "cleft" mitral valve is also usually present. Complete AV canal defects result from maldevelopment of the endocardial cushions, producing a single, common AV valve and ventricular septal defect (VSD) in addition to an ostium primum ASD. Pathophysiology results from left-to-right shunting at the atrial and/or ventricular levels as well as AV valve insufficiency, producing pulmonary overcirculation and congestive heart failure, particularly during early infancy.

Clinical Features: Significant left-to-right shunting leads to congestive heart failure. Neonates/infants with complete AV canal defects develop symptomatic congestive failure earlier than those with the partial form. Chest radiograph reveals

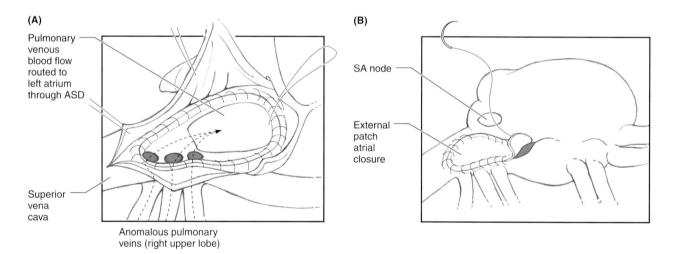

(A)

Pulmonary venous blood flow routed to left atrium through ASD

Superior vena cava

Anomalous pulmonary veins (right upper lobe)

(B)

SA node

External patch atrial closure

FIGURE 8–1.3.   Repair of sinus venosus ASD associated with anomalous drainage of the right superior pulmonary veins. *(A)* After cardiopulmonary bypass has been established, a cavoatrial incision is made along the posterolateral aspect of the superior vena cava, extending across the sinoatrial junction; care must be taken to stay well posterior to the sinoatrial node. An autologous pericardial baffle is then sutured within the vena cava and right atrium to encompass the anomalous pulmonary venous connections and the ASD. The baffle is shaped and positioned in such a way as to divert the anomalous pulmonary venous drainage across the ASD into the left atrium. *(B)* A second patch may be used to close the cavoatrial incision to avoid lumenal narrowing at the cavoatrial junction.

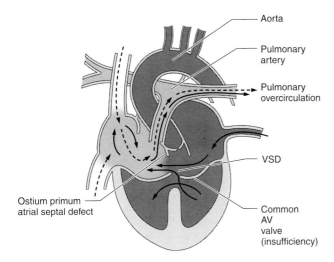

Complete AV-canal
(atrial and ventricular level left-to-right shunting)

FIGURE 8–2. Schematic drawing of AV septal defect (ostium primum and complete AV canal). (■)——➤, Oxygenated; (□)---➤, Deoxygenated; (▨)---➤, mixed.

cardiomegaly and increased pulmonary vascularity. The electrocardiogram characteristically shows left axis deviation, prominent P waves (atrial enlargement), and a prolonged P-R interval (first-degree AV block). Two-dimensional echocardiography with Doppler is diagnostic; it visualizes all components of AV canal defects. Angiography reveals a "gooseneck" deformity of the left ventricular outflow tract and the extent of AV valve incompetence.

Concepts of Correction: Correction of partial AV canal defects involves patch closure of the ostium primum ASD and repair of the cleft left-sided (mitral) valve. Complete AV canal repair involves patch closure of the ostium primum ASD and ventral septal defect, partitioning of the common AV valve into left- and right-sided valves, and repair of the cleft left-sided valve.

Corrective Operation(s):

- Partial AV septal defect-pericardial patch ASD closure and repair of cleft mitral valve
- Complete AV septal defect-single- or two-patch repair involving ASD and ventral septal defect patch closure, common AV valve partitioning, and repair of cleft mitral valve

General Considerations

AV septal (AV canal) defects comprise about 5% of congenital cardiac anomalies and account for 30% to 40% of the cardiac defects observed in Down's, syndrome patients. Basically, AV canal defects are caused by maldevelopment of the endocardial cushions resulting in morphologic abnormalities of the atrial and ventricular septa as well as the AV valves. The ventricular septum is also attenuated ("scooped out"), causing the AV valves to be positioned abnormally close to the cardiac apex. The left ventricular outflow tract is longer and narrower than usual, since the aortic valve is not in its normally "couched" position between the AV valve

annuli. This "gooseneck" deformity of the left ventricular outflow tract may result in varying degrees of left ventricular outflow tract obstruction. Finally, downward displacement of the coronary sinus, AV node, and bundle of His is another common characteristic of this defect.

Partial AV canal defects, also known as *ostium primum* atrial septal defects (ASDs), occur when the superior aspects of the endocardial cushions fail to develop and close the ostium primum portion of the interatrial septum. Ostium primum ASDs are also associated with a maldeveloped mitral valve in which there is a "cleft" in the anterior leaflet; this malformation predisposes to mitral insufficiency. **Complete AV canal defects** (Fig. 8–2.1) comprise a VSD in addition to an ostium primum ASD; the VSD is produced by a failure of the inferior extension of the endocardial cushions to close the interventricular septum. Moreover, the right and left AV valves are, in effect, fused into a single common AV valve common to both right and left ventricular chambers. The common AV valve is usually composed of six leaflets (left superior, left lateral, left inferior, right inferior, right lateral, and right superior) and is downwardly displaced toward the cardiac apex. The common valve may be centered over both, usually normally developed, ventricular chambers, thereby facilitating a biventricular reconstruction. However, if the valve is displaced predominantly over one ventricle, the other ventricle is often hypoplastic, making a biventricular repair more difficult. In such cases, a univentricular repair may be necessary. AV valvar insufficiency is frequently observed in both partial and complete defects. Although AV canal defects are broadly classified as "partial" or "complete," they are actually composed of a broad spectrum of lesions involving the atrial, ventricular, and valvar components of the AV canal. Many complex variations on this theme occur, but with less frequency.

The pathophysiology of AV canal defects is related to left-to-right shunting at the atrial and/or ventricular levels through the septal defects and AV valvar insufficiency, producing pulmonary hypertension and congestive heart failure, particularly during early infancy. The early development of congestive heart failure and rapidly progressive pulmonary vascular occlusive disease is more frequent with complete AV canal defects versus the partial form, due to the large left-to-right ventricular shunt and regurgitant AV valve. Left untreated, mortality is high in infants with complete AV canal defects; life expectancy is <2 years in 80% of these patients. Other cardiac anomalies infrequently associated with AV canal defects include patent ductus arteriosus, anomalous pulmonary venous connection, left ventricular outflow tract obstruction, double-outlet right ventricle, transposition of the great arteries, and tetralogy of Fallot.

Diagnostic Keys

The signs and symptoms associated with AV canal defects depend on the magnitude of left-to-right shunting and AV valve insufficiency. In turn, the degree of left-to-right shunt

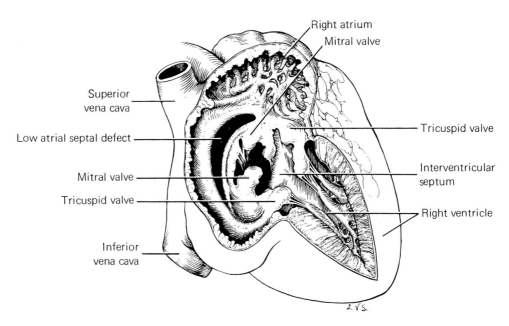

FIGURE 8–2.1.   Complete AV canal defect. The most common forms of complete AV canal defects are a VSD, a single common AV valve overriding both ventricles, and an ostium secundum ASD. Reproduced with permission. Verrier ED: The Heart: II. Congenital Diseases. In: *Current Surgical Diagnosis and Treatment*, Norwalk, Appleton & Lange, 1994, p. 394.

is determined by the sizes of the atrial and ventricular septal defects, the relative ventricular compliances, and the relative resistances of the systemic and pulmonary vascular beds. A significant left-to-right shunt leads to pulmonary hypertension and congestive heart failure. Dyspnea, fatigue, failure to thrive, and recurrent pulmonary infections appear in the first few months of life in patients with complete AV septal defects. Patients with partial AV septal defects usually present with less severe heart failure symptoms that tend to present beyond the first year of life. Significant AV valve insufficiency can accentuate symptoms in both forms of this defect. A prominent pulmonic flow murmur and wide fixed splitting of S2 are present with the partial form. A loud holosystolic murmur along the left lower sternal border (VSD), loud S2, apical middiastolic murmur (across the common AV valve), hyperactive precordium, and hepatomegaly are consistent physical findings in complete AV septal defects. Radiograpic findings of four-chamber enlargement and increased pulmonary vascular markings are observed with these defects and are directly related to the degree of left-to-right shunting. Electrocardiography characteristically shows left axis deviation, prominent P waves (atrial enlargement), and a prolonged P-R interval (first-degree AV block). Two-dimensional echocardiography with Doppler permits assessment of all components of AV septal defects including the septal and valvular components. Cardiac catheterization and angiography are necessary when significant pulmonary hypertension is suspected from physical exam and prior radiologic studies, in order to assess pulmonary-to-systemic blood flow ratios and pulmonary vascular resistances accurately. Significant preoperative AV valve regurgitation and elevated pulmonary vascular resistance are both associated with increased operative risk. Ventriculography reveals the characteristic "gooseneck" deformity of the left ventricular outflow tract and the extent of AV valvar regurgitation.

Operative Correction

In general, surgical correction of AV canal defects is indicated in the setting of symptomatic, refractory congestive heart failure. In asymptomatic patients, elective repair may be undertaken by 6 months of age for complete AV canal defects and by 1 to 2 years for partial defects. Early complete repair is advocated in order to avoid the development of irreversible pulmonary vascular occlusive disease; palliative pulmonary artery banding to reduce pulmonary blood flow may be considered if severe congestive heart failure is further complicated by other factors precluding immediate definitive repair (e.g., acute respiratory infection, associated uncorrectable cardiac malformations). In general, surgically correctable cardiac anomalies should also be addressed during the AV canal repair.

A median sternotomy and cardiopulmonary bypass with bicaval venous cannulation and cardiopulmonary bypass and/or deep hypothermic circulatory arrest (infants ≤4 kg) is employed for repair of both partial and complete AV canal defects. For partial AV canal defects, the ostium primum

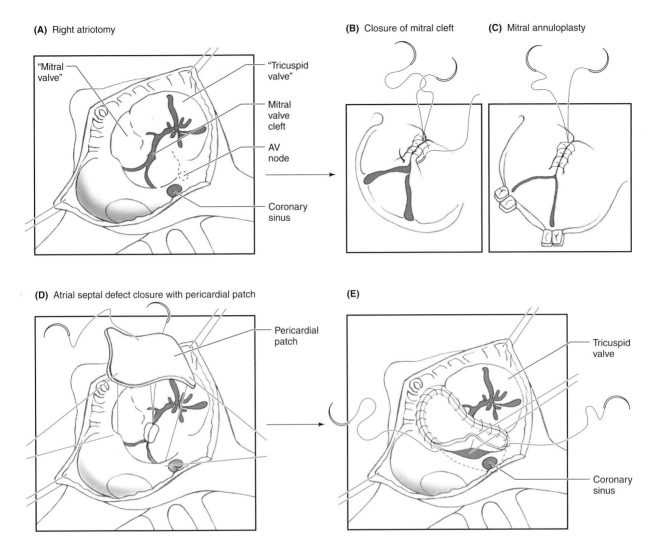

(A) Right atriotomy

"Mitral valve"

"Tricuspid valve"

Mitral valve cleft

AV node

Coronary sinus

(B) Closure of mitral cleft

(C) Mitral annuloplasty

(D) Atrial septal defect closure with pericardial patch

Pericardial patch

(E)

Tricuspid valve

Coronary sinus

FIGURE 8–2.2. Repair of partial AV canal defect. *(A)* After cardiopulmonary bypass has been established, the ostium primum ASD and "cleft" mitral valve are accessed through a right atriotomy, which runs close and parallel to the AV groove. *(B)* The cleft in the anterior mitral valve leaflet is closed with interrupted 3-0 or 4-0 Prolene™ sutures beginning peripherally and moving centrally. Mitral valve competence is tested by filling the left ventricle with cold saline. *(C)* If mitral insufficiency persists centrally after closure of the cleft, an annuloplasty may be used reduce the annular circumference and reduce or eliminate the central regurgitation. This is performed with pledgeted mattress sutures placed in the annulus at the bases of the two commissures. *(D)* A pericardial patch is used to close the ASD. *(E)* The pericardial patch is sutured to the ventricular septal crest located between the AV valves and carried inferior to the coronary sinus. The coronary sinus will drain into the left atrium.

ASD and cleft mitral valve are accessed through a right atriotomy. The repair consists of closure of the cleft in the anterior mitral valve leaflet accessed through the ASD followed by pericardial patch closure of the ASD (Fig. 8–2.2). The cleft in the anterior mitral valve leaflet is closed with interrupted 3-0 or 4-0 Prolene™ sutures, beginning peripherally and moving centrally. Mitral valve competence is repeatedly tested during its repair by filling the left ventricle with cold saline. If the mitral valve is still centrally regurgitant after the cleft repair, mitral annuloplasty with pledgeted mattress sutures placed in the annulus at the bases of both valve commissures can be performed to reduce the annular circumference and thereby bring the leaflets into complete central coaptation. The ostium primum ASD is then closed with an autologous pericardial patch secured with a continuous 5-0 Prolene™ suture beginning at the base of the mitral cleft. Care must be taken to avoid placing sutures in the proximal conduction bundles running along the underlying ventricular septal crest and potentially causing AV block. The low-lying coronary sinus is also incorporated underneath the patch so that it will drain into the left atrium; this takes the suture line away from the AV node and bundle of His. Closure of the atriotomy and separation from cardiopulmonary bypass follows.

The principles of complete AV canal repair include closure of both the ventricular and atrial components of the septal defect, dividing the common AV valve in the left-sided "mitral" and right-sided "tricuspid" valves with attachment of these new valves to the top of the ventricular septal defect (VSD) patch, and closure of the septal commissure ("cleft") in the left-sided valve. Once cardiopulmonary bypass or deep hypothermic circulatory arrest has been established, the right atrium is opened along a line parallel and close to the AV groove, exposing the ostium primum defect and the common AV valve. The competence and conformation of the AV valve is assessed by filling the ventricles with cold saline. The repair is then effected with either a single- or a two-patch technique. In the single-patch technique, developed at the Mayo clinic, the crest of the interventricular septum is exposed (Fig. 8–2.3). It is sometimes necessary to incise "bridging" valve leaflets, which overlie the crest. A tailored GoreTex™ patch is then attached to the interventricular septum at its midpoint, about 3 to 5 mm to the right of the crest, with a double-armed 4-0 or 5-0 Prolene™ suture. A continuous suture line is then carried superiorly and inferiorly along the septal crest, securing the patch to it. The leaflet edges on either side of the patch are attached to the patch with interrupted pledgeted 5-0 or 6-0 Prolene™ sutures. The cleft between the left (mitral) inferior and superior leaflets is then closed with interrupted 5-0 or 6-0 Prolene™ sutures. Competence of the mitral valve is tested by filling the left ventricle with cold saline. The superior aspect of the GoreTex™ patch is used to close the ostium primum defect; the coronary sinus is included under the patch, leav-

ing it to drain into the right atrium. The right atriotomy is closed, and separation from cardiopulmonary bypass is commenced.

The two-patch technique, proposed by Carpentier, involves closure of the VSD with a Dacron™ patch and use of an autologous pericardial patch for closure of the ostium primum ASD (Fig. 8–2.4). The common AV valve and ostium primum ASD are accessed in the same manner as for the one-patch technique. The VSD is closed with a Dacron™ patch secured to the right side of the interventricular septum using a continuous 4-0 or 5-0 Prolene™ suture. The midpoints of the bridging valve leaflets are then attached to the crest of this Dacron™ "neoseptum" and a second autologous pericardial patch with a 5-0 Prolene™ suture. A series of interrupted 5-0 Prolene™ mattress sutures is then used to secure these leaflets to both patches. The cleft between the left (mitral) inferior and superior leaflets is then closed with interrupted 5-0 or 6-0 Prolene™ sutures. Mitral valve competence is then tested as in the single-patch technique. The remainder of the pericardial patch is then folded back and secured over the ostium primum ASD with the free ends of the suture used to secure the Dacron™ patch. We tend to suture the atrial patch inferior to the ostium of the coronary sinus, allowing it to drain into the left atrium; this is to avoid suture placement into the AV node or bundle of His. If, however, a left superior vena cava drains into the coronary sinus, the atrial patch must be placed such that the coronary sinus flow returns normally to the right atrium to avoid significant arterial desaturation.

Transesophageal echocardiography is an invaluable tool for intraoperative evaluation of AV septal defects prior to and following repair. Careful assessment of AV valve regurgitation or stenosis, intraventricular or atrial shunting, left ventricular outflow, and ventricular function should be made immediately following repair.

The operative mortality rates after repair of partial AV canal defects is <2%, with the most significant recognized complication being injury to the conduction system resulting in AV block. Mortality rates after complete AV canal repair range optimally range between 1.5% and 4.5%. Postoperative complications include complete heart block (1% to 2%), residual interventricular shunt (5% to 7%), and left AV valve insufficiency requiring subsequent repair or replacement (5% to 10%). The long-term prognosis in patients undergoing partial and complete AV canal repair depends largely on the development and severity of mitral insufficiency over time.

8.3   Ventricular Septal Defect (Fig. 8–3)

Incidence: Comprise 20% of congenital heart defects

Pathophysiology: Defect in interventricular septum permits left-to-right shunting of blood. Right ventricular volume overload and pulmonary overcirculation can produce congestive heart failure in infancy and irreversible pulmonary

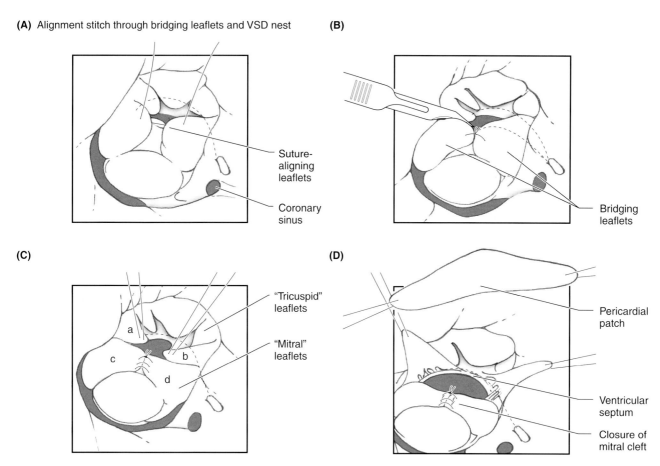

(A) Alignment stitch through bridging leaflets and VSD nest

Suture-aligning leaflets

Coronary sinus

(B)

Bridging leaflets

(C)

"Tricuspid" leaflets

"Mitral" leaflets

a
c
b
d

(D)

Pericardial patch

Ventricular septum

Closure of mitral cleft

FIGURE 8–2.3. "One-patch" repair of complete AV canal defect. *(A)* After cardiopulmonary bypass has been established, the common AV valve, VSD, ostium primum ASD, and "cleft" mitral valve are accessed through a right atriotomy, which runs close and parallel to the AV groove. An alignment stitch is brought through the bridging leaflets and ventricular septal crest. *(B)* The bridging leaflets are divided over the ventricular crest, creating six leaflets *(C)*. *(D)* The VSD crest is exposed and the cleft in the anterior mitral valve leaflet is closed with interrupted 3-0 or 4-0 Prolene™ sutures. *(E)* A Dacron or pericardial patch is sutured to the VSD crest. *(F)* The central "tricuspid" leaflets are attached to the patch. *(G)* The suture line is continued circumferentially around the patch, closing the ASD.

hypertension later in life. Shunt reversal (right-to-left) due to elevated pulmonary vascular resistances leads to systemic hypoxemia (Eisenmenger's syndrome).

Clinical Features: Small VSDs are usually asymptomatic; larger defects may lead to symptomatic congestive heart failure at 6 to 8 weeks of age. Eisenmenger's syndrome with congestive symptoms and cyanosis usually presents after the second decade. A loud pansystolic ejection murmur at the left lower sternal border is characteristic. Radiographic findings are revealing of pulmonary congestion. Electrocardiography often reveals right and left ventricular hyper-

trophy. Two-dimensional echocardiography with Doppler is diagnostic with localization and measurement of the defect.

Concepts of Correction: Many VSDs close spontaneously and are therefore observed for up to 1 year. Indications for early surgical closure include (1) large VSDs that do not spontaneously close within 1 year, (2) congestive symptoms refractory to medical treatment, (3) elevated pulmonary vascular resistances in infants older than 6 months, and (4) inlet and conal VSDs.

Corrective Operation(s): Patch VSD closure

(E)   **(F)**

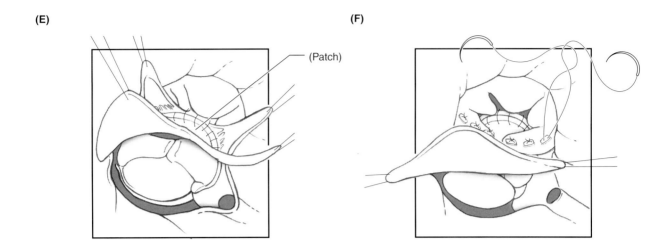

(G) Closure of ostium primum ASD

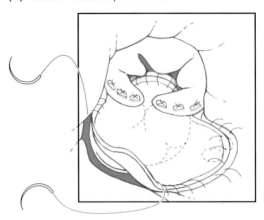

FIGURE 8–2.3.   (Continued)

FIGURE 8–2.4.   "Two-patch" repair of complete AV canal defect. *(A)* After cardiopulmonary bypass has been established, the common AV valve, VSD, ostium primum ASD, and "cleft" mitral valve are accessed through a right atriotomy, which runs close and parallel to the AV groove. *(B)* A Dacron™ patch is secured to the right side of the interventricular septum using a continuous 4-0 to 5-0 Prolene™ suture, closing the VSD. *(C)* The bridging valve leaflets are attached to the crest of this Dacron™ "neoseptum" and a second autologous pericardial patch with interrupted 5-0 Prolene™ sutures. *(D)* A series of mattress sutures are passed through the bridging valve leaflets, the neoseptum, and a second patch (pericardial). This patch will be used for the ASD closure. *(E)* The cleft in the anterior mitral valve leaflet is closed with interrupted 3-0 or 4-0 Prolene™ sutures beginning peripherally and moving centrally. Mitral valve competence is then tested by filling the left ventricle with cold saline. The remainder of the pericardial patch is then folded back and secured over the ostium primum ASD with the free ends of the suture used to secure the Dacron™ patch. *(F)* The atrial patch is usually sutured inferior to the coronary sinus, allowing it to drain into the left atrium. This keeps the suture line away from the AV node and the bundle of His.

(A) Right atriotomy

(B) Patch closure of VSD

Ventricular septal defect

Bundle of His

Retracted AV valve leaflet, exposing VSD

Superior vena cava

Coronary sinus

Inferior vena cava

(D) Mattress sutures passed through valve leaflets, neoseptum, and pericardial patch (for ASD closure)

(C) Stitch approximating bridging leaflets of common AV valve and crest of Dacron "neoseptum"

VSD patch

ASD

ASD patch

VSD patch

(E) Suture end from VSD closure

Suture closure of mitral cleft

ASD closure

Tricuspid valve

Coronary sinus

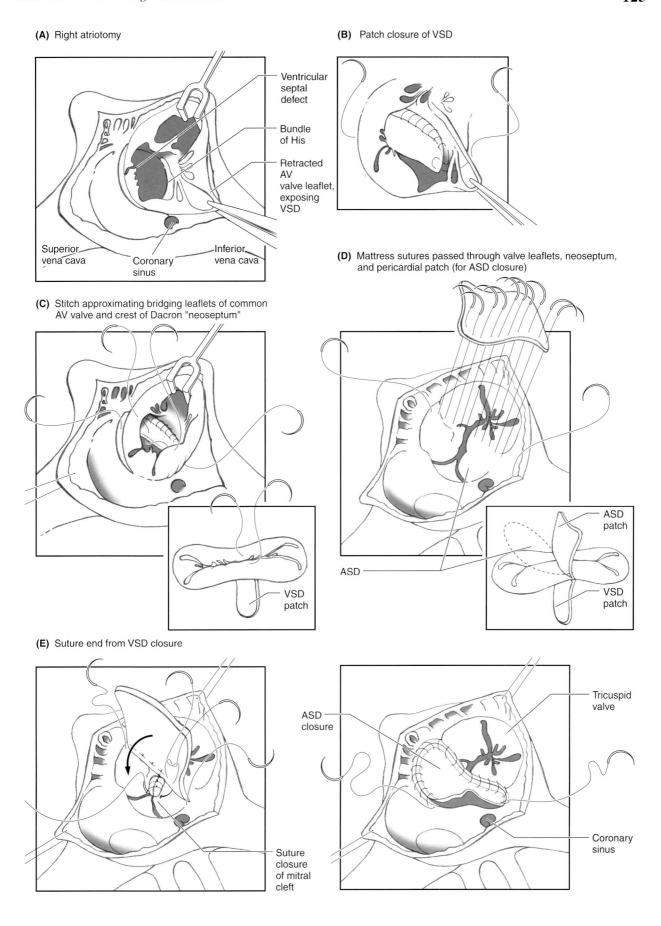

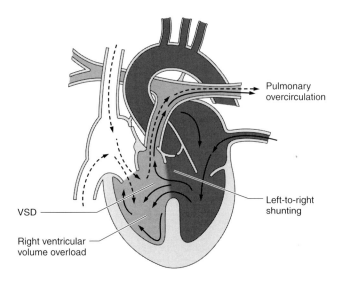

FIGURE 8–3. Schematic drawing of VSD. (■)———►, Oxygenated; (□)---►, Deoxygenated; (▨)═══►, mixed.

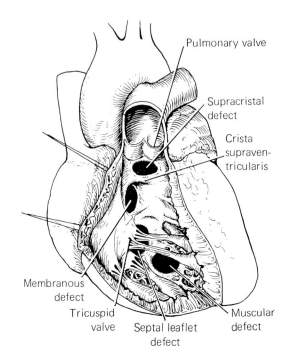

FIGURE 8–3.1. Anatomic locations of the four major types of VSDs, including perimembranous, muscular, inlet (AV canal-type), and conal defects. Reproduced with permission. Verrier ED: The Heart: II. Congenital Diseases. In *Current Surgical Diagnosis and Treatment*, Norwalk, Appleton & Lange, 1994, p. 395.

General Considerations

VSDs represent one or more holes in the interventricular septum that separates the right and left ventricles. VSDs are the most common congenital heart defects, accounting for about 20% of all defects. The interventricular septum is divided into several different anatomic subsections: (1) the membranous septum, (2) the muscular (trabecular) septum, (3) the inlet (AV canal) septum, and (4) the conal (outlet) septum. Four major anatomic types of VSDs have been derived from these septal divisions: **perimembranous, muscular, inlet, and conal** (Fig. 8–3.1). The most common type are perimembranous VSDs (70% to 80%), which are usually located within the membranous septum between the conal and muscular septa. Perimembranous VSDs may be located solely within the membranous septum but may also extend into any of the other regions of the interventricular septum. Furthermore, this form may extend to the tricuspid valve annulus near the anteroseptal commissure; if the anterior and septal leaflets adhere to the edge of the VSD, a left ventricle-to-right atrial shunt may ensue. Aortic regurgitation may result if the perimembranous VSD extends to the base of the noncoronary leaflet of the aortic valve. Muscular VSDs (10%) are located within the membranous septum and are often composed of multiple holes. Inlet (6%) VSDs are located in the AV canal, just beneath the tricuspid valve. Conal (4%) VSDs lie within the conal septum, just inferior to the pulmonary valve. In conal VSDs, the right coronary or noncoronary leaflets of the aortic valve may prolapse through the VSD from the Venturi effect, leading to valvular damage and aortic insufficiency. VSDs are often components of more complex cardiac anomalies (e.g., complete AV canal, tetralogy of Fallot) and often coexist with a patent ductus arteriosus or coarctation of the aorta.

The differential pressures between the left and right ventricles results in a left-to-right shunt across the VSD, leading to increased pulmonary blood flow. The magnitude of the shunt is a function of the defect size and the pulmonary and systemic vascular resistances. Large defects are termed nonrestrictive if the cross-sectional area of the defect is greater than or equal to that of the aortic annulus. There is little to no resistance to blood flow across the defect, and the right ventricular systolic pressure approaches that of the left ventricular pressure; the pulmonary-to-systemic flow ratio (Q_p/Q_s) is inversely proportional to the ratio of the pulmonary-to-systemic vascular resistances. Nonrestrictive defects are less likely to close spontaneously and generally result in congestive heart failure early in life. Small defects are termed *restrictive*, since they present significant resistance to flow across the defect. Consequently, the right ventricular pressure is, at most, only mildly elevated and the $Q_p/Q_s \leq 1.5$. Moderately sized VSDs represent an intermediate group of defects in which the right ventricular systolic pressure is indeed elevated, but not beyond 50% of the left ventricular pressure; the Q_p/Q_s ranges between 2.5 and 3.0.

The two major physiologic consequences of VSDs are congestive heart failure and pulmonary overcirculation. Although small increases in pulmonary blood flow are generally well tolerated, large increases to more than twice systemic flow may lead to congestive heart failure, severe pulmonary congestion and respiratory tract infections, and poor growth during infancy. Persistently elevated pulmonary blood flow also leads to irreversible pulmonary hypertension, produced by medial and intimal proliferation of the pulmonary arterioles. If this process is untreated, pulmonary vascular resistance will continue to rise to a point where there is a reversal of flow across the defect (right-to-left shunting), producing arterial hypoxemia. This phenomenon is referred to as Eisenmenger's syndrome and occurs in 10% of untreated nonrestrictive VSDs.

Thirty percent to 40% of all VSDs close spontaneously. The probability of spontaneous closure is inversely related to the VSD size and age of the patient. Sixty percent to 70% of small VSDs, particularly perimembranous and muscular VSDs, close spontaneously in early life. Furthermore, 80%, 50%, and 25% of large VSDs discovered at the age of 1, 6, and 12 months, respectively, eventually close spontaneously. Conversely, inlet and conal VSDs generally do not close spontaneously, and early surgical closure is generally recommended. VSDs that appear likely to close spontaneously are generally observed for about 1 year. Moderate to large VSDs that remain open after a 1-year interval should be closed. Other indications for early VSD repair include (1) severe, congestive heart failure that is refractory to aggressive medical decongestive therapy (i.e., digoxin, diuretics) or (2) elevated pulmonary vascular resistances in infants older than 6 months of age.

Diagnostic Keys

Infants with small VSDs are usually asymptomatic, displaying normal growth and development. Physical examination often reveals a loud pansystolic ejection murmur at the left lower sternal border. Larger defects result in congestive symptoms including dyspnea on exertion, hepatomegaly, rales, and frequent pulmonary infections at 6 to 8 weeks of age. Patients who develop Eisenmenger's syndrome generally present later in life (after the second decade) when cyanosis is evident. The P2 is increased with significant pulmonary hypertension. Radiographic findings are usually associated with larger defects and include enlargement of the heart and pulmonary arteries with signs of pulmonary congestion (i.e., increased pulmonary vascular markings). Electrocardiography shows signs of left and right ventricular hypertrophy. Two-dimensional echocardiography is diagnostic, with localization of the defect and estimation of the degree of interventricular shunting. Doppler studies of the pulmonary artery and the VSD may be used to assess right ventricular and pulmonary artery pressures indirectly. Although not routinely employed, cardiac catheterization is useful for the measurement of pulmonary artery pressures, pulmonary vascular resistance, and calculation of shunt size in patients suspected of fixed pulmonary resistance. Catheterization is also useful in cases of multiple

cardiac defects and multiple complex muscular septal defects.

Operative Correction

VSD repair is performed through a median sternotomy on cardiopulmonary bypass (Fig. 8–3.2). Deep hypothermic circulatory arrest may be preferred in infants weighing <8 kg. Most VSDs can be repaired through a right atriotomy. The atriotomy is extended from the inferior vena cava toward the right atrial appendage, being careful to avoid the sinus node. The VSD is exposed by retracting the septal and anterior leaflets of the tricuspid valve. A prosthetic patch (Dacron™ or GoreTex™) is placed over the VSD using pledgetted, interrupted 5-0 or 6-0 Prolene™ sutures, taking care not to place sutures through the adjacent conduction fiber bundles.

Conal defects are more easily accessed through the pulmonary valve via a pulmonary arteriotomy. A right ventriculotomy or left apical ventriculotomy may be required for closure of some inferiorly located muscular VSDs.

The overall operative mortality for isolated VSD repair is <3%. Permanent, complete AV heart block is a rare but recognized complication following VSD repair; pacemaker placement may be required in these cases. The long-term prognosis in survivors is generally excellent.

8.4 Patent Ductus Arteriosus (Fig. 8–4)

Incidence: Comprises 12% to 15% of congenital heart defects; 1:2 male:female.

Pathophysiology: Left-to-right shunt from the thoracic aorta to the pulmonary artery leads to augmented pulmonary blood flow, pulmonary hypertension, and congestive heart failure.

Clincal Features: Most patients are asymptomatic, but congestive heart failure may present early in life. Physical exam reveals a characteristic continuous harsh flow murmur at the left second intercostal space with wide pulse pressure and bounding peripheral pulses. The electrocardiogram is normal in small shunts but may reveal left ventricular hypertrophy in large shunts. Chest radiograph may reveal cardiomegaly with a prominent pulmonary artery and overall vascularity. Echocardiography is diagnostic, demonstrating blood from across the ductus with associated left ventricular hypertrophy and left atrial enlargement.

Concept of Correction: Correction involves ductal closure with indomethacin, coil embolization, or surgical ligation.

Corrective Operation(s): Patent ductus arteriosus ligation

General Considerations

Patent ductus arteriosus (PDA) represents the persistent patency of the fetal ductus arteriosus, a communication between the upper descending thoracic aorta and the main

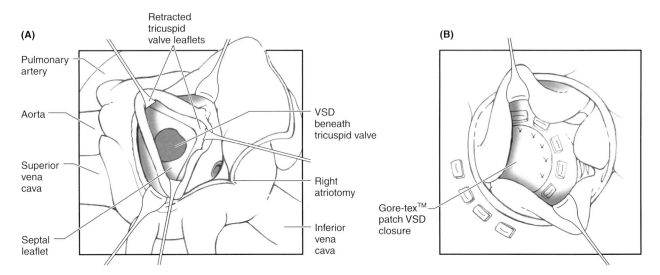

(A)

Retracted
tricuspid
valve leaflets

Pulmonary
artery

Aorta

Superior
vena
cava

Septal
leaflet

VSD
beneath
tricuspid valve

Right
atriotomy

Inferior
vena
cava

(B)

Gore-tex™
patch VSD
closure

FIGURE 8–3.2. Transatrial repair of perimembranous VSD. *(A)* After cardiopulmonary bypass has been established, a right atriotomy extending from the interior vena cava toward the right atrial appendage is performed. The VSD is exposed by retracting the septal and anterior tricuspid valve leaflets. *(B)* The VSD is closed by securing a prosthetic patch (Dacron™ or GoreTex™) over the VSD, using interrupted pledgetted 5-0 or 6-0 Prolene™ sutures. Care must be taken to avoid placing sutures through the adjacent conduction fiber bundles. Also, it may be necessary to place some of the securing sutures through the tricuspid valve annulus, to avoid damaging the nearby aortic valve.

pulmonary artery. In fetal life, the ductus arteriosus, derived from the sixth aortic arch, shunts blood from the pulmonary artery to the aorta, bypassing the still immature pulmonary vasculature. Lung expansion during the first

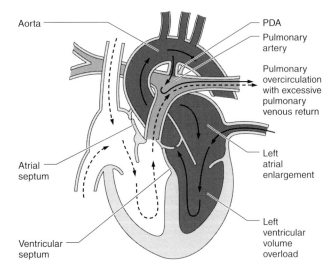

Aorta

Atrial
septum

Ventricular
septum

PDA

Pulmonary
artery

Pulmonary
overcirculation
with excessive
pulmonary
venous return

Left
atrial
enlargement

Left
ventricular
volume
overload

FIGURE 8–4. Schematic drawing of PDA. (■)——➤, Oxygenated; (□)----➤, Deoxygenated; (▨)⇉➤, mixed.

hours after birth leads to a rapid fall in pulmonary vascular resistance and corresponding increase in pulmonary blood flow. The resultant rise in arterial PO_2 and fall in circulating prostaglandins promotes contraction of the smooth muscle in the wall of the ductus arteriosus and ductal closure. In some cases, however, the ductus remains open for several weeks or even longer, resulting in left-to-right shunts of varying degrees depending on the size of the ductus and the pulmonary vascular resistance. This anomaly, comprising 12% to 15% of congenital heart defects (30% in premature infants), may be well tolerated for years in some patients; however, a persistent shunt can produce heart failure early in life as well as progressive pulmonary hypertension later on. Risk factors include hypoxia, high altitudes, prematurity, respiratory distress syndrome, and associated cardiac malformations.

Diagnostic Keys

Many patients with isolated PDA are asymptomatic, but congestive heart failure may present early in life. Physical exam reveals a characteristic continuous harsh flow murmur heard most easily in the left second intercostal space. A wide pulse pressure results in bounding peripheral pulses. Electrocardiography may be normal in cases of small shunts, but will reveal some degree of left ventricular hypertrophy in large shunts. Similarly, chest radiography may be normal in small shunts, but if the shunt is large, mild cardiomegaly with a prominent pulmonary artery may present. Increased pulmonary vascularity and left ventricular hypertrophy may also be evident on chest film. Echocardiography is diagnostic, demonstrating blood flow from the aorta to the pulmonary artery with associated left ventricular hypertrophy and left atrial enlargement. Cardiac catheterization is not required for isolated PDA evaluation.

Operative Correction

Early administration of indomethacin may cause ductal closure in many premature infants, obviating surgical treatment. Indomethacin therapy, however, is generally contraindicated if renal insufficiency or intracranial bleeding is present. Small PDAs that do not spontaneously close within the first 3 months of life or larger PDAs that lead to symptoms of congestive failure should undergo surgical closure. Ductal closure for bacterial endocarditis prophylaxis is generally indicated for smaller PDAs. In most cases, adequate exposure of the ductus is achieved through a small left posterolateral thoracotomy in the third or fourth intercostal space (Fig. 8–4.1). The left lung is retracted anteromedially and the parietal pleura overlying the ductus is incised. The ductus is identified and dissected, taking care not to injure the phrenic and left recurrent laryngeal nerves nearby. The ductus is interrupted with a surgical clip in neonates. In older children, the ductus is divided between appropriate vascular clamps with oversewing of the ends. Multiple suture ligation is an alternative method of ligation but is associated with a higher incidence of residual patency.

Percutaneous coil embolization has produced satisfactory results in selected cases and may emerge as the treatment of choice in the future. Some centers have achieved good results with clip ligation of PDAs using a video-assisted thoracoscopic approach.

For isolated PDA ligation, the operative mortality is well below 1%. The operative risk is somewhat greater in the older patient with preexisting pulmonary hypertension. Complications, albeit rare, include hemorrhage and damage to the recurrent laryngeal and phrenic nerves. Immediate improvement in pulmonary vascularity and heart size is often seen after PDA ligation in infants with congestive heart failure. Long-term results are generally excellent.

8.5 Partial Anomalous Pulmonary Venous Connection (Fig. 8–5)

Incidence: Comprises <1% of congenital heart defects

Pathophysiology: One or more, but not all, of the pulmonary veins drain into the right atrium or its venous tributaries; ASDs are commonly associated. This anomaly results in a left-to-right shunt leading to pulmonary hypertension, pulmonary vascular disease, and congestive heart failure if left untreated.

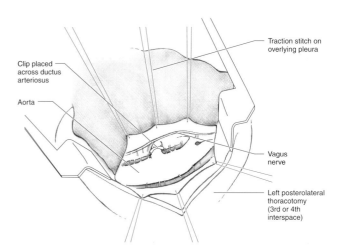

Clip placed across ductus arteriosus

Aorta

Traction stitch on overlying pleura

Vagus nerve

Left posterolateral thoracotomy (3rd or 4th interspace)

FIGURE 8–4.1.   Ligation of PDA. The pleural space is entered through a left posterolateral thoracotomy incision through the third or fourth intercostal space. The left lung is retracted anteromedially, and the parietal pleura overlying the ductus and descending aorta is incised lateral to the vagus and recurrent laryngeal nerves. These nerves are reflected anteromedially with the pleural flap. The ductus is then carefully dissected free. In premature infants, the ductus is closed with Hemoclips or a single ligature. In term infants or older patients, ductal closure is accomplished with double ligation at the aortic and pulmonary arterial ends. Alternatively, the ductus may be divided between two Potts' clamps followed by oversewing the cut ends with 5-0 Prolene™; this requires a more complete full-length dissection of the ductus.

Clinical Features: Physical manifestations resemble those of ASD, including signs and symptoms of congestive heart failure by the third or fourth decades. The S2 is widely split and fixed if it is associated with an ASD; the S2 is normal if it is an isolated defect. The electrocardiogram may reveal right ventricular hypertrophy. Chest radiography may reveal right atrial and ventricular enlargement with increased pulmonary vascularity. Echocardiography is diagnostic. Angiography is not usually required, but it can define right lung arterial blood supply in scimitar syndrome.

Concepts of Correction: Redirect anomalous pulmonary venous return into the left atrium.

Corrective Operation(s):   Patch baffling of anomalous pulmonary venous drainage into the left atrium

General Considerations

Partial anomalous pulmonary venous connection (PAPVC) is a rare congenital anomaly in which one or more, but not

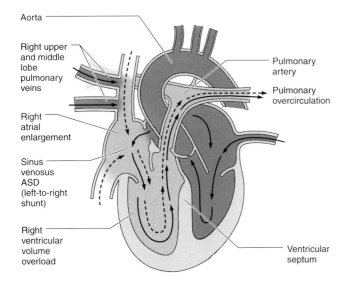

FIGURE 8–5. Schematic drawing of partial anomalous pulmonary venous connection. (■)——▶, Oxygenated; (□)----▶, Deoxygenated; (▨)----▶, mixed.

all, pulmonary veins drain into the right atrium or its venous tributaries (e.g., superior/inferior vena cava, coronary sinus, left innominate vein). Typically, the right pulmonary veins tend to drain into the right atrium or vena cavae; the left pulmonary veins drain into the coronary sinus or left innominate vein. This defect is commonly associated with ASDs. Although numerous variations have been described, two specific syndromes have been defined: (1) **sinus venosus ASD** and (2) **scimitar syndrome** (Fig. 8–5.1). In patients with a sinus venosus ASD, the right upper and middle lobe pulmonary veins drain into the superior vena cava at or below the azygous vein or at its junction with the right atrium. In the scimitar syndrome, the right pulmonary vein drains into the inferior vena cava. The name of this variation refers to a crescent-shaped density seen adjacent to the right heart border on chest radiography. This syndrome is associated with right lung hypoplasia, sometimes leading to rightward mediastinal shift.

The pathophysiology of these defects resembles that of an ostium secundum ASD, namely, a left-to-right shunt leading to pulmonary hypertension and pulmonary vascular disease. Extensive anomalous venous connections lead to hemodynamics resembling total anomalous pulmonary venous connection (see Total Anomalous Pulmonary Venous Return section in Chapter 9).

Diagnostic Keys

Physical manifestations of this anomaly resemble that of an ASD, specifically, signs and symptoms of congestive heart failure, usually by the third and fourth decades. When associated with an ASD, the S2 is widely split and fixed; when no

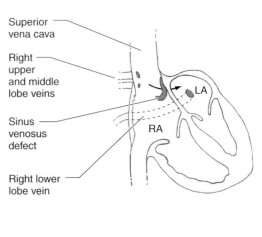

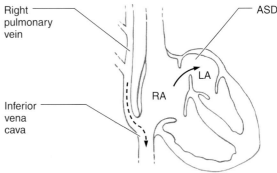

FIGURE 8–5.1. Two forms of partial anomalous pulmonary venous connections. *(A)* Sinus venosus ASD. The right upper and middle lobe pulmonary veins enter the superior vena cava. *(B)* In the scimitar syndrome, the right pulmonary vein drains into the inferior vena cava. RA = right atrium; LA = left atrium.

ASD is present, the S2 is normal. Electrocardiography may reveal right ventricular hypertrophy. Chest radiography may reveal right atrial and right ventricular enlargement with increased pulmonary vascular markings. Two-dimensional echocardiography diagnostic. Angiography is usually not required, but it may be useful in defining the right lung arterial blood supply in the scimitar syndrome.

Operative Correction

Surgical correction of partial anomalous pulmonary venous return is usually performed electively between the ages of 2 and 5 years. A significant left-to-right shunt ($Q_p/Q_s > 1.5:1$) is an indication for repair. Surgical repair is performed through a median sternotomy under cardiopulmonary bypass and is directed toward restoring normal pulmonary venous drainage into the left atrium. During repair of a sinus venosus ASD, a pericardial patch is placed anterior to the associated anomalous pulmonary vein orifices,

(A) Right atriotomy

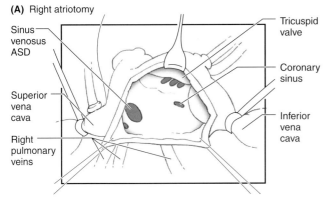

(B)

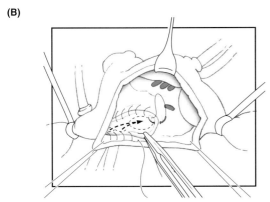

FIGURE 8–5.2.   Operative correction of sinus venosus ASD. *(A)* After cardiopulmonary bypass has been established, an oblique right atriotomy is performed. *(B)* An autologous pericardial patch is then secured over the anomalous right pulmonary vein orifice and the ASD, with a continuous 4-0 or 5-0 Prolene™ suture, to baffle the anomalous pulmonary venous drainage through the ASD into the left atrium.

(A) Right atriotomy

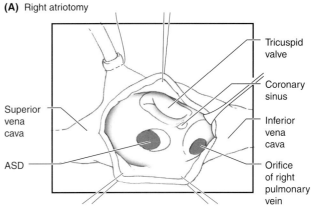

(B)

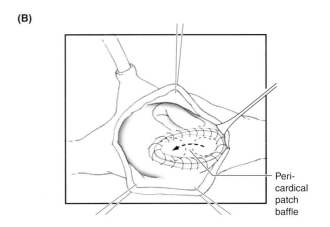

FIGURE 8–5.3.   Operative correction of the scimitar syndrome. *(A)* After cardiopulmonary bypass has been established, an oblique right atriotomy is performed. *(B)* An autologous pericardial patch is then secured over the anomalous right pulmonary vein orifices and the ASD, with a continuous 4-0 or 5-0 Prolene™ suture, to baffle the anomalous pulmonary venous drainage through the ASD into the left atrium. Care is taken to avoid obstructing the superior vena caval orifice.

directing the pulmonary venous return into the left atrium (Fig. 8–5.2).

In the scimitar syndrome, PAPVC is repaired by resecting the atrial septum and baffling the pulmonary venous return to the left atrium with a pericardial patch (Fig. 8–5.3). Once cardiopulmonary bypass has been established, a right atriotomy is created directly over the inferior vena caval orifice. Through this incision, an ASD is created by excising a portion of the interatrial septum at the foramen ovale. An autologous pericardial patch is then secured over the anomalous right pulmonary vein orifice and ASD with a continuous 4-0 or 5-0 Prolene™ suture in order to baffle

the pulmonary venous drainage through the ASD into the left atrium. Care is taken to avoid obstruction of the inferior vena caval orifice and to carry the suture line to the right of the coronary sinus, staying clear of the AV node. The right atriotomy is then closed, completing the operation.

Surgical correction of PAPVC is associated with a very low morbidity and mortality, with generally excellent long-term prognoses.

CHAPTER 9

Cyanotic Defects

David D. Yuh, MD, and Bruce A. Reitz, MD

Introduction

Cyanotic defects are lesions that result in **reduced pulmonary arterial blood flow,** usually due to shunting of desaturated systemic venous blood to the systemic arterial circulation without traversing the pulmonary vascular bed. This **right-to-left shunting** usually results from obstruction of right ventricular outflow combined with an anatomic defect between the right and left heart chambers (i.e., septal defect). Clinically, this results in cyanosis; the degree of cyanosis is proportional to the magnitude of right-to-left shunting and inversely proportionate to the amount of pulmonary arterial blood flow. Often, the ductus arteriosus and/or bronchial and mediastinal collateral vessels provide a substantial proportion of pulmonary blood flow in cases of severe right ventricular outflow tract obstruction. Intravenous prostaglandin E_1 is often used in the early postnatal period to maintain ductal patency and pulmonary blood flow, which allows time for the neonate to be stabilized prior to definitive corrective measures.

Surgical therapy consists of operations designed to augment pulmonary blood flow. Palliative shunts divert systemic arterial or venous blood to the pulmonary arterial circulation. Definitive correction generally consists of eliminating or bypassing the existing obstruction to pulmonary arterial flow.

9.1 Tetralogy of Fallot (Fig. 9–1)

Incidence: Comprises 10% of congenital heart defects; most common cyanotic defect (50%).

Pathophysiology: Tetralogy of Fallot (ToF) consists of a large ventricular septal defect (VSD), right ventricular outflow tract obstruction (RVOTO), aorta overriding the VSD, and right ventricular hypertrophy. RVOTO leads to right-to-left shunting across a nonrestrictive VSD, resulting in inadequate pulmonary blood flow and varying degrees of cyanosis.

Clinical Features: Most ToF patients are symptomatic, present-ing with cyanosis, clubbing, dyspnea on exertion, and hypercyanotic spells. "Squatting" is an adaptive behavior, seen in untreated older children, that augments pulmonary blood flow. A systolic ejection murmur along the upper left sternal border represents flow across the RVOTO. The electrocardiogram reveals right ventricular hypertrophy, and chest radiograph reveals a characteristic "boot-shaped" heart and diminished pulmonary vascularity. Echocardiography and cardiac catheterization with angiography are used to identify and characterize the ToF lesions and to plan surgical repair.

Concepts of Correction: Early total correction is generally preferred and is performed by widening the right ventricular outflow tract and closing the VSD. Cyanotic ToF infants with unfavorable anatomy for safe repair can undergo a palliative systemic-to-pulmonary artery shunt to increase pulmonary blood flow until definitive repair can be performed. Severely hypoplastic or atretic right ventricular outflow tracts may be reconstructed with a homograft or prosthetic valved conduit.

Corrective Operation(s):

- *Blalock-Taussig Shunt* (palliative)
- *Standard Complete Repair:* (1) VSD patch closure and (2) widening of the RVOTO
- *Rastelli Operation:* (1) VSD patch closure and (2) right ventricular outflow tract reconstruction with homograft or prosthetic valved conduit

General Considerations

The Tetralogy of Fallot (ToF) is the most common cyanotic congenital cardiac anomaly, constituting over 50% of all cases of cyanotic congenital heart disease and approximately 10% of all congenital defects. The four related defects comprising the tetralogy as defined by Fallot[1] in 1888 are (1) a large **VSD;** (2) **RVOTO;** (3) a **rightward-displaced aorta** (dextroposition), which overrides the VSD; and (4) **right ventricular hypertrophy.** Although the embryologic derivation of this constellation of defects is controversial to this day, the tetralogy is generally believed

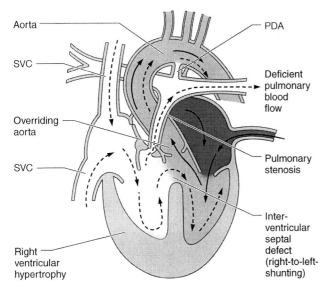

Aorta

SVC

Overriding aorta

SVC

Right ventricular hypertrophy

PDA

Deficient pulmonary blood flow

Pulmonary stenosis

Inter-ventricular septal defect (right-to-left-shunting)

FIGURE 9–1. Schematic drawing of ToF. (■)——▶, Oxygenated; (□)----▶, Deoxygenated; (▣)▭▭▶, mixed.

to be caused by the anterosuperior malalignment of the infundibular ventricular septum during fetal cardiac development. The septal (leftward) end of the infundibular septum inserts in an abnormally anterior and leftward position, lying in front of the septal band rather than between its left anterosuperior and right posteroinferior limbs; this has the effect of "crowding" the right ventricular outflow tract. The VSD in ToF is typically large and of the perimembranous variety (in 75% to 80%). The aorta overrides the VSD, deriving blood flow from both ventricles, and is rotated in a clockwise direction. The RVOTO results from malalignment of the infundibular septum and secondary trabecular hypertrophy and, in 75% of cases, some degree of pulmonary valve maldevelopment (i.e., stenosis, atresia, bicuspid valve). Associated cardiac defects are common, including left superior vena cava, atrioventricular (AV) septal defect, patent ductus arteriosus (PDA), and atrial septal defect (ASD). A right aortic arch occurs in about 25% of these patients. Varying degrees of pulmonary artery hypoplasia are almost always seen in ToF. Five percent of patients have coronary artery anomalies, the most important of which is a right coronary artery origin from the left anterior descending artery, which, in turn, courses across the right ventricular outflow tract to reach the left ventricle.

The pathophysiologic manifestations of ToF stem from RVOTO and consequent **right-to-left shunting** of deoxygenated blood across a large, nonrestrictive VSD into the left ventricle, the aorta, and the systemic circulation. The diminished pulmonary blood flow and ventricular right-to-left shunting in TOF results in **cyanosis,** the severity of which depends on the ratio of the combined resistance to blood flow derived from the RVOTO and pulmonary vascular bed (normally very low) to the resistance of the systemic

vascular bed. With the large VSD, the two ventricles can be thought of as a single pumping chamber that distributes the total cardiac output to the pulmonic and systemic circulations in proportion to the resistances presented to it by the RVOTO and the systemic vascular bed. Cyanosis is usually ameliorated at birth due to collateral blood flow supplied to the pulmonary circulation by a patent ductus arteriosus and/or bronchial arteries. If the RVOTO is severe enough, however, closure of the ductus over the ensuing days or weeks after birth leads to significant cyanosis. If this condition is allowed to progress, right ventricular hypertrophy increases, leading to progressive RVOTO and worsening cyanosis. Most of the mortalities during the first year of life in these patients are due to cerebral infarction and cardiac arrest from thrombosis or anoxia. It bears mentioning that there is a small subset of patients with minimal RVOTO in whom no shunt or even a left-to-right shunt is present and who consequently do not develop cyanosis in infancy or early childhood; this variant form is known as **acyanotic ToF.**

Diagnostic Keys

Although acyanotic ToF patients remain asymptomatic for quite some time, <10% of patients with ToF survive to the age of 21 without surgical treatment. Indeed, most ToF patients develop signs and symptoms, specifically cyanosis, clubbing, and dyspnea on exertion, by 6 weeks to 6 months of age; earlier presentation in the newborn period may result from pulmonary atresia with ductal dependency. **Hypercyanotic spells,** or sudden episodes of intense cyanosis followed by unconsciousness, are prevalent between 2 and 6 months of age. "**Squatting**" to relieve dyspnea is another aspect of this syndrome observed in older children and represents an adapted maneuver to increase systemic venous return and systemic vascular resistance, thereby augmenting pulmonary blood flow across the obstructed right ventricular outflow tract. This phenomenon is seldom observed in the United States since most cases of ToF are diagnosed and treated early in life. A crescendo-decrescendo systolic ejection murmur auscultated along the upper left sternal border usually represents flow across the RVOTO. Electrocardiography reveals right ventricular hypertrophy and right axis deviation. Chest radiography characteristically reveals a "boot-shaped" heart (*coeur en sabot:* concave pulmonary artery segment, right ventricular hypertrophy, and small left ventricle) and diminished pulmonary vascularity (pulmonary oligemia). Two-dimensional echocardiography with Doppler is extremely helpful, revealing the characteristic components of ToF; the severity of RVOTO can also be assessed. Cardiac catheterization and angiography are usually performed, since accurate assessment of coronary artery anatomy, complex VSDs, anomalous pulmonary artery arborization, ventricular function, and hemodynamic data are necessary to plan operative repair.

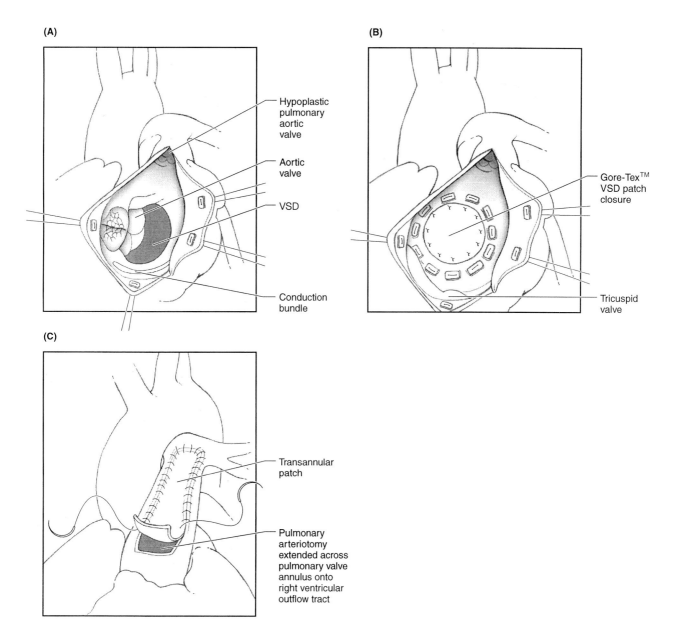

(A)

Hypoplastic pulmonary aortic valve

Aortic valve

VSD

Conduction bundle

(B)

Gore-Tex™ VSD patch closure

Tricuspid valve

(C)

Transannular patch

Pulmonary arteriotomy extended across pulmonary valve annulus onto right ventricular outflow tract

FIGURE 9–1.1. Totally corrective repair of ToF with pulmonary stenosis. *(A)* Once cardiopulmonary bypass has been established, the right ventricular outflow tract is opened with a vertical right ventriculotomy. This incision is created along the free wall of the infundibulum, originating at the level of the infundibular septum, and carried across the pulmonary valve annulus onto the main pulmonary artery. If necessary, a pulmonary valvotomy (valvar pulmonic stenosis) and/or resection of hypertrophied infundibular myocardium (subvalvar pulmonic stenosis) is performed to widen the right ventricular outflow tract. *(B)* The ventricular septal defect is accessed by retracting the anterior and septal leaflets of the tricuspid valve and closed with a Dacron™ patch using 5-0 or 6-0 Prolene™ sutures in a continuous or horizontal mattress (pledgeted) pattern. *(C)* If the pulmonary valve annulus is hypoplastic, a transannular patch (autologous pericardium, Dacron™, or GoreTex™) closure of the right ventriculotomy and pulmonary arteriotomy is performed, further widening the right ventricular outflow tract. If the pulmonary valve annulus is of normal caliber, the pulmonary arteriotomy is closed primarily, and the ventriculotomy is closed with a patch.

Operative Correction

The timing of operative correction of ToF is somewhat controversial, although presently there is a trend toward **early total correction** between 3 and 12 months of age for most cases of ToF. The **modified Blalock-Taussig shunt** (systemic-to-pulmonary artery) is performed in cyanotic infants whose anatomy is not yet amenable to total repair (see Pulmonary Atresia with Intact Ventricular Septum section in Chapter 8). These include cases of extremely hypoplastic pulmonary arteries, an anomalous coronary artery crossing the right ventricular outflow tract, and associated complex cardiac lesions. This palliative measure is designed to augment pulmonary blood flow and relieve cyanosis until definitive repair can be effected.

The totally corrective operation is performed through a median sternotomy on cardiopulmonary bypass (Fig. 9–1.1). If present, the modified Blalock-Taussig shunt is ligated and divided during cooling, and the ductus arteriosus is ligated if patent. The right ventricular outflow tract is accessed through a **vertical right ventriculotomy** originating at the level of the infundibular septum and carried along the free wall of the infundibulum; the incision is extended distally across the pulmonary valve annulus up to the pulmonary artery bifurcation if the annulus is hypoplastic. This incision may be carried even further along the right and/or left pulmonary arteries if their orifices are stenotic. If the pulmonary valve is stenotic (e.g., bicuspid valve), a pulmonary valvotomy is performed (see Pulmonary Stenosis with Intact Ventricular Septum section in Chapter 7); severely dysplastic or thickened valve leaflets may be excised. Subvalvar pulmonary stenosis is relieved by wedge resection of hypertrophied infundibular myocardial bundles. The large VSD is exposed by retracting the tricuspid valve leaflets, and **VSD closure** is performed with a Dacron™ patch secured with 5-0 or 6-0 Prolene™ sutures in a continuous or horizontal mattress (pledgeted) pattern (see Ventricular Septal Defect section in Chapter 9). Along the superior edge of the defect, the anchoring sutures are placed to the right of the aortic valve annulus in the crista supraventricularis to correct the dextroposition of the aorta. If the pulmonary valve annulus is of normal size, the right ventriculotomy is closed with an autologous pericardial patch, and the pulmonary arteriotomy is closed primarily, completing the operation. If the annulus is hypoplastic, an autologous pericardial (or prosthetic Dacron™, GoreTex™) **transannular patch** is used to close the right ventriculotomy and pulmonary arteriotomy, effectively widening the right ventricular outflow tract (see Pulmonary Atresia with Intact Ventricular Septum section in Chapter 7).

In patients with severe hypoplasia or atresia of the right ventricular outflow tract or in patients with an anomalous origin of the left anterior descending coronary artery from the right coronary artery, a **Rastelli operation** is performed

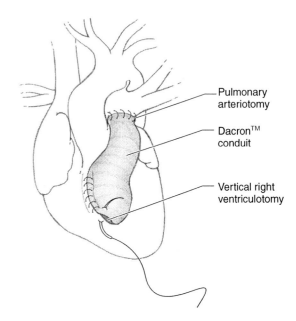

— Pulmonary arteriotomy

— Dacron™ conduit

— Vertical right ventriculotomy

FIGURE 9–1.2.   Rastelli operation for ToF with severe hypoplasia or atresia of the right ventricular outflow tract. After cardiopulmonary bypass has been established, a right atriotomy is created, and the VSD is closed with a Dacron™ patch as described previously. An aortic or pulmonary homograft (or valved prosthetic conduit) is then anastomosed (end to side) between a transverse right ventriculotomy and longitudinal pulmonary arteriotomy.

(Fig. 9–1.2). After cardiopulmonary bypass has been established, a right atriotomy is created, and a vent is placed across the foramen ovale into the left atrium to keep the left ventricle decompressed during the operation. A short vertical ventriculotomy is made in the midportion of the free wall of the right ventricle. The ventriculotomy is placed as close to the VSD as possible, avoiding the major right ventricular branches of the right coronary artery; stay stiches are placed at the ventriculotomy edges to expose the VSD adequately. The VSD is then closed with a Dacron™ patch as described above. A longitudinal arteriotomy is created at the confluence of the right and left pulmonary arteries, and the distal end of a 7- to 10-mm aortic or pulmonary homograft (or valved prosthetic conduit) is anastomosed to the arteriotomy in an end-to-side fashion with a continuous 7-0 polydioxanone continuous suture line. The proximal end of the conduit is then beveled and anastomosed to the right ventriculotomy in an end-to-side fashion using a continuous 4-0 or 5-0 Prolene™ suture line. Care must be taken to avoid compression of the coronary arteries between the graft and the surface of the right ventricle. The right atriotomy is closed, completing the operation.

In patients with favorable anatomy, the operative mortality of total ToF repair is about 0.4% to 3%, with generally good long-term results. Postrepair survival reported by Kirklin and associates[2] has been 94%, 92%, 91%, 90%, and 87% at 1 month and 1, 5, 10, and 20 years, respectively. Varying degrees of right ventricular failure in the early postoperative period and mild, well-tolerated pulmonary insufficiency are commonly observed. Residual right ventricular outflow tract obstruction requiring reoperation occurs in approximately 5% of cases. Long-term ventricular tachyarrhythmias requiring antiarrhythmic and/or pacemaker therapy can occur in 3% to 5% of cases.

9.2 *D*-Transposition of the Great Arteries (Fig. 9–2)

Incidence: Comprises approximately 5% of congenital heart defects with a 3:1 male/female predominance.

Pathophysiology: Venticuloarterial discordance, whereby the aorta arises from the right ventricle and the pulmonary artery arises from the left ventricle. Transposition of the great arteries (TGA) is associated with an intact ventricular septum (TGA/IVS) or a VSD (TGA/VSD). Systemic and pulmonary circulations are placed in parallel (normally in series). A "left-to-right" shunt (i.e., ASD, VSD, PDA) is required to permit oxygenated blood from the left heart to enter the right-sided systemic circulation. In neonates with inadequate "mixing" between the two circuits, progressive cyanosis and acidosis results in an early demise.

Clinical Features: Neonates with TGA/IVS present with severe cyanosis refractory to supplemental oxygen. Neonates with TGA/VSD are less cyanotic but are more likely to develop pulmonary hypertension and congestive heart failure in infancy

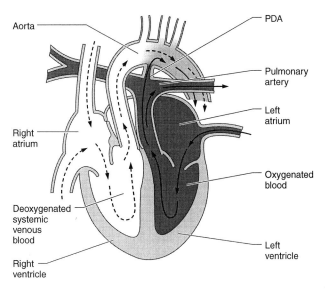

FIGURE 9–2. *D*-transposition of the great arteries. (■)——▸, Oxygenated; (□)----▸, Deoxygenated; (□)----▸, mixed.

due to pulmonary overcirculation. Electrocardiographic findings are consistent with right ventricular hypertrophy and, in cases of TGA/VSD, left ventricular hypertrophy. Chest radiograph characteristically reveals an "egg-on-a-string" cardiac silhouette with or without accenuated pulmonary vascularity. Echocardiography is diagnostic, revealing ventriculoarterial discordance and associated cardiac malformations.

Concepts of Correction: Atrial switch operations are designed to redirect systemic and pulmonary venous return to the appropriate ventricles. Arterial switch operations involve "retransposition" of the great vessels by constructing a "neoaorta" and "neopulmonary artery."

Corrective Operation(s):

- Mustard or Senning atrial switch operations
- Jatene arterial switch operation
- Rastelli operation for TGA/VSD and pulmonic stenosis
- Damus-Kaye-Stansel operation for TGA/VSD and subaortic stenosis

General Considerations

TGA is a congenital cardiac defect in which the aorta arises from the right ventricle and the pulmonary artery arises from the left ventricle; this situation is termed *ventriculoarterial discordance*. This defect accounts for approximately 5% of congenital heart defects with 3:1 male:female predominance. Embryologically, it is felt that TGA results from perturbations in the differential growth rates of the subpulmonic and subaortic conal musculature. By far the most common form of TGA (90%) is identified as *D*-TGA: the transposed aorta is located anteriorly and to the right of the pulmonary artery. In the less common *L*-TGA form (10%), the aorta lies to the left of the pulmonary artery. Approximately 70% of patients with TGA will have an IVS with no other significant cardiac malformations other than a PDA. A VSD is present in the remaining 30% of TGA cases. Variable coronary artery patterns are seen in TGA; however, they usually (>99%) originate from the sinuses of Valsalva that face the pulmonary artery; these "facing sinuses" are usually oriented in the leftward/anterior and rightward/posterior directions. The two most common coronary artery patterns observed in *D*-TGA are illustrated in Fig. 9–2.1. Other associated cardiac anomalies include pulmonic stenosis, which occurs in 30% to 35% of patients with TGA/VSD, and LVOTO, which occurs in up to 10% of all patients with TGA.

TGA results in several important physiologic and anatomic derangements: First, the pulmonary and systemic circulations are in *parallel* with each other instead of in series; the two circuits are separated from each other. Therefore, oxygenated blood circulates through the lungs and left side of the heart while deoxygenated blood circulates through the systemic circulation and the right side of the heart. Without a functional "left-to-right" shunt (i.e., ASD, VSD, PDA) between the two circuits to allow oxygenated

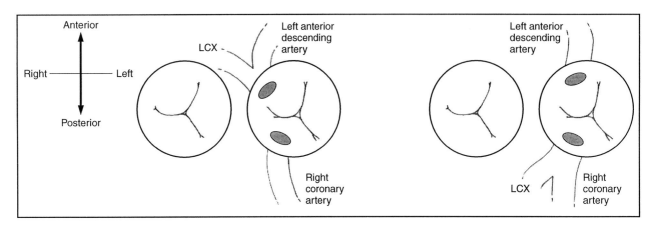

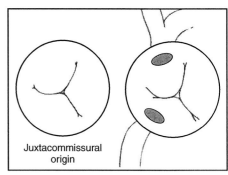

FIGURE 9–2.1. The two most common coronary artery patterns in *D*-TGA. (*Left*) Left main coronary artery arises from the left/anterior coronary sinus "facing" the main pulmonary artery and gives rise to the left anterior descending and circumflex coronary arteries. The right coronary artery arises from the rightward/posterior facing sinus (68%). (*Right*) The right coronary artery arises from the right/posterior facing sinus and gives rise to the circumflex (Cx) coronary artery. The left anterior descending coronary artery arises alone from the leftward/anterior facing sinus. (Reproduced with permission. Castaneda AR et al: *D*-transposition of the great arteries. In: *Cardiac Surgery of the Neonate and Infant*, Philadelphia, W.B. Saunders, 1994, p. 413.)

blood from the left heart to enter the right-sided systemic circulation, this derangement is incompatible with life. In *D*-TGA/VSD, there is a right-to-left shunt across the VSD during the systolic phase of the cardiac cycle due to the higher right-sided systemic pressures.

Conversely, there is an equivalent left-to-right shunt across the VSD during the diastolic phase, due to the increased venous return to the left atrium and subsequent increase in left ventricular end-diastolic pressure over that of the right ventricle. In neonates with inadequate "mixing" between the two circuits, progressive **cyanosis** and acidosis results in an early demise. Second, since pulmonary blood flow is generally greater than systemic blood flow due to (1) the lower pulmonary vascular resistance and

(2) systemic-to-pulmonary circulation shunting, pulmonary hypertension, obstructive pulmonary vascular disease, and congestive heart failure develop over time in untreated patients. Third, in untreated *D*-TGA/IVS, the left ventricle fails to develop normally (i.e., chamber dimensions and wall thickness) since it is presented with the low-resistance pulmonary vascular circulation. Hence, in as short a period as several weeks, the left ventricle loses its capacity to sustain an adequate cardiac output against a normal systemic vascular resistance; this has significant ramifications with respect to surgical correction. In patients with *D*-TGA/VSD, a large septal defect maintains systemic left ventricular pressure, and the left ventricle appears to develop normally during the first year of life.

Left untreated, the overall long-term life expectancy of patients with *D*-TGA is poor, with 1-month, 6-month, and 1-year survival rates of approximately 55%, 15%, and 10%, respectively. The prognosis is particularly poor in untreated patients with *D*-TGA/IVS, with survival rates of 17% and 4% at 2 months and 1 year, respectively. Early palliative maneuvers for patients with *D*-TGA/IVS include prostaglandin E_1 infusion and/or Rashkind atrial balloon septostomy to promote left-to-right shunting. Infants with *D*-TGA/VSD or *D*-TGA with a large PDA are less cyanotic than patients with *D*-TGA/IVS; however, they are more likely to develop pulmonary hypertension and congestive heart failure as early as 3 to 4 months of age.

Diagnostic Keys

Neonates with *D*-TGA commonly present with varying degrees of cyanosis and congestive heart failure. The severity of these symptoms depends largely on the extent of communication and mixing between the two parallel circulations. Patients with *D*-TGA/IVS usually have poor mixing through a patent foramen ovale or ASD and develop a rapidly progressive cyanosis refractory to supplemental oxygen, beginning in the first hours of life; without treatment, early death usually occurs. Conversely, patients with *D*-TGA/VSD generally have good mixing, are less cyanotic, and do not present in congestive failure until the end of the first month of life, when the pulmonary vascular resistance begins to fall and less oxygenated blood is shunted to the systemic circulation. Auscultation is often unrevealing except for a systolic flow murmur when a VSD or pulmonic stenosis is present. Electrocardiographic changes consistent with right ventricular hypertrophy are usually observed with *D*-TGA/IVS. Changes associated with left ventricular hypertrophy also tend to occur in cases of *D*-TGA associated with a VSD, PDA, and/or pulmonic stenosis.

Characteristic changes on chest radiography include an oval cardiac silhouette on the end of a very narrow vascular pedicle constituting the superior mediastinum, resembling an "egg-on-a-string." This is sometimes associated with prominent pulmonary vascular markings due to augmented pulmonary blood flow. Two-dimensional echocardiography with Doppler is usually diagnostic, revealing the ventriculoarterial discordance. Furthermore, associated malformations including pulmonic stenosis, atrial and ventricular septal defects, LVOTO, aortic arch obstruction, and coronary artery anomalies are consistently well detailed with echocardiography. Cardiac catheterization is not routinely performed to diagnose TGA; however, useful information can be obtained from such studies, including calculation of pulmonary vascular resistance, the precise locations of intracardiac shunts and great vessel relationships, the size and function of the AV valves, the condition of both ventricles, coronary artery distribution, and the presence of other cardiac anomalies.

Operative Correction

Corrective operations for *D*-TGA are divided into two major categories: **atrial switch** and **arterial switch** operations. Performed under cardiopulmonary bypass, atrial switch operations are designed (1) to redirect systemic venous return to the mitral valve, left ventricle, and pulmonary artery and (2) to transpose pulmonary venous return to the tricuspid valve, right ventricle, and aorta. The **Mustard** and **Senning** operations utilize baffles to achieve this transposition of venous return. Although often successful initially, several significant late complications have arisen from these operations including long-term atrial arrhythmias, tricuspid regurgitation, baffle obstruction of pulmonary or systemic venous return, and baffle leaks. Moreover, since the tricuspid valve and right ventricle are committed to support the systemic circulation after atrial switch operations, poor right ventricular function has been noted on follow-up catheterizations, prompting concerns about premature right ventricular failure. These problems have led to the development of a more "anatomic" correction, the **Jatene arterial switch** operation.

The Jatene arterial switch operation has become the preferred technique for treatment of *D*-TGA in most cardiac centers. This type of correction has the benefit of placing the systemic circulatory workload on the more powerful left ventricle and is generally associated with fewer complications. Early performance of the arterial switch operation within the first days to weeks of life is now recommended, particularly with *D*-TGA/IVS, because significant delay may result in a "deconditioned" left ventricle, which will be unable to support the systemic circulation. The risk of postoperative acute left ventricular failure as the left ventricle is suddenly called on to support the systemic circulation may increase with postponement. Early repair is also recommended for *D*-TGA/VSD; although the left ventricle may be sufficiently conditioned to support the systemic circulation, significant delay risks the development of irreversible pulmonary vascular occlusive disease, frequent respiratory tract infections, and failure to thrive. Furthermore, the VSD may partially close spontaneously, limiting exposure of the left ventricle to systemic pressures and retarding its normal development.

The Jatene operation is performed through a median sternotomy under cardiopulmonary bypass (Fig. 9–2.2). Periods of deep hypothermic circulatory arrest may also be used, particularly during repair of complex associated lesions. The ascending aorta and pulmonary trunk are first dissected away from each other, and the ductus arteriosus is divided between ligatures. The ascending aorta is then transected at its midportion, and the pulmonary trunk is transected just proximal to its bifurcation. Two buttons of "neopulmonary artery" (former aortic root) containing the origins of the left and right coronary arteries are transposed and anastomosed to the "neoaorta" (former pulmonary trunk) using continuous 7-0 Prolene™ sutures. The

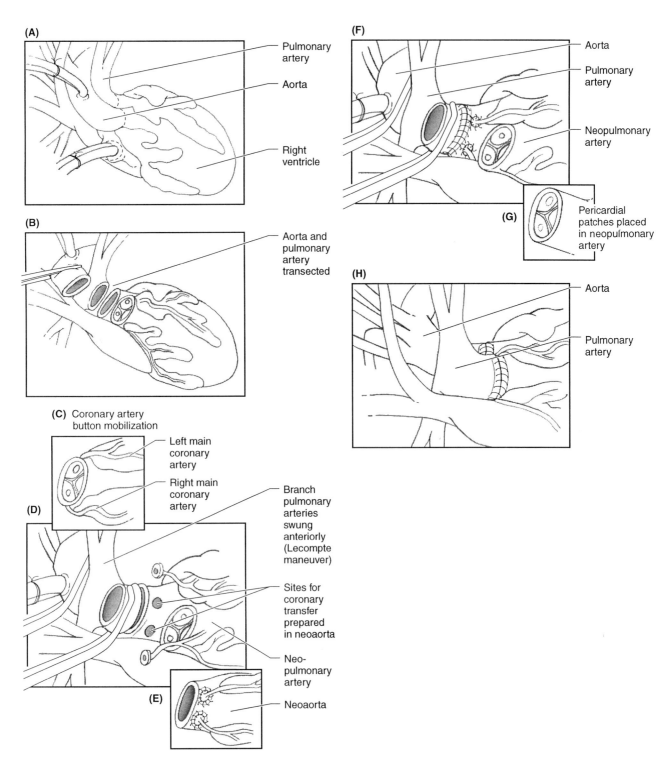

FIGURE 9–2.2. Jatene arterial switch operation. *(A)* Through a median sternotomy, cardiopulmonary bypass is established, and the ductus arteriosus is divided between ligatures. *(B)* The ascending aorta and pulmonary trunk are divided. *(C)* "Buttons" of the aortic root containing the left and right coronary artery ostia are excised. *(D)* The pulmonary artery bifurcation is swung anteriorly, beneath the distal aortic segment (Lecompte maneuver) and anastomosed to the neoaorta with a continuous 6-0 Prolene™ suture. *(E)* The coronary buttons are anastomosed to the "neoaorta" (former pulmonary trunk) using continuous 7-0 Prolene™ sutures. *(F)* The neoaorta is anastomosed to the distal aortic segment. *(G)* The defects in the "neopulmonary artery" (former aortic root) are repaired with autologous pericardium. *(H)* The distal pulmonary artery segment is anastomosed to the neopulmonary artery with a continuous 6-0 Prolene™ suture.

resulting defects in the neopulmonary artery are repaired with glutaraldehyde-treated autologous pericardium. The pulmonary artery bifurcation is swung anteriorly, beneath the distal ascending aorta/aortic arch (**Lecompte maneuver**). The distal aortic segment is anastomosed end-to-end to the neoaorta with a continuous 6-0 polydioxanone suture. The distal, bifurcated pulmonary artery segment is similarly anastomosed to the neopulmonary artery. Associated lesions such as a VSD (see Ventricular Septal Defect section in Chapter 8) and aortic arch anomalies (see Coarctation of the Aorta and Interrupted Aortic Arch sections in Chapter 7) are concomitantly repaired.

Perioperative mortality for arterial switch operations in experienced cardiac centers ranges between 2% and 5%. Mortality is most often due to ventricular failure secondary to imperfect coronary artery transfers to the neoaorta or right ventricular dysfunction in the setting of severe pulmonary vascular disease. The most common complication following arterial switch operations is supravalvar pulmonary artery stenosis. Excellent ventricular function is to be expected following arterial switches, and significant incompetence of the neoaortic valve has not been observed. Long-term survival rates have been estimated to be around 90%.

The **Rastelli procedure** is indicated for *D*-TGA/VSD with pulmonary stenosis or atresia. The procedure is performed as described previously (see Tetralogy of Fallot section above); however, the VSD patch serves as a baffle, directing the left ventricular outflow through the VSD (usually a perimembranous subaortic VSD) toward the aortic valve (Fig. 9–2.3). In a series of 117 patients with *D*-TGA/VSD and pulmonic stenosis who underwent the Rastelli opera-

tion at the Mayo Clinic, overall surgical mortality was 16%, with the best results in patients with "typical" VSDs located high in the perimembranous septum, in proximity to the subaortic area.[3] Causes of early hospital deaths included low cardiac output, myocardial infarction, and pulmonary hypertension. Causes of late deaths included sudden death, pulmonary hypertension, and left ventricular dysfunction. Ten- and 18-year survival rates were 61% and 58%, respectively. Reoperation rates after 5, 10, and 18 years were 31%, 70%, and 84%, respectively, with the most common cause being obstruction of the extracardiac conduit between the right ventricle and pulmonary arterial confluence.

The **Damus-Kaye-Stansel** procedure is indicated for patients with *D*-TGA/VSD with subaortic stenosis (Fig. 9–2.4). In this procedure, the left ventricular output

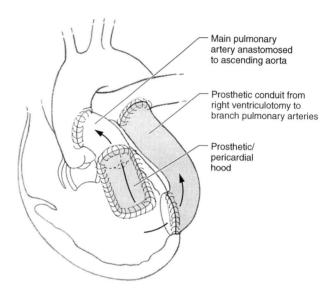

Main pulmonary artery anastomosed to ascending aorta

Prosthetic conduit from right ventriculotomy to branch pulmonary arteries

Prosthetic/ pericardial hood

FIGURE 9–2.4. The Damus-Kaye-Stansel procedure for *D*-TGA/VSD with subaortic stenosis. After cardiopulmonary bypass has been established, a vertical right ventriculotomy is created, and the VSD is closed with a Dacron™ patch as described (see Ventricular Septal Defect Section in Chapter 9. The main pulmonary trunk is then transected just proximal to the bifurcation, and a matching aortotomy is made in the adjacent ascending aorta. The proximal end of the transected pulmonary artery is anastomosed end to side to the aorta using a continuous 5-0 Prolene™ suture; a pericardial or prosthetic hood is usually interposed in this anastomosis to prevent distortion of the great arteries or semilunar valves. An aortic or pulmonary homograft (or prosthetic valved-conduit) is interposed between the distal pulmonary segment and the right ventriculotomy using 4-0 or 5-0 Prolene™ continuous sutures.

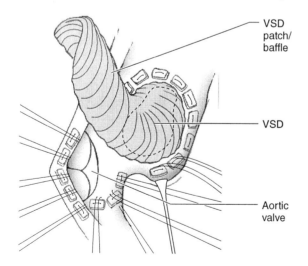

VSD patch/ baffle

VSD

Aortic valve

FIGURE 9–2.3. The Rastelli procedure for *(D*-TGA/VSD with pulmonary stenosis or atresia. The procedure is performed as previously described for ToF except that the Dacron™ patch placed over the VSD is fashioned as a baffle to direct the left ventricular outflow through the VSD and toward the aortic valve.

is directed to the aorta by way of the pulmonary outflow tract. Performed through a median sternotomy under cardiopulmonary bypass, a short vertical ventriculotomy is made in the midportion of the free wall of the right ventricle. The ventriculotomy is placed as close to the VSD as possible, avoiding the major right ventricular branches of the right coronary artery; stay stitches are placed at the ventriculotomy edges to expose the VSD adequately. The VSD is then closed with a Dacron™ patch as described previously (see Ventricular Septal Defect section in Chapter 9). The main pulmonary artery is transected about 5 mm proximal to its bifurcation, and a matching aortotomy is made in the adjacent ascending aorta. The proximal end of the transected pulmonary artery is anastomosed to the aorta in an end-to-side fashion using a continuous 5-0 Prolene™ suture; a pericardial or prosthetic (Dacron™, GoreTex™) hood is usually incorporated into this anastomosis to avoid distortion of the great arteries or semilunar valves. Finally, an aortic or pulmonary homograft (or valved prosthetic conduit) is anastomosed to the distal end of the transected pulmonary artery in an end-to-end fashion with a continuous 7-0 polydioxanone continuous suture line. The proximal end of the conduit is then beveled and anastomosed to the right ventriculotomy in an end-to-side fashion using a continuous 4-0 or 5-0 Prolene™ suture line.

9.3 Congenitally Corrected Transposition of the Great Arteries (Fig. 9–3)

Incidence: Comprises less than 1% of congenital heart defects.

Pathophysiology: Combined AV and ventriculoarterial discordance resulting in "corrected" transposition of systemic and pulmonary circulations. There is a high incidence of associated intracardiac anomalies including VSD, pulmonary out-

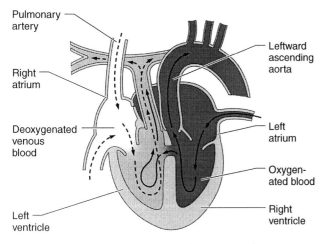

FIGURE 9–3.   Schematic drawing of congenitally corrected TGAs. (■)——▶, Oxygenated; (□)----▶, Deoxygenated; (▨)----▶, mixed.

flow tract obstruction, tricuspid insufficiency, and AV conduction anomalies.

Clinical Features: Isolated CC-TGA may remain asymptomatic for decades. Late sequelae include tricuspid insufficiency, AV block, and congestive heart failure. Earlier symptoms are related to associated congenital cardiac anomalies: cyanosis with VSD and pulmonic stenosis, or congestive heart failure with large VSDs. Likewise, electrocardiographic and radiographic findings correlate with associated cardiac defects. Echocardiography is diagnostic and identifies the associated defects.

Concepts of Correction: Corrective procedures correspond to the associated anomalies and include VSD closure, relief of pulmonary outflow tract obstruction, and tricuspid valve replacement. Recently, a "double-switch" approach, with combined atrial and arterial switch procedures, has been used with early success.

Corrective Operation(s):
- VSD repair
- left ventricle-to-pulmonary artery homograft conduit to relieve pulmonary outflow tract obstruction
- tricuspid valve replacement
- "double-switch" procedure (combined arterial and atrial switch)

General Considerations

Also referred to as *L*-TGA or *ventricular inversion,* congenitally corrected transposition of the great arteries (CC-TGA) is a rare congenital cardiac anomaly, constituting less than 1% of congenital cardiac disease. In this anomaly, systemic venous return entering the right atrium empties into a morphologic left ventricle through the mitral valve; the left ventricle delivers this blood into the pulmonary artery. Pulmonary venous return entering the left atrium empties into a morphologic right ventricle via the tricuspid valve; the right ventricle delivers blood into the aorta. The left ventricle and the mitral valve lie to the *right* of the right ventricle and tricuspid valve, hence the term "ventricular inversion." The aorta lies to the left and anterior to the pulmonary artery, as the *L*-TGA designation infers, in contrast to the more common form of *D*-TGA. Therefore, AV discordance is functionally corrected with concomitant transposition of the great arteries. The coronary circulation corresponds to the morphology of the ventricles as do the AV valves: the left-sided right ventricle is supplied by a morphologic right coronary artery, and the right-sided left ventricle is supplied by a morphologic left coronary artery system. The course of AV conduction bundle fibers is abnormal in CC-TGA: with respect to VSDs, the bundle of His courses along the anterosuperior and anteroinferior borders of the VSD on the anatomic left side of the septum instead of its usual course along the posteroinferior VSD margins.

Associated cardiac anomalies are present in most cases of CC-TGA and influence the clinical course of these patients. A VSD is present in 70% to 80% of patients with

CC-TGA. The VSD is usually perimembranous in location and lies behind the posterior leaflet of the right-sided mitral valve. **Valvar or subvalvar pulmonary stenosis** (45% to 60%) commonly occurs with CC-TGA. **Tricuspid insufficiency** is also common (30%) in these patients and is generally associated with an Ebstein's type of valve deformity. Furthermore, a variety of AV conduction abnormalities are observed in these patients with an increasing incidence of first-, second-, and third-degree AV block (up to 30%) and supraventricular tachycardia as they age.

Diagnostic Keys

Isolated CC-TGA without any associated defects may remain asymptomatic until the third or fourth decade of life. Complications at this late stage include tricuspid insufficiency (40%), spontaneous complete AV block (40%), or congestive heart failure due to a progressive deterioration of systemic right ventricular function. In most cases of CC-TGA, however, associated cardiac anomalies lead to symptoms during the first few months of life and determine the clinical course. Cyanosis is common with a VSD and pulmonic stenosis. Congestive heart failure is seen with large VSDs. A harsh holosystolic murmur detected along the left lower sternal border may indicate a VSD or tricuspid regurgitation. A systolic ejection murmur at the upper left sternal border may suggest pulmonic stenosis. Chest radiography reveals a characteristic anterior and leftward position of the aorta. Radiographic evidence of pulmonary overcirculation may be noted in patients with a VSD; pulmonary congestion may be seen in patients with tricuspid regurgitation. Varying patterns of AV conduction abnormalities may be observed with electrocardiography. Two-dimensional echocardiography is diagnostic and reliably identifies the anatomic features of CC-TGA as well as associated anomalies. Cardiac catheterization and angiography may be necessary to define pulmonary artery anatomy more clearly and to measure intracardiac pressures and pulmonary vascular resistance.

Operative Correction

Operative intervention in cases of CC-TGA is based on the associated defects. The timing of VSD closure is the same as for other patients; however, there is an increased incidence of complete AV block following VSD repair in these patients due to the anomalous course of the bundle of His. Typically perimembranous, the VSD is most frequently approached through the right atrium and right-sided mitral valve. A Dacron™ patch is secured over the VSD using pledgeted mattress sutures placed through the defect and placed within the left-sided right ventricular surface along its anterosuperior border to minimize the incidence of AV block. The remaining edges of the patch may be sutured to the right-sided left ventricular surface of the VSD. Alternatively, the VSD may be approached via the aortic valve annulus, if it is large enough. This approach permits placement of all repair sutures directly on the left-sided right ventricular surface circumscribing the VSD, avoiding the right-sided conduction bundles.

Relief of pulmonary outflow tract stenosis generally requires the placement of a homograft conduit between the morphologic left ventricle and the pulmonary artery since the posterior location of the outflow tract and its proximity to the conduction bundles predisposes to complete AV block with resection of subvalvar tissue and transannular patching. Significant tricuspid insufficiency in CC-TGA generally requires valve replacement.

Left-sided "right" ventricular failure occurs in some patients with CC-TGA as a result of long-term work against systemic vascular resistances. Aggressive afterload reduction may be beneficial, with cardiac transplantation reserved for medical failures. The use of the Jatene arterial switch operation in conjunction with an atrial switch procedure has been used with early success in selected patients with CC-TGA. This "double-switch" operation is appropriate for patients with nonobstructed ventriculoarterial connections and a robust right-sided "left" ventricle that has been conditioned by functioning at systemic pressures (usually from pulmonary outflow tract obstruction). This approach possesses several theoretical advantages including the use of the right-sided "left" ventricle to support the systemic circulation, minimizing the hemodynamic consequences of tricuspid valve insufficiency, and decreasing the incidence of iatrogenic AV block. Long-term results with this new approach are not yet available as experience is still accumulating.

The overall operative mortality for intracardiac repair in patients with CC-TGA is approximately 10% to 20%. The incidence of perioperative heart block is also 10% to 20%. Approximately 25% of these patients will require reoperation, usually for progressive left-sided tricuspid valve insufficiency.

9.4 Tricuspid Atresia (Fig. 9–4)

Incidence: Comprises 1% to 3% of congenital heart defects

Pathophysiology: Atretic tricuspid valve, hypoplastic right ventricle, ASD, and restricted pulmonary blood flow (70%) lead to right-to-left shunting and cyanosis. In patients with unrestricted pulmonary blood flow (30%), pulmonary overcirculation and congestive heart failure develop. Manifestations of left ventricular volume overload (e.g., ventricular dilation, mitral regurgitation, ventricular dysfunction) result from combined systemic and pulmonary venous return.

Clincial Features: Most patients are cyanotic, presenting with a harsh systolic ejection murmur at the left lower sternal border (VSD). The electrocardiogram reveals a characteristic notched P wave and evidence of left ventricular hypertrophy. The chest radiograph is variable but may display a "boot-shaped" or "egg-on-a-string" (*D*-TGA) cardiac silhouette; increased or diminished pulmonary vascularity is present depending on

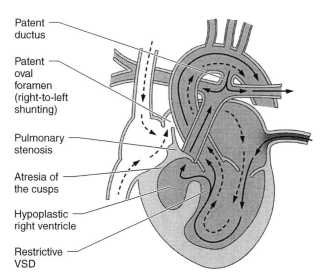

FIGURE 9–4. Schematic drawing of tricuspid atresia. (■)⟶, Oxygenated; (□)---⟶, Deoxygenated; (▨)---⟶, mixed.

Patent ductus
Patent oval foramen (right-to-left shunting)
Pulmonary stenosis
Atresia of the cusps
Hypoplastic right ventricle
Restrictive VSD

pulmonary blood flow. Two-dimensional echocardiography is diagnostic, revealing an atretic tricuspid valve, disparate ventricular sizes, and an ASD.

Concepts of Correction: Initial palliation consists of a Blalock-Taussig systemic-to-pulmonary artery shunt for cyanotic infants or pulmonary artery banding in infants with pulmonary overcirculation. This is generally followed by a bidirectional Glenn shunt at 12 to 18 months and then a modified Fontan operation performed at 2 to 4 years of age. The Fontan operation creates a total cavopulmonary connection, directing systemic venous return directly to the pulmonary artery.

Corrective Operation(s):

- Stage 1: Palliation by a Blalock-Taussig systemic-to-pulmonary artery shunt or pulmonary artery band
- Stage 2: Pre-Fontan operation, using a bidirectional Glenn shunt or hemi-Fontan operation
- Stage 3: Definitive correction, using a modified Fontan operation

General Considerations

Tricuspid atresia results from the development failure of the AV valve between the right atrium and right ventricle. It is the third most common form of cyanotic congenital heart disease after the tetralogy of Fallot and *D*-transposition of the great arteries and comprises 1% to 3% of congenital heart defects. Tricuspid atresia is classified into three types based on the relationship of the great vessels to the ventricles, otherwise known as *ventriculoarterial concordance*. The most common type, **type I** (60% to 80%), consists of normal ventriculoarterial concordance. **Type II** (15% to 25%) consists of *D*-transposition, and **type III** (3%) consists of *L*-transposition. These groups are further stratified into subgroups based on the degree of obstruction to pulmonary blood flow. Subtypes A, B, and C denote

(A) Tricuspid atresia with no transposition (69%–83%)

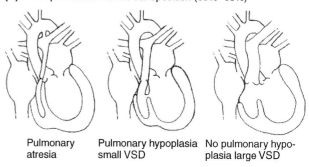

Pulmonary atresia | Pulmonary hypoplasia small VSD | No pulmonary hypoplasia large VSD

(B) Tricuspid atresia with *D*-transposition (17%–27%)

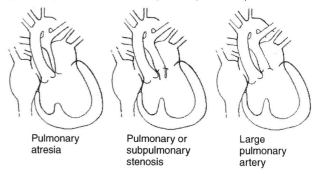

Pulmonary atresia | Pulmonary or subpulmonary stenosis | Large pulmonary artery

(C) Tricuspid atresia with *L*-transposition (3%)

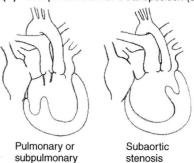

Pulmonary or subpulmonary stenosis | Subaortic stenosis

FIGURE 9–4.1. Anatomic classification of tricuspid atresia. *(A)* Type I, normal ventriculoarterial concordance. *(B).* Type II, *D*-transposition of the great arteries. *(C)* *L*-transposition of the great arteries. Subtypes A, B, and C denote pulmonary atresia, pulmonary stenosis, and no obstruction, respectively. (Reproduced with permission. Pearl JM et al.: Tricuspid atresia. In Baue AE et al. (eds): *Glenn's Cardiovascular and Thoracic Surgery*, 6/e. Stamford, Appleton & Lange, 1996, p. 1433.)

pulmonary atresia, pulmonary stenosis, and no obstruction, respectively (Fig. 9–4.1). Type IB tricuspid atresia, with normal ventriculoarterial concordance, pulmonary arterial hypoplasia, and a small, restrictive VSD, is the most common form, with an occurrence of about 65%. All forms of tricuspid atresia ASD and a **right-to-left shunt** across it, permitting egress of blood from the right atrium; the right atrium is usually dilated and hypertrophied. Also characteristic of tricuspid atresia is a markedly **hypoplastic right ventricle** and a **VSD** that usually communicates with the right ventricular outflow tract (infundibulum). Commonly, the VSD is restrictive and the infundibulum may be narrow, presenting varying degrees of obstruction to pulmonary flow. About 70% of patients with tricuspid atresia have **restricted pulmonary blood flow** resulting in **cyanosis.** In addition to a restrictive VSD and/or narrow infundibulum, this restriction to pulmonary blood flow may also stem from valvar pulmonary stenosis or atresia and pulmonary artery stenosis or hypoplasia. Neonates with pulmonary atresia and, hence, ductal-dependent pulmonary blood flow, develop severe cyanosis as the ductus arteriosus closes. Conversely, in patients with tricuspid atresia with *unobstructed* blood flow (30%), neither the VSD nor the right ventricular outflow tract is particularly restrictive, often resulting in pulmonary overcirculation. In these patients, cyanosis is mild or absent; however, they commonly develop pulmonary hypertension and, if left untreated, congestive heart failure.

The left atrium and ventricle are subject to chronic volume overload, since these chambers receive both systemic and pulmonary venous return. This condition leads to left ventricular dilation and hypertrophy, which, in turn, often leads to mitral insufficiency and a diminished ejection fraction. Obstruction to systemic blood flow in the forms of coarctation of the aorta, interrupted aortic arch, and subaortic stenosis are also commonly associated with tricuspid atresia.

Diagnostic Keys

Most patients with tricuspid atresia present with some degree of cyanosis. Patients with type I tricuspid atresia tend to become cyanotic in the first month of life and may have a history of **hypercyanotic spells.** Patients with type II tricuspid atresia are less cyanotic and present later in life with signs and symptoms of **congestive heart failure,** including dyspnea, recurrent respiratory infections, failure to thrive, and hepatomegaly. Cardiac auscultation reveals a harsh systolic ejection murmur at the left lower sternal border, which stems from flow across the VSD. Electrocardiography usually reveals a characteristic notched P wave and evidence of left ventricular hypertrophy. The cardiac silhouette on chest radiography is quite variable in tricuspid atresia; a "boot-shaped" heart (disparate ventricles, pulmonic hypoplasia) or "egg-on-a-string" (transposition of the great arteries) may be noted. Increased or decreased pulmonary vascularity may be observed, depending on the degree of pulmonary blood flow. Two-dimensional echocardiography with Doppler is often diagnostic, revealing the atretic tricuspid valve, disparate ventricular sizes (i.e., small right ventricle, large left ventricle), and ASD.

The relationship of the great arteries, VSD, PDA, and coarctation of the aorta, if present, can also be visualized. Although the diagnosis of tricuspid atresia can be made with echocardiography, cardiac catheterization and angiography are usually necessary in planning operative repair. Parameters that should be accurately assessed include pulmonary arterial and left ventricular pressures, shunt fractions, pulmonary vascular resistance, and pulmonary artery anatomy.

Operative Correction

The strategy of operative correction of tricuspid atresia is composed of (1) an early palliative procedure(s) that *establishes adequate pulmonary blood flow* and, if necessary, relieves systemic outflow obstruction and (2) a subsequent definitive procedure(s) that diverts systemic venous return directly to the pulmonary arteries. Infants with tricuspid atresia and a restrictive ASD usually undergo a **Rashkind procedure** (balloon atrial septostomy) as part of the initial cardiac catheterization to improve the right-to-left atrial shunt. Patients with obstruction to pulmonary blood flow and cyanosis require a modified **Blalock-Taussig shunt** (systemic-to-pulmonary artery) in the newborn period to augment pulmonary blood flow and ameliorate the cyanosis (see Pulmonary Atresia with Intact Ventricular Septum section in Chapter 7). Conversely, patients with unrestricted pulmonary blood flow, pulmonary overcirculation, and congestive heart failure may require **pulmonary artery banding** to reduce pulmonary blood flow, thereby treating the congestive heart failure and avoiding the development of subsequent irreversible pulmonary vascular occlusive disease. Pulmonary artery banding may be performed through a median sternotomy; cardiopulmonary bypass is not required (Fig. 9–4.2). After limited dissection between the main pulmonary artery and the aorta, a prosthetic band (e.g., Dacron™) is passed around and fixed to the main pulmonary artery, just proximal to its bifurcation. The circumference and "tightness" of the band is adjusted such that the distal pulmonary artery pressure is reduced to one-third of the systemic pressure with an arterial oxygen saturation ≤75%.

Subsequent to the initial palliative procedure(s), most patients with tricuspid atresia are tracked toward a definitive modified **Fontan procedure.** This tracking process usually begins with a palliative bidirectional **Glenn shunt** (superior vena cava (SVC)-to-pulmonary artery anastomosis), with takedown of the Blalock-Taussig shunt, if present, at 4 to 6 months of age. The Glenn shunt serves to provide reasonable pulmonary blood flow and relieves the volume overload on the left ventricle. This palliative procedure is particularly useful in young infants deemed to be at increased risk for a Fontan procedure or in those infants whose associated defects require correction before the Fontan repair. A bidirectional Glenn shunt is performed via a median sternotomy on cardiopulmonary bypass (Fig. 9–4.3).

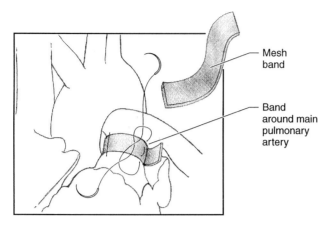

FIGURE 9–4.2. Pulmonary artery banding. After separating the ascending aorta and main pulmonary artery, a prosthetic band (e.g., Dacron™) is passed around and fixed to the main pulmonary artery, just proximal to the bifurcation. The circumference and "tightness" of the band are adjusted such that the distal pulmonary artery pressure is reduced to one-third of the systemic pressure with an arterial oxygen saturation ≤75%.

After any existing systemic-to-pulmonary artery shunts are taken down, the azygous vein is ligated and divided. The SVC is then divided, and its cranial end is anastomosed to the superior surface of the right pulmonary artery in an end-to-side fashion using a continuous 6-0 Prolene™ suture. The cardiac end of the SVC is oversewn, completing the procedure. An important variant of this procedure is the so-called **"hemi-Fontan" procedure,** in which both cranial and cardiac ends of the transected SVC are anastomosed to the superior and inferior surfaces of the right pulmonary artery, respectively, followed by patch occlusion of the SVC-right atrial orifice (Fig. 9–4.4). The hemi-Fontan procedure facilitates a subsequent completion Fontan operation, which would entail removal of the occluding patch and the placement of an intraatrial tunnel to divert the venous return from the inferior vena cava to the SVC-right atrial orifice. The overall operative mortality for the Glenn shunt is approximately 4% to 5%, and adequate palliation, with improved arterial oxygen saturations, may be sustained for 5 to 7 years. Over time, venous collaterals develop

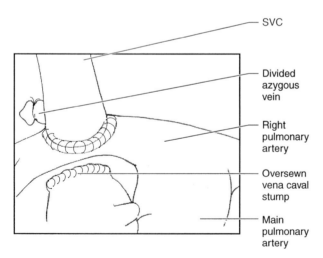

FIGURE 9–4.3. Bidirectional Glenn shunt. Through a median sternotomy, utilizing cardiopulmonary bypass, any prior systemic-to-pulmonary artery shunt is taken down, and the azygous vein is ligated and divided. The SVC is divided, and its cranial end is anastomosed end to side to the superior surface of the right pulmonary artery with a continuous 6-0 Prolene™ suture. The cardiac end of the SVC is oversewn.

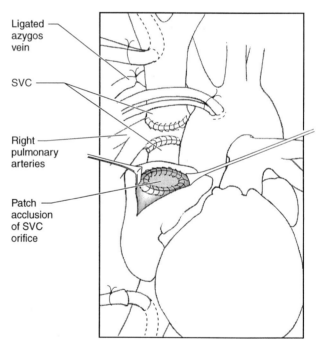

FIGURE 9–4.4. Hemi-Fontan procedure. Through a median sternotomy, utilizing cardiopulmonary bypass, a Glenn shunt is performed (see Fig. 10–4.3). In addition, the cardiac end of the transected SVC is anastomosed to the inferior surface of the right pulmonary artery. Through a right atriotomy, a GoreTex™ patch is sewn over the SVC-right atrial orifice with a continuous 6-0 Prolene™ suture.

between the SVC to the inferior vena cava (IVC), resulting in the reestablishment of right-to-left shunting and cyanosis to varying degrees.

The modified Fontan procedure, usually performed at approximately 2 to 4 years of age, is the definitive repair for patients with tricuspid atresia. The Fontan operation and its variants serve to direct systemic venous return to the pulmonary artery, bypassing the right ventricle. Optimal preconditions for a successful Fontan repair include a normal pulmonary vascular resistance and pulmonary artery pressures (mean pressure <15 mm Hg), adequate pulmonary artery caliber, and normal left ventricular function (ejection fraction >60%). Contraindications for this procedure include small or stenotic pulmonary arteries and an elevated pulmonary vascular resistance.

Originally described by Fontan in 1971,[4] the Fontan procedure has subsequently undergone many modifications. The modified Fontan procedure is performed via a median sternotomy using cardiopulmonary bypass (Fig. 9–4.5). After the azygous vein is ligated and divided, the SVC is transected, and its cranial and cardiac ends are anastomosed to the superior and inferior surfaces of the right pulmonary artery in an end-to-side fashion using running 6-0 Prolene™ sutures. Through a right atriotomy,

the atrial septum is excised within the borders of the limbus of the fossa ovalis. A "lateral tunnel" is then created that directs the venous return from the IVC orifice up to the SVC orifice. This baffle is fashioned from a GoreTex™ tube graft and is sutured to the lateral wall of the right atrium using a continuous 6-0 Prolene™ suture. The right atriotomy is closed, and separation from cardiopulmonary bypass is commenced. At Stanford, we prefer an extracardiac IVC-to-pulmonary artery connection instead of the intraatrial tunnel (Fig. 9–4.6). In this variation, the IVC is transected at its right atrial junction, and a GoreTex™ tube graft is interposed end to end between the IVC and the inferior surface of the right pulmonary artery. This operation, in conjunction with a previously performed bidirectional Glenn shunt, establishes a total cavopulmonary connection. In some cases, a "fenestration" or hole is created in the intraatrial tunnel, serving as a residual right-to-left atrial shunt. In the extracardiac technique, the fenestration takes the form of a small GoreTex™ tube graft interposed between the extracardiac conduit and the right atrial appendage. This option is useful in decompressing high systemic venous pressures in the setting of transient increases in pulmonary vascular resistance during the early postoperative period. Such fenestrations may be electively closed at

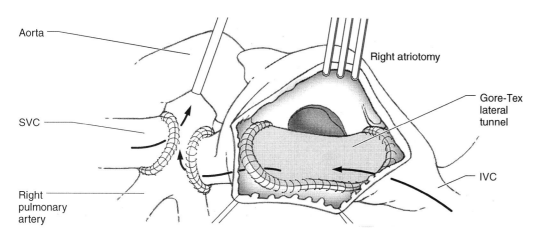

FIGURE 9–4.5. Modified Fontan procedure, lateral tunnel technique. The modified Fontan procedure is performed via a median sternotomy using cardiopulmonary bypass. After the azygous vein is ligated and divided, the SVC is transected, and its cranial and cardiac ends are anastomosed to the superior and inferior surfaces of the right pulmonary artery in an end-to-side fashion using running 6-0 Prolene™ sutures. Through a right atriotomy, the atrial septum is excised within the borders of the limbus of the fossa ovalis. A "lateral tunnel" is then created that directs the venous return from the IVC orifice up to the SVC orifice. This baffle is fashioned from a GoreTex™ tube graft and is sutured to the lateral wall of the right atrium using a continuous 6-0 Prolene™ suture.

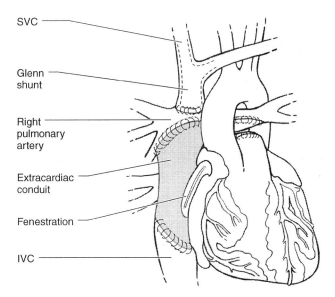

SVC

Glenn
shunt

Right
pulmonary
artery

Extracardiac
conduit

Fenestration

IVC

FIGURE 9–4.6. Modified Fontan procedure—Extracardiac technique. This modification of the Fontan procedure involves the interposition of an extracardiac GoreTex™ conduit between the IVC and the inferior surface of the right pulmonary artery. A previously constructed Glenn shunt is also illustrated. A fenestration placed between the conduit and the right atrial appendage serves to reduce systemic venous pressure in the early postoperative period.

a later date with a patch deployed by a transvenous catheter. Fenestration of the Fontan circuit may be used in high-risk patients but is generally not required in patients with tricuspid atresia and good left ventricular function.

The overall operative mortality through all stages leading to the Fontan operation is <10%. Low cardiac output and/or congestive heart failure are potential early postoperative complications, particularly in patients with long-standing cyanosis and left ventricular volume overload. Persistent pleural effusions are commonly seen after the Fontan procedure; however, their incidence has fallen significantly (10% to 15%) with the use of fenestrations.

In patients with *D*-transposition of the great arteries, a VSD, and subaortic stenosis, the Damus-Kaye-Stansel procedure (see *D*-Transposition of the Great Arteries section above) may be combined with the bidirectional Glenn shunt. In the Damus-Kaye-Stansel procedure, the main pulmonary artery is transected just proximal to its bifurcation. The proximal cut end of the main pulmonary artery is anastomosed end-to-side to the proximal ascending aorta, directing left ventricular blood to the aorta. The VSD is closed through a right ventriculotomy, and a valved conduit is placed between the right ventricle and the distal

pulmonary artery bifurcation, directing right ventricular blood to the pulmonary artery.

9.5 Total Anomalous Pulmonary Venous Connection (Fig. 9–5)

Incidence: Comprises 1% to 2% of congenital heart defects

Pathophysiology: Entire pulmonary venous return drains into the right atrium, usually via a common pulmonary vein confluence, resulting in complete pulmonary and systemic venous mixing. Oxygenated blood reaches the left heart via an interatrial connection (i.e., ASD, patent foramen ovale). Mechanical or functional obstruction of pulmonary venous return leads to cyanosis, pulmonary hypertension, and congestion.

Clinical Features: Neonates with obstructed TAPVC present with profound cyanosis and severe respiratory distress. Auscultation reveals a loud S2 (pulmonary hypertension). The electrocardiogram reveals right atrial enlargement and right ventricular hypertrophy. Chest radiograph reveals a normal cardiac silhouette with pulmonary edema. Infants with

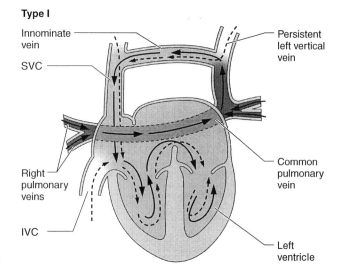

FIGURE 9–5. Schematic drawing of total anomalous pulmonary venous connection. (■)——▶, Oxygenated; (□)---▶, Deoxygenated; (▨)---▶, mixed.

unobstructed TAPVC usually present several months later with mild cyanosis, congestive heart failure, recurrent pulmonary infections, and failure to thrive. Auscultation reveals widely split, fixed S2, hyperactive precordium, and pulmonary outflow murmur. The electrocardiogram reveals right atrial enlargement and right ventricular hypertrophy. Chest radiograph reveals cardiomegaly and increased pulmonary vascularity. In both obstructed and unobstructed TAPVC, echocardiography is usually diagnostic, revealing a common pulmonary venous confluence without connection to the left atrium and an interatrial communication.

Concepts of Correction: The goal of operative repair is to redirect the entire pulmonary venous return to the left atrium.

Corrective Operation(s):

- *supra- and infracardiac TAPVC:* Direct anastomosis of the common pulmonary venous confluence to the left atrium, ASD patch closure, and ligation of persistent vertical vein
- *cardiac TAPVC:* Open coronary sinus into the left atrium and ASD patch (baffle) closure, directing coronary sinus and pulmonary venous return into the left atrium.

General Considerations

Total anomalous pulmonary venous connection (TAPVC) is a congenital cardiac anomaly in which the entire pulmonary venous return to the heart drains into the right atrium instead of the left atrium. TAPVC is a rare defect, comprising 1% to 2% of congenital cardiac defects. The classification of four forms of TAPVC, by Darling and associates,[5] is based on the anatomic connection of the pulmonary veins to the right atrium and includes **supracardiac** (45%), **cardiac** (25%), **infracardiac** (25%), and **mixed** (5%) patterns of venous drainage (Fig. 9–5.1). In most cases of TAPVC, the pulmonary venous return converges into a **common pulmonary vein confluence** located posterior to the left atrium. In the supracardiac configuration, the common pulmonary vein confluence drains into the right atrium via an ascending vertical vein leading into the left innominate vein or into the SVC. In the cardiac pattern, the common pulmonary vein connects to the coronary sinus or directly with the right atrium. In the infracardiac variety, the common pulmonary vein drains through the diaphragm into the portal vein or ductus venosus. The mixed type consists of combinations of the other three varieties of TAPVC.

The pathway of pulmonary venous return to the right atrium is **obstructed** or **unobstructed.** The obstruction may be *mechanical* (e.g., compression of the common pulmonary vein by local structures) or *functional* (e.g., inadequate pulmonary venous capacitance). The infracardiac type is most commonly obstructed, and the cardiac type is rarely obstructed. Since pulmonary blood flow empties into the right atrium, an **interatrial right-to-left shunt** (i.e., ASD, patent foramen ovale) is needed to maintain systemic output and, therefore, is necessary for survival. A PDA is also common with TAPVC. Since all pulmonary venous

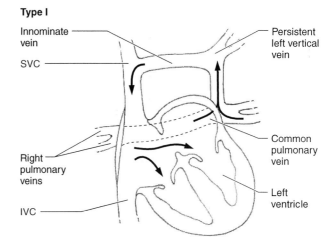

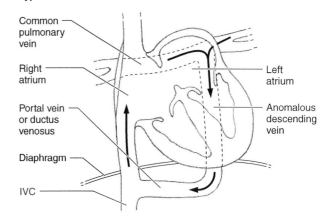

FIGURE 9–5.1. Types of total anomalous pulmonary venous connection. (*Top*) Supracardiac; the common pulmonary vein drains into the right atrium via an ascending left vertical vein, innominate vein, and SVC. (*Middle*) Cardiac; the common pulmonary vein connects directly to the coronary sinus. (*Bottom*) Infracardiac; the common pulmonary vein drains into the right atrium by way of a descending vertical vein, portal vein or ductus venosus, and IVC. (Reproduced with permission. Verrier ED: The heart: II. Congenital diseases. In Way LW: *Current Surgical Diagnosis and Treatment*, 10/e, Norwalk, Appleton & Lange, p. 398).

return is delivered to the right atrium, there is complete mixing of pulmonary and systemic venous blood within the right heart. The distribution of this mixed venous return to the left atrium and right ventricle depends on the size of the interatrial communication. If it is restrictive, minimal venous return will reach the left heart, resulting in decreased cardiac output and elevated right atrial pressures. In most cases of TAPVC, however, the interatrial communication is large and nonrestrictive, and the distribution of blood flow between the right and left hearts depends on the relative compliances of the ventricles and the relative pulmonary and systemic vascular resistances. As pulmonary vascular resistance decreases during the neonatal period, the ratio of pulmonary to systemic blood flow (Q_p/Q_s) increases and may reach values as high as 5:1. Left uncorrected, this pulmonary overcirculation leads to pulmonary hypertension.

When pulmonary venous return is obstructed (e.g., infracardiac type), a paucity of oxygenated blood reaches the left heart, and the patients become extremely cyanotic. Furthermore, elevated pulmonary venous pressures leads to pulmonary edema, pulmonary hypertension, and suprasystemic right ventricular pressures. In the absence of pulmonary venous obstruction (e.g., supracardiac and cardiac types), a large amount of oxygenated blood reaches the left heart, and minimal arterial desaturation is noted.

Diagnostic Keys

The clinical presentation of TAPVC depends on the presence and level of pulmonary venous obstruction. Neonates with obstructive TAPVC present in respiratory distress and profound cyanosis in the first few hours of life. Cardiac auscultation reveals a loud S2, consistent with pulmonary hypertension. Electrocardiographic criteria for right atrial enlargement and right ventricular hypertrophy are usually noted. Chest radiography usually reveals a normal cardiac silhouette; however, pulmonary edema is evident. Two-dimensional echocardiography is usually diagnostic, revealing a common pulmonary venous confluence without connection to the left atrium and the interatrial communication. Doppler reveals pulmonary venous flow patterns moving away from the heart as well as the site of venous obstruction. Cardiac catheterization may be detrimental in the critically ill acidotic neonate and should therefore be reserved for cases of the more complex mixed variety or when echocardiography is equivocal. Patients without significant pulmonary venous obstruction often present beyond the newborn period during the first few months of life with signs and symptoms of mild cyanosis, growth retardation, recurrent pulmonary infections, and congestive heart failure. Auscultation usually reveals a widely split and fixed S2, a hyperactive precordium, and a pulmonary outflow murmur at the upper left sternal border. Electrocardiography reveals right atrial enlargement and right ventricular hypertrophy. Chest radiography typically reveals cardiomegaly (primarily from right atrial and ventricular enlargement) and increased pulmonary vascularity. Again, as in cases with obstructed pulmonary venous return, two-dimensional echocardiography with Doppler is usually

diagnostic. The common pulmonary venous confluence without connection to the left atrium is characteristic. A dilated coronary sinus (cardiac type) or dilated left innominate vein and SVC (supracardiac type) may be visualized in addition to the interatrial communication. Cardiac catheterization may be indicated in these patients to define the anomalous venous connections better.

Operative Correction

All cases of TAPVC are treated with operative repair. Unlike most of the other congenital cardiac anomalies, there is no effective means of medical treatment for this condition, palliative or otherwise. The timing of the repair is related to the degree of obstruction to pulmonary venous return. Critically ill neonates with severely obstructed pulmonary venous return require emergency correction after they have been stabilized (i.e., intubation/ventilation, diuretics). Patients with unobstructed TAPVC should undergo elective repair soon after diagnosis (4 to 12 months of age) to diminish the adverse effects of cyanosis, pulmonary hypertension, and right heart volume overload.

The goal of operative repair is to redirect the entire pulmonary venous return to the left atrium. All repairs are performed through a median sternotomy, utilizing cardiopulmonary bypass. The technique used for repair of supra- and infracardiac TAPVC involves the direct anastomosis of the posteriorly located pulmonary venous confluence to the left atrium, ligation of the vertical vein (supracardiac), and autologous pericardial patch closure of the ASD (Fig. 9–5.2). For the supracardiac and infracardiac forms of TAPVC, a right atriotomy is created, exposing the interatrial septum. The foramen ovale is completely excised, exposing the posterior left atrial wall. Parallel incisions are then made in the common pulmonary vein and the left atrium, and a side-to-side anastomosis between these two structures is created using a running 6-0 or 7-0 Prolene™ or polydioxanone suture. Special attention must be paid to avoid narrowing this anastomosis; interrupted sutures may be helpful in this regard. The interatrial defect is closed with an autologous pericardial patch followed by closure of the right atriotomy and separation from cardiopulmonary bypass. For supracardiac TAPVC, the ascending vertical vein is ligated as it exits the pericardium or at its junction with the left innominate vein. For infracardiac TAPVC, the descending vertical vein is ligated at the level of the diaphragm.

The cardiac type of TAPVC is repaired by opening the coronary sinus into the left atrium followed by placement of an autologous pericardial patch placed over the ASD and the coronary sinus ostium in such a way as to baffle the pulmonary venous return into the left atrium (Fig. 9–5.3). The coronary sinus is accessed through a right atriotomy. The foramen ovale is excised, and the common wall of the coronary sinus and the left atrium is incised, permitting free

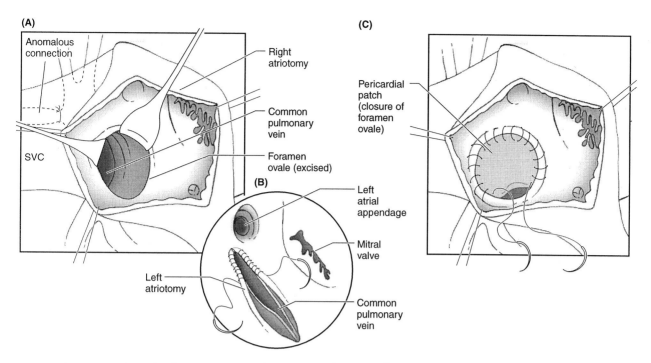

FIGURE 9–5.2. Surgical correction of supracardiac total anomalous pulmonary venous connection. *(A)* Once cardiopulmonary bypass has been established, a right atriotomy is created, exposing the interatrial septum. The foramen ovale is completely excised, exposing the posterior left atrial wall. *(B)* Parallel incisions are then made in the common pulmonary vein and the left atrium, and a side-to-side anastomosis between these two structures is created using a running 6-0 or 7-0 Prolene™ or polydioxanone suture. Special attention must be paid to avoid narrowing this anastomosis; interrupted sutures may be helpful in this regard. The ascending vertical vein is ligated as it exits the pericardium. *(C)* The interatrial defect is closed with an autologous pericardial patch followed by closure of the right atriotomy and separation from cardiopulmonary bypass. Operative correction of infracardiac total anomalous pulmonary venous connection is similar except that the descending vertical vein is ligated at the level of the diaphragm.

drainage of the coronary sinus (composed of pulmonary venous and coronary sinus blood) into the left atrium. An autologous pericardial patch is secured over the interatrial defects with a continuous 4-0 or 5-0 Prolene™ suture, taking care to avoid the AV node by taking the suture line within the coronary sinus orifice. The right atriotomy is then closed, followed by separation from cardiopulmonary bypass.

Placement of a transthoracic pulmonary artery catheter is frequently helpful for the postoperative management of patients with obstructed TAPVC since pulmonary artery pressures of systemic magnitude are not unusual in this subset of patients. Hyperventilation, sedation, and inhaled nitric oxide, as a pulmonary dilator, are generally effective in lowering pulmonary vascular resistance in the postoperative period.

The current overall operative mortality for TAPVC repair is under 10%. Preoperative acidosis, pulmonary venous obstruction, and the infracardiac type of TAPVC are negative prognostic factors. The most common cause of postoperative death is persistent pulmonary hypertension. The late development of pulmonary venous obstruction, usually within the first year following repair, occurs in 5% to 10% of patients and is associated with an extremely poor prognosis. The site of obstruction is at the anastomosis or within the pulmonary veins themselves. Long-term results are generally excellent after successful TAPVC repair.

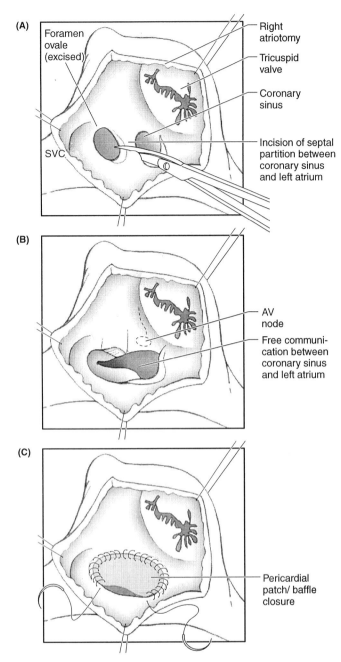

FIGURE 9–5.3. Surgical correction of cardiac total anomalous pulmonary venous connection. *(A)* Once cardiopulmonary bypass has been established, the coronary sinus is accessed through a right atriotomy, and the foramen ovale is excised. *(B)* The common wall of the coronary sinus and the left atrium is incised, permitting free drainage of the coronary sinus (composed of pulmonary venous and coronary sinus blood) into the left atrium. Care must be taken to avoid injury to the AV node. *(C)* An autologous pericardial patch is secured over

9.6 Truncus Arteriosus (Fig. 9–6)

Incidence: Comprises less than 1% of congenital heart defects

Pathophysiology: A single common artery, or truncus, overlying the ventricular septum and a nonrestrictive VSD gives rise to the coronary arteries, pulmonary arteries, and ascending aorta. Complete mixing of systemic and pulmonary venous return at the VSD and truncal valve levels results in moderate cyanosis. As the pulmonary vascular resistance decreases after birth, significant left-to-right shunting at the truncal level leads to excessive pulmonary blood flow, pulmonary hypertension, and congestive heart failure.

Clinical Features: Neonates with truncus defects usually present in congestive heart failure due to excessive pulmonary blood flow. Cyanosis develops due to pulmonary vascular occlusive disease. Flow across the VSD results in a systolic murmur along the left sternal border. The electrocardiogram reveals biventricular hypertrophy. Chest radiograph reveals cardiomegaly and increased pulmonary vascularity. Echocardiography is diagnostic, revealing the large truncus, an absent pulmonary valve, and a VSD.

Concepts of Correction: Early total correction is indicated, entailing the separation of the pulmonary trunk away from the main truncus, closing the VSD, and placing an extracardiac conduit between a right ventriculotomy and distal pulmonary artery trunk, reconstructing the right ventricular outflow tract.

Corrective Operation(s):

*   truncal repair
*   truncal repair with truncal valve replacement (truncal valve insufficiency)
*   truncal repair with ascending aortoplasty (associated interrupted aortic arch)

General Considerations

Truncus arteriosus is a rare cardiac anomaly in which a single large arterial trunk arises from the base of the heart, overrides the ventricular septum, and gives rise to the coronary arteries, pulmonary arteries, and the ascending aorta in varying configurations. At the origin of the artery in question is a single semilunar truncal valve comprising two to six cusps. The anomaly is thought to result from the developmental failure of the aorticopulmonary septum and subpulmonary infundibulum. This failure of septation almost always results in an associated nonrestrictive VSD. Four types of truncus configurations have been identified by the **Collett-Edwards classification** (Fig. 9–6.1). In **type I** truncus (60%), a single arterial trunk gives rise to the aorta

the interatrial defects with a continuous 4-0 or 5-0 Prolene™ suture, taking care to avoid the AV node by taking the suture line within the coronary sinus orifice. The right atriotomy is then closed, followed by separation from cardiopulmonary bypass.

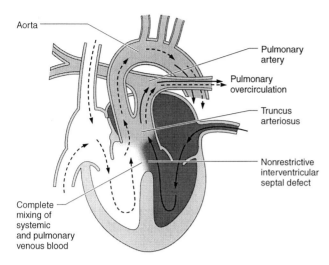

FIGURE 9–6. Schematic drawing of truncus arteriosus. (■)——▶, Oxygenated; (□)----▶, Deoxygenated; (▨)--▶, mixed.

and main pulmonary artery. **Type II** defects (20%) refer to those cases in which the pulmonary arteries arise separately from the posterolateral aspect of the truncus. In **type III** truncus (10%), the two pulmonary arteries also originate from the posterior aspect of the truncus, but their orifices are widely separated. In **type IV** truncus (10%), the pulmonary artery branches are absent, with pulmonary blood flow derived from aortopulmonary collaterals. Most clinical cases consist of type I or II defects or an intermediate variant. Associated cardiac anomalies are quite common with

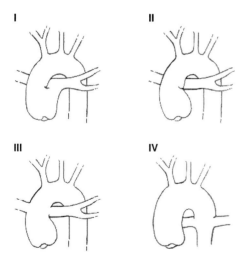

FIGURE 9–6.1. Collett and Edwards classification of truncus arteriosus. (Reproduced with permission. Hermanz-Schulman M, Fellows KE: Persistent truncus arteriosus: Pathologic, diagnostic and therapeutic considerations. Semin Roentgenol 20:121–129, 1985.)

truncus arteriosus. Of particular consequence are coronary artery (50%) and aortic arch anomalies (10% to 30%) including coarctation, interrupted aortic arch, and right aortic arch. DiGeorge syndrome is present in 30% of truncus patients.

Physiologically, complete mixing of systemic and pulmonary venous blood at the levels of the nonrestrictive VSD and single truncal valve results in moderate cyanosis, with arterial oxygen saturations ranging from 85% to 90%. The level of systemic oxygen saturation depends on the magnitude of pulmonary blood flow, which, in turn, is dependent on the pulmonary vascular resistance. During the first few days after birth, the relatively high pulmonary vascular resistance restricts pulmonary blood flow; hence cyanosis may be noted immediately after birth. As the pulmonary vascular resistance falls, the **left-to-right shunt** at the level of the great vessels increases significantly. Although this serves to increase pulmonary blood flow and reduce the cyanosis to some degree, it leads to pulmonary overcirculation, pulmonary hypertension, and congestive heart failure. Furthermore, dysfunction of the malformed truncal valve often proves to be detrimental. Truncal valve insufficiency leads to ventricular dilation and low diastolic coronary perfusion pressures, which may result in myocardial ischemia. Stenosis of the truncal valve predisposes to ventricular hypertrophy, increased myocardial oxygen consumption, and reduced coronary and systemic perfusion.

Left untreated, over 80% of infants born with truncus arteriosus die within the first year of life, primarily due to severe congestive heart failure. Those infants surviving beyond the first year usually develop the sequelae of pulmonary vascular obstructive disease, including Eisenmenger's syndrome, and die during the third and fourth decades of life.

Diagnostic Keys

Neonates with truncus defects typically present in varying degrees of congestive heart failure due to excessive pulmonary blood flow. Cyanosis becomes evident after the development of significant pulmonary vascular occlusive disease. Cardiac auscultation reveals a regurgitant systolic murmur along the left sternal border resulting from flow across the VSD. Electrocardiography often reveals right and left ventricular hypertrophy. Chest radiography reveals cardiomegaly, from biventricular and left atrial enlargement, and increased pulmonary vascularity. Two-dimensional echocardiography with Doppler is diagnostic, revealing the telltale truncus overriding the ventricular septum, an absent pulmonary valve, and VSD. Other important aspects can be identified, including the pulmonary artery anatomy and function of the truncal valve (i.e., stenosis or insufficiency). Cardiac catheterization with angiography is indicated in selected cases when further definition of the pulmonary artery anatomy, pulmonary vascular resistance, and aortic arch anatomy is required.

Operative Correction

All diagnosed cases of truncus arteriosus should undergo operative repair as early in life as possible, since about 50% of truncus patients managed medically with digitalis and diuretics die during the first month of life. Operative repair may be contraindicated in older patients with prohibitively high pulmonary vascular resistances. Complete repair consists of the separation of the pulmonary arteries from the main truncus and repair of the resultant defect in the aorta, VSD closure, and reconstruction of the right ventricular outflow tract using an extracardiac conduit.

Through a median sternotomy under cardiopulmonary bypass, the pulmonary arteries are excised from the main truncus, and the resultant aortic defect is closed with a pericardial patch (Fig. 8–6.2). A right vertical ventriculotomy is then performed, and the VSD is identified and closed with a Dacron™ or GoreTex™ patch (see Ventricular Septal Defect section in Chapter 9). A cryopreserved aortic or pulmonary homograft is then anastomosed between the right ventriculotomy and the distal pulmonary artery trunk with continuous 4-0 or 5-0 Prolene™ sutures, thereby directing right ventricular outflow into the pulmonary arteries. A pericardial hood is frequently used at the ventricular anastomosis to avoid anastomotic distortion. The patient is then weaned from cardiopulmonary bypass.

Several technical modifications to the basic repair are necessary in cases with associated anomalies. Significant truncal valve insufficiency usually necessitates valve replacement using a cryopreserved aortic or pulmonary homograft (Fig. 9–6.3). The ascending aorta is transected just

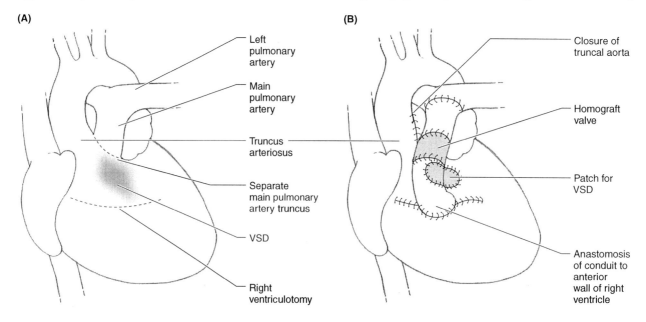

FIGURE 9–6.2.   Standard repair of truncus arteriosus. *(A)* Through a median sternotomy under cardiopulmonary bypass, the pulmonary arteries are excised from the main truncus, and the resultant aortic defect is closed; a pericardial patch may be required to close the defect to avoid excessive distortion of the truncal valve or coronary arteries. A right ventriculotomy is then performed, exposing the VSD. The VSD is identified and closed with a Dacron™ or GoreTex™ patch. *(B)* A cryopreserved aortic or pulmonary homograft is then anastomosed between the right ventriculotomy and the distal pulmonary artery trunk with continuous 4-0 or 5-0 sutures, thereby directing right ventricular outflow into the pulmonary arteries. A pericardial hood is frequently used at the ventricular anastomosis to avoid anastomotic distortion. (Reproduced with permission. Verrier ED: The heart: II. Congenital diseases. In Way LW: *Current Surgical Diagnosis and Treatment*, 10/e, Norwalk, Appleton & Lange, p. 399.)

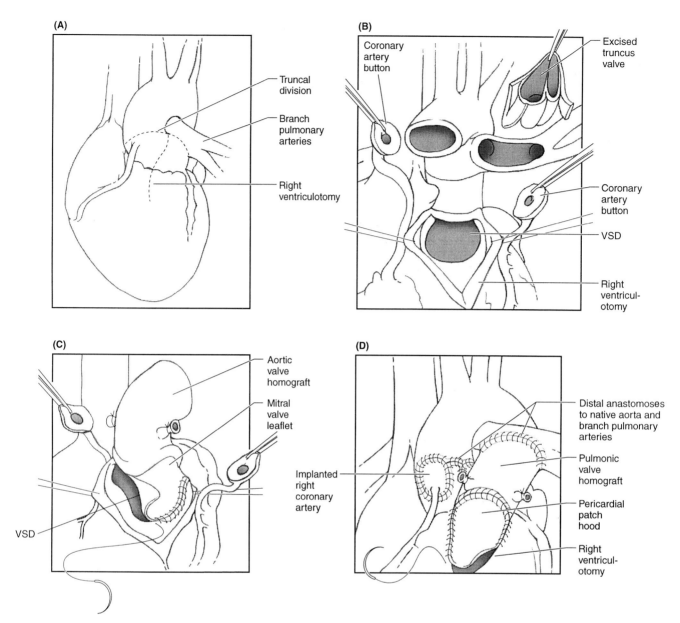

FIGURE 9–6.3. Repair of truncus arteriosus including truncal valve replacement. *(A, B)* The ascending aorta is transected just distal to the pulmonary artery origin, and the truncal valve is excised. The coronary arteries are excised from the truncal wall. *(C)* Through a right ventriculotomy, the proximal end of an aortic homograft is anastomosed end to end to the truncal valve annulus with a continuous 4-0 or 5-0 Prolene™ suture, using the anterior mitral leaflet to close the VSD. *(D)* The coronary ostia are then reimplanted to this homograft, and the distal end is anastomosed end to end to the ascending aorta with a continuous 4-0 or 5-0 Prolene™ suture. The right ventricular outflow tract is reconstructed between the right ventriculotomy and the pulmonary artery bifurcation, as previously described (see Fig. 9–6.2).

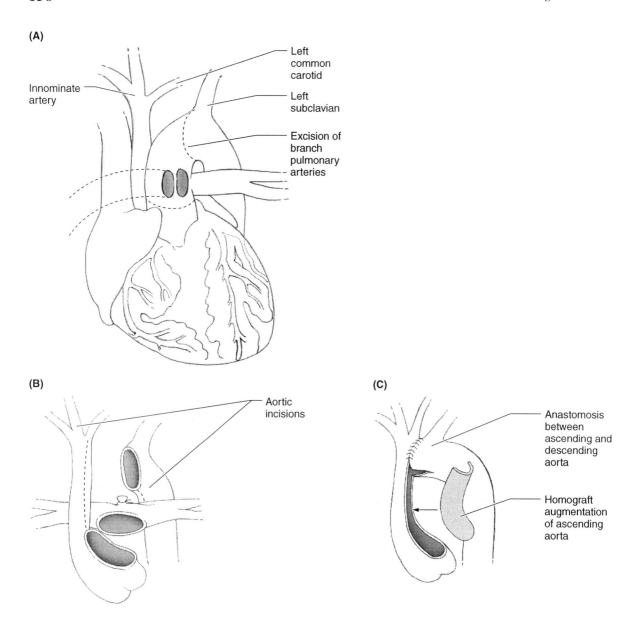

(A)

Innominate
artery

Left
common
carotid

Left
subclavian

Excision of
branch
pulmonary
arteries

(B)

Aortic
incisions

(C)

Anastomosis
between
ascending and
descending
aorta

Homograft
augmentation
of ascending
aorta

FIGURE 9–6.4.   Repair of truncus arteriosus with an associated
interrupted aortic arch. *(A, B)* The branch pulmonary arteries are
excised, and the ductus arteriosus is divided. The remainder of
the ascending aorta is then opened along its medial surface.
(C) A primary end-to-end anastomosis of the ascending and
descending aorta is performed using a continuous 4-0 or 5-0
Prolene™ suture. The remaining defect along the inferior aspect
of the aortic arch is repaired with an allograft. This serves to
augment the ascending aorta, eliminating any residual stenosis
between the truncal valve and the aortic arch anastomosis. The
right ventricular outflow tract is reconstructed with a valved
homograft as in Fig. 9–6.2.

distal to the pulmonary artery origin, and the truncal valve is excised. The coronary arteries are excised from the truncal wall. Through a right ventriculotomy, the proximal end of an aortic homograft is anastomosed end to end to the truncal valve annulus with a continuous 4-0 or 5-0 Prolene™ suture, using the anterior mitral leaflet to close the VSD. The coronary ostia are then reimplanted to this homograft, and the distal end is anastomosed end to end to the ascending aorta with a continuous 4-0 or 5-0 Prolene™ suture. The right ventricular outflow tract is reconstructed as described for the standard truncus repair.

In the event of an associated interrupted aortic arch, the branch pulmonary arteries are excised, and the ductus arteriosus is divided (Fig. 9–6.4). The remainder of the ascending aorta is opened along its medial surface, and a primary end-to-end anastomosis of the ascending and descending aorta is performed with a continuous 4-0 or 5-0 Prolene™ suture. The remaining defect along the inferior aspect of the aortic arch is repaired with an allograft. This serves to augment the ascending aorta, eliminating any residual stenosis between the truncal valve and the aortic arch anastomosis.

Early mortality following truncus repair ranges between 10% and 20% and is largely dependent on associated anatomic anomalies, pulmonary vascular resistance, and the preoperative condition of the infant. Patients undergoing early repair usually require reoperation for conduit replacement as the child grows.

References

1. FALLOT A. Contribution al'Anatomic pathologique de la Maladie Bleue (Cyanose Cardiaque). Marseille, Barlatier-Feissat, 1888.

2. KIRKLIN JW, BARRATT-BOYES BG. Ventricular septal defect and pulmonary stenosis or atresia. In: *Cardiac Surgery*. Churchill – Livingstone. New York, 1993, 2/e, p. 919.

3. PUGA FJ. The Rastelli procedure for transposition of the great vessels, pulmonary stenosis, and ventricular septal defect. In: *Glenn's Thoracic and Cardiovascular Surgery*. ed. Baue AE, et al. Appleton & Lange, Stamford, 6/e, p. 1384.

4. FONTAN F, BAUDET E. Surgical repair of tricospic atresia. *Thorax* 1971;26:240.

5. DARLING RC, ROTHNEY WB, CRAIG JM. Total pulmonary venous drainage into the right side of the heart. *Lab Invest* 1957;6:44.

CHAPTER 10

Miscellaneous Defects

David D. Yuh, MD, and Bruce A. Reitz, MD

Introduction

This section describes some of the rarer congenital cardiac defects that cannot be classified in the categories given in previous chapters.

10.1 Congenital Mitral Valve Disease (Fig. 10.1)

Incidence: Comprises less than <1% of congenital heart defects

Pathophysiology: Malformation of the mitral valve apparatus results in mitral stenosis, insufficiency, or both. Significant flow obstruction or regurgitation of the mitral valve results in elevated pulmonary venous pressures and pulmonary congestion. Left untreated, pulmonary vascular occlusive changes and pulmonary hypertension lead to right ventricular hypertrophy and right heart failure.

Clinical Features: Patients may present with signs and symptoms of pulmonary hypertension and congestion and congestive heart failure. Congenital mitral stenosis is associated with a right ventricular lift, prominent S2, and middiastolic flow murmur. Congenital mitral insufficiency results in an apical pansystolic murmur. The electrocardiogram reveals left atrial enlargement and right ventricular hypertrophy. Chest radiograph reveals cardiomegaly and signs of pulmonary venous hypertension. Echocardiography is diagnostic, defining abnormal mitral valve morphology.

Concepts of Correction: Valve repair is preferred to valve replacement in infants and children with congenital mitral valve disease (CMVD). Varied repair techniques have been described, depending on the particular lesion.

Corrective Operation(s):

- *mitral insufficiency:* Mitral annuloplasty, leaflet resection/plication, cleft repair, and chordal repair
- *mitral stenosis:* Supravalvar ring resection, commissurotomy, chordal fenestration, and papillary muscle splitting

General Considerations

CMVD comprises a spectrum of rare malformations of one or more components of the mitral valve apparatus including portions of the left atrial wall adjacent to the mitral annulus. These malformations generally result in congenital mitral valve **stenosis, incompetence**, or degrees of both. Congenital mitral stenosis is caused by narrowing at the level of the valve orifice (i.e., mitral annulus and leaflets) and/or levels above or below the valve (e.g., chordae tendinae, papillary muscles, supravalvar ring). Congenital mitral incompetence may be caused by prolapse or dysplasia (e.g., clefts, hypoplasia) of one or both of the valve leaflets as well as mitral annular dilation (e.g., cardiomyopathy). Significant flow obstruction or regurgitation of the mitral valve results in elevated pulmonary venous pressures and pulmonary congestion. Pulmonary vascular occlusive changes and pulmonary hypertension lead to right ventricular hypertrophy and right heart failure. CMVD is commonly associated with other cardiac anomalies including atrial septal defect (ASD), ventricular septal defect (VSD), aortic stenosis, and coarctation of the aorta.

Diagnostic Keys

The clinical signs and symptoms of isolated CMVD are identical to those present in acquired mitral valve disease, with the natural history dependent on the severity of mitral stenosis or incompetence and any coexisting lesions. Symptoms of pulmonary hypertension and congestive heart failure including dyspnea, orthopnea, paroxysmal noctural dyspnea, and recurrent pulmonary infections occur in 75% of patients with CMVD before 1 year of age. Physical signs of congenital mitral stenosis include a right ventricular lift and prominent S2, suggestive of pulmonary hypertension as well as a middiastolic flow murmur. Signs of congenital mitral insufficiency include an apical pansystolic

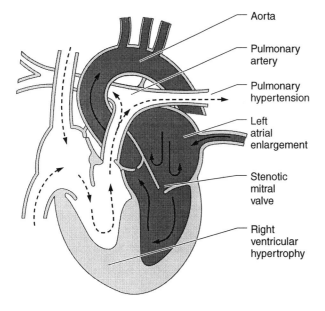

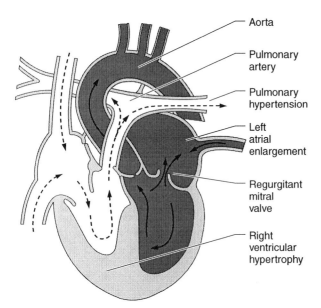

FIGURE **10–1.**   Schematic drawing of
CMVD. (■)———▶, Oxygenated; (□)----▶,
Deoxygenated; (▨)----▶, mixed.

murmur and laterally displaced left ventricular apical
impulse.

Isolated congenital mitral stenosis is usually severe and
presents in the first months to years of life. Isolated mitral incompetence usually presents somewhat later in life
with moderately severe symptoms. In both cases, symptoms and the need for correction come earlier when other
cardiac anomalies exist. Electrocardiographic evidence of
left atrial enlargement and right ventricular hypertrophy
is typically present with CMVD. Cardiomegaly, particularly left atrial enlargement, is the foremost radiographic
sign. Signs of pulmonary venous hypertension may also be

present. Two-dimensional echocardiography with Doppler
is usually diagnostic of CMVD, defining mitral annular size,
leaflet morphology, and chordae tendinae/papillary muscle
malformation. Transvalvar gradient and chamber pressure
magnitudes may also be estimated; associated anomalies are
also revealed. Cardiac catheterization and cineangiography
may be useful in defining equivocal or complex cases.

Operative Correction

Severe pulmonary venous hypertension refractory to medical management warrants early operation in patients with
CMVD, particularly when it is associated with signs and
symptoms of congestive heart failure. Approximately 40%
of patients diagnosed with congenital mitral stenosis have
obstruction severe enough to warrant surgical intervention;
most patients with untreated severe congenital mitral stenosis die within the first 5 years of life. Isolated mitral insufficiency often manifests later in childhood and is often managed medically, with surgery reserved for refractory cases.
Surgical techniques of repair and replacement for the many
types of CMVD closely resemble those used for acquired
valvular disease in adults. Valve repair is usually preferred
in the neonatal and pediatric populations, since valve replacement in these young patients requires placement of
a mechanical prosthesis; tissue valves are subject to rapid
deterioration in children.

Repairs for congenital mitral insufficiency are varied
and depend on the particular valvar malformation encountered. Operations are performed using a median sternotomy
and cardiopulmonary bypass. The mitral valve is usually
exposed through a right atriotomy and a vertical incision
in the interatrial septum. **Mitral annuloplasty** is indicated
for isolated annular dilation. In this procedure, the annular
diameter is reduced by plicating the annulus with one or
more heavy pledgeted sutures placed through the annulus
at the valve commissures. **Valve leaflet resection/plication**
is indicated to repair an incompetent leaflet that is unsup-
ported by chordae tendinae. In these procedures, the surface
area of the incompetent valve leaflet is reduced by partial
resection or imbricating using interrupted sutures. Leaflet
prolapse and incompetence due to chordal elongation can
be treated with **chordal shortening**. Cleft leaflets may be
repaired with interrupted sutures.

Repairs for congenital mitral stenosis, like those for
mitral insufficiency, are varied. Supravalvar rings may
be resected. **Commissurotomy** is indicated when the valve
commissures are absent or fused. Valve leaflets that are
excessively tethered by shortened chordae tendinae and/or
dysplastic papillary muscles, leading to valvar stenosis, may
be mobilized with **papillary muscle splitting**. Recently,
balloon dilation of congenitally stenotic mitral valves has
been employed with varying success rates.

Prosthetic valve replacement in infants may be required
for complex or severe CMVD. Supraannular insertion of

mitral prostheses is frequently required in infants and young children because of the small annulus diameter. In older childrens with annular diameters >20 mm, prosthetic mitral valve replacement is technically similar to the adult procedure. In all cases of mitral valve repair or replacement, the technical success of the repair should be assessed with intraoperative transesophageal echocardiography with Doppler.

Perioperative mortality for surgical treatment of CMVD is highly variable considering the wide spectrum of clinical presentations and valve anomalies. Satisfactory results can usually be achieved with valve repair when feasible. However, high early mortality frequently results from the technical difficulties associated with mitral valve replacement in children under 1 year of age. Many patients who undergo early correction of CMVD will require reoperation at some later point in life for valve replacement or correction of residual mitral valve incompetence.

10.2 Cor Triatriatum (Fig. 10.2)

General Considerations: Cor triatriatum comprises <1% of congenital heart defects

Pathophysiology: Persistence of a common pulmonary vein forms an "accessory" left atrial chamber that communicates with the "true" left atrium via a restrictive fibromuscular diaphragm. Pulmonary venous return is restricted, resulting in pulmonary venous congestion and hypertension, right ventricular hypertrophy, and congestive heart failure.

Clinical Features: Depending on the degree of pulmonary venous obstruction, patients may present in congestive heart failure in early infancy or later in life. The electrocardiogram reveals right ventricular hypertrophy. Chest radiograph reveals

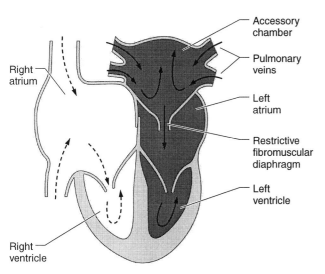

FIGURE 10–2. Schematic drawing of cor triatriatum. (■)——▶, Oxygenated; (□)---▶, Deoxygenated; (▦)==▶, mixed.

signs of right heart enlargement and pulmonary congestion. Echocardiography is diagnostic, demonstrating the accessory chamber and anomalous membrane.

Concepts of Correction: Operative correction entails complete excision of the restrictive membrane.

Corrective Operation(s):

• Excision of anomalous membrane

General Considerations

Cor triatriatum is an exceedingly rare congenital cardiac anomaly in which a persistent common pulmonary vein forms an "accessory" left atrial chamber that is separated from the "true" left atrium by a thick-walled fibromuscular diaphragm. Outflow from the common pulmonary venous chamber into the true left atrium consists of one or more small ostia in the diaphragm, which are generally restrictive. Pressure gradients between the venous sinus and the true left atrium may approach 20 to 25 mm Hg. The resultant obstruction to pulmonary venous return leads to severe pulmonary hypertension and congestion, right ventricular hypertrophy, and congestive heart failure. There are three basic anatomic configurations of cor triatriatum, based on the communication of the accessory chamber with the right atrium (Fig. 10–2.1): (1) intact atrial septum with no communication between the pulmonary venous chamber and the right atrium (65%), (2) ASD above the obstructing membrane with communication of the accessory chamber with the right and left atria, and (3) ASD below the obstructing membrane.

The size of the ostia draining the accessory chamber into the true left atrium determines the degree of pulmonary venous obstruction and clinical course of patients with cor triatriatum. If the aperture(s) is small and severely restrictive, as in about 75% of patients born with classical cor triatriatum, the newborn infant becomes critically ill during the first few months of life and, without surgical treatment, dies at an early age. Conversely, if the communication is larger and less restrictive, or if the accessory chamber communicates with the right atrium through an ASD, the patient presents later in childhood or young adulthood with a clinical picture resembling mitral stenosis. An ASD between the accessory chamber and the right atrium imposes a **significant left-to-right shunt**; this serves to exacerbate pulmonary congestion and to decrease left ventricular preload and systemic cardiac output. An ASD between the right atrium and the low-pressure true left atrium results in **right-to-left shunting** and varying degrees of cyanosis.

Cor triatriatum is commonly associated with other anomalies; isolated cor triatriatum occurs in only 30% of cases. The most common associated cardiac anomalies include patent ductus arteriosus (PDA), partial anomalous pulmonary venous connection, unroofed coronary sinus with left superior vena cava, VSD, coarctation of the aorta, and tetralogy of Fallot.

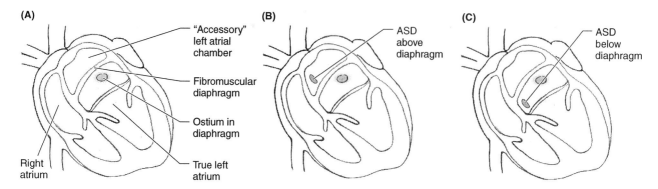

FIGURE 10–2.1. Three basic anatomic variations of cor triatriatum. The three configurations of cor triatriatum are based on the communication of the accessory chamber with the *right* atrium. *(A)* Intact atrial septum with no communication between the pulmonary venous chamber and the right atrium. *(B)* ASD above the fibromuscular diaphragm with communication of the accessory chamber with the right and left atria. *(C)* ASD below the obstructing membrane.

Diagnostic Keys

Infants with restrictive cor triatriatum typically present in a low cardiac output state with pallor, tachypnea, poor peripheral perfusion, and failure to thrive. If a significant left-to-right shunt exists, signs and symptoms of pulmonary congestion may also be present. Varying degrees of cyanosis may be associated with right-to-left shunting. Children and young adults with cor triatriatum who present later in life typically display the signs and symptoms of pulmonary venous hypertension and right heart failure. Electrocardiography may show evidence of right ventricular hypertrophy. Chest radiography displays evidence of pulmonary venous congestion and right-sided cardiac enlargement. Two-dimensional echocardiography is diagnostic, with demonstration of the bipartite left atrium and obstructing membrane. Careful assessment of the drainage of all four pulmonary veins into the accessory chamber is mandatory. Identification of an ASD or other anomalies is also reliably achieved with echocardiography.

Operative Correction

Surgical correction of restrictive cor triatriatum is indicated in the first year of life. Through a median sternotomy under cardiopulmonary bypass, a right atriotomy is made, and an incision is made in the interatrial septum through the foramen ovale (Fig. 10–2.2). The partitioning diaphragm between the pulmonary venous sinus and the true left atrium is identified, exposed, and completely excised back to the wall of the atrial septum. Complete excision of the anomalous membrane is tantamount to a successful operation. The atrial septum is then reconstructed with a GoreTex™ or autologous pericardial patch. Alternatively, a left atrial

approach is possible, particularly in older children. In this approach, a left atriotomy is made posterior to the atrioventricular groove. The anomalous membrane is exposed by retracting the interatrial septum anteriorly and is excised completely. If present, the ASD is closed in the standard fashion.

Mortality after surgical correction of isolated cor triatriatum is extremely low, except when the infant is critically ill prior to repair. When associated with other anomalies, operative mortality is related to the severity of these anomalies. The life expectancy after repair, especially when performed in infancy, approaches that of the general population.

10.3 Aortopulmonary Window (Fig. 10.3)

Incidence: Comprises <0.5% of congenital heart defects

Pathophysiology: A large, nonrestrictive communication exists between the proximal ascending aorta and the main pulmonary artery, resulting in a high-flow arterial-level left-to-right shunt. This condition leads to pulmonary overcirculation, rapidly progressive congestive heart failure, and pulmonary hypertension.

Clinical Features: Infants usually present with signs and symptoms of congestive heart failure early in life. Those few patients who survive past infancy rapidly develop Eisenmenger's syndrome. Physical examination reveals a systolic flow murmur and wide pulse pressures. The electrocardiogram reveals left and right ventricular hypertrophy as well as left atrial enlargement due to augmented pulmonary flow. Chest radiograph reveals cardiomegaly as well as signs of pulmonary congestion. Echocardiography is usually diagnostic, demonstrating the aortopulmonary (AP) window position and degree of shunting.

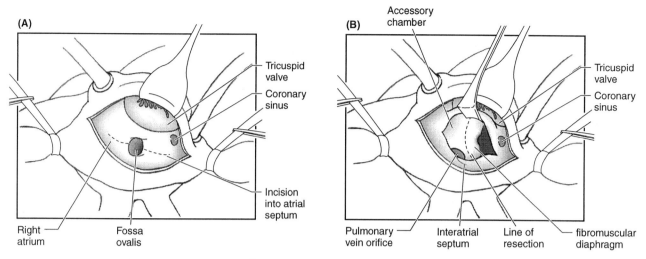

FIGURE 10–2.2. Operative repair of cor triatriatum. *(A)* Through a median sternotomy under cardiopulmonary bypass, a right atriotomy is performed, and in incision is made in the interatrial septum through the fossa ovalis. *(B)* The partitioning diaphragm between the pulmonary venous sinus and the true left atrium is identified, exposed, and completely excised back to the wall of the atrial septum. Complete excision of the anomalous membrane is tantamount to a successful operation. The atrial septum is then reconstructed with a GoreTex™ or autologous pericardial patch.

Concepts of Correction: Early closure is indicated in all patients with AP window except cases of advanced pulmonary hypertension.

Corrective Operation(s):

• Primary AP window closure

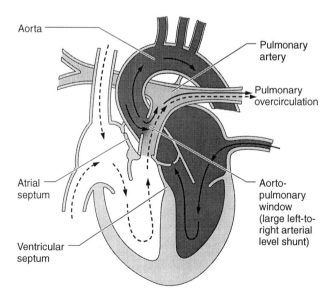

FIGURE 10–3. Schematic drawing of AP window. (■)——➤, Oxygenated; (□)---➤, Deoxygenated; (▨)--➤, mixed.

• AP window closure with a Dacron™ or autologous pericardial patch.

Pathophysiology

AP window represents a rare congenital anomaly in which a large communication exists between the proximal ascending aorta and the main pulmonary artery. This defect arises from incomplete separation of the aorta and pulmonary arteries during embryologic conotruncal development. There are three major morphologic types of AP window (Fig. 10–3.1): In type I, the defect is located between the left posterolateral wall of the proximal ascending aorta and the anterolateral wall of the main pulmonary trunk. In type II, the defect is located between the posterolateral aspect of the ascending aorta and the origin of the right pulmonary artery. In type III, the origin of the right pulmonary artery arises anomalously from the ascending aorta. Physiologically, this defect results in a high-flow arterial-level **left-to-right shunt** leading to pulmonary overcirculation and rapidly progressive congestive heart failure after birth, as the pulmonary vascular resistance falls. Moreover, left uncorrected, the augmented pulmonary artery flow may lead to the rapid development of pulmonary vascular occlusive disease. Most of the shunts in AP window are large and nonrestrictive to blood flow; hence there is no tendency for spontaneous closure of this defect. Left untreated, many

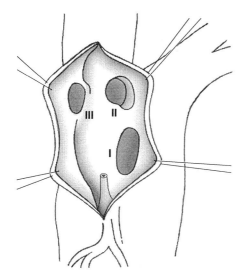

FIGURE 10–3.1.   Three major morphologic types of AP window. *Type I:* The defect is located between the left posterolateral wall of the proximal ascending aorta and the anterolateral wall of the main pulmonary trunk. *Type II:* The defect is located between the posterolateral aspect of the ascending aorta and the origin of the right pulmonary artery. *Type III:* The origin of the right pulmonary artery arises anomalously from the ascending aorta. (Reproduced with permission. Haas G: Patent ductus arteriosus and aortopulmonary window. In Baue AE et al. (eds): *Glenn's Cardiovascular and Thoracic Surgery,* 6th ed. Stamford, Appleton & Lange, 1996, p. 1153.)

infants expire from severe congestive heart failure. Eisenmenger's syndrome develops rapidly in the few infants who survive past the early postnatal period. Smaller, restrictive shunts result in less severe congestive symptoms. From 30% to 50% of patients with AP window have coexisting cardiac anomalies including VSD, tetralogy of Fallot, subaortic stenosis, ASD, right aortic arch, and PDA. Palliative medical management consists of digoxin and diuretics for congestive failure, with mechanical ventilation and inotropic support reserved for the critically ill infant.

Diagnostic Keys

AP window is a highly lethal defect, and its clinical presentation is often dramatic. Infants with isolated AP window typically present early in life with signs and symptoms of severe congestive heart failure including tachypnea, failure to thrive, and recurrent respiratory infections. Physical examination reveals a systolic flow murmur of varying intensity accompanied by wide pulse pressures. Findings on electrocardiography and chest radiography typically indicate left and right ventricular hypertrophy as well as left atrial enlargement due to pulmonary overcirculation; prominent pulmonary vascularity is also present. Two-dimensional echocardiography with Doppler is usually sufficient for diagnosis, demonstrating the position of the AP window and the extent of blood flow across it. Cardiac catheterization with angiography is usually not required for diagnosis, but it may be useful in cases of advanced pulmonary vascular disease, pulmonary hypertension, and associated cardiac defects.

Operative Correction

AP windows in symptomatic infants should be closed early after the diagnosis is made, preferably before 3 months of age. Since congestive heart failure and pulmonary vascular changes are usually severe with this anomaly, corrective surgery is recommended for all patients with AP window except in advanced cases with very high pulmonary vascular resistances. Through a median sternotomy, employing cardiopulmonary bypass, the defect may be accessed through a transverse arteriotomy made in the aorta or the main pulmonary artery (Fig. 10–3.2). The aortic root, including the aortic valve cusps and coronary artery ostia, should be inspected, since anomalies of these structures are associated with AP window. Small windows may be closed primarily with sutures alone, whereas larger defects may be patched from within the aorta using a Dacron patch or autologous pericardium. The arteriotomy is then closed, and the patient is weaned from cardiopulmonary bypass.

Mortality after early AP window repair is exceedingly low, with an excellent long-term prognosis. Repairs performed later in life are often subject to the effects of severe pulmonary vascular occlusive disease.

10.4 Aneurysm of the Sinus of Valsalva (Fig. 10.4)

Incidence: Comprises <1% of congenital cardiac defects

Pathophysiology: Thinning of the aortic medial layer in the wall of a sinus of Valsalva results in an aneurysmal dilation, which may extend and rupture into a corresponding cardiac chamber, forming an aortocardiac fistula. Aneurysms usually arise from the right coronary sinus and extend into the right ventricle or right atrium. Aneurysmal rupture into the right heart results in a large left-to-right shunt, which, in turn, can lead to congestive heart failure. Unruptured aneurysms extending into the right heart may cause tricuspid valve stenosis/incompetence, right ventricular outflow tract obstruction, or complete heart block.

Clinical Features: Aneurysms of the sinus of Valsalva are usually asymptomatic prior to rupture. Rupture results in a sudden

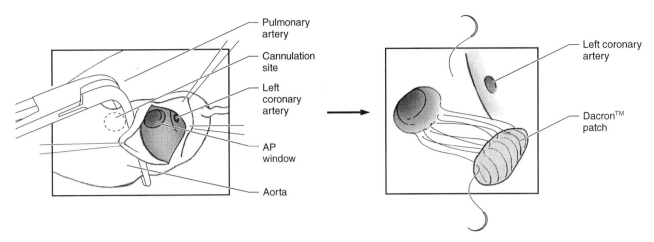

FIGURE 10–3.2. Operative repair of type I AP window. Through a median sternotomy, employing cardiopulmonary bypass, the defect may be accessed through a transverse arteriotomy made in the aorta or the main pulmonary artery. The aortic root, including the aortic valve cusps and coronary artery ostia, should be inspected, since anomalies of these structures are associated with AP window. Small windows may be closed primarily with sutures alone, and larger defects may be patched from within the aorta using a Dacron™ patch or autologous pericardium.

onset of chest pain, dyspnea, and palpitations or more gradual signs and symptoms of congestive heart failure. A parasternal continuous murmur is characteristic. Electrocardiography and chest radiography often reveal left or biventricular hypertrophy and signs of pulmonary congestion. Echocardiography is diagnostic, revealing the aneurysmal origin. Cardiac catheterization with angiography pinpoints the aneurysmal origin, involved cardiac chambers, degree of left-to-right shunting, and associated defects (i.e., VSD, coarctation of the aorta, aortic valve prolapse).

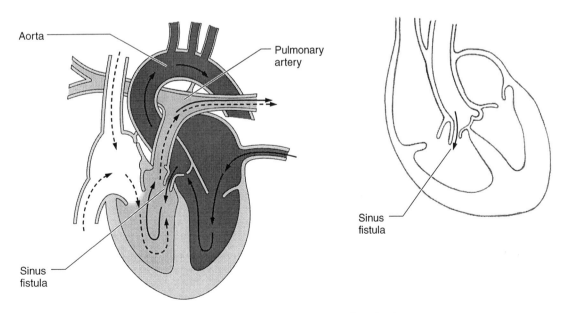

FIGURE 10–4. Schematic drawing of the sinus of Valsalva. (■)———▶, Oxygenated; (□)---▶, Deoxygenated; (▨)---▶, mixed.

Concepts of Correction: Operative correction entails excision of the aneurysmal sac back to its aortic origin and patch closure of the defect

Corrective Operations(s):

• aneurysmorrhaphy

General Considerations

Aneurysms arising from the sinus of Valsalva are caused by a thinning of the aortic media layer in the sinus wall. Aneurysms arising from the right coronary sinus are the most common (67%) and usually extend and rupture into the right ventricle or right atrium. The noncoronary sinus is involved less frequently (25%) and usually ruptures into the right atrium. Aneurysms arising from the left coronary sinus are infrequent (8%); they generally rupture into the left atrium. Morphologically, these aneurysms resemble a windsock, with a wide base at the aortic origin and tapered tip extending into the chamber in which they may rupture. Physiologically, aneurysmal rupture into the right heart creates an aortocardiac fistula and large **left-to-right shunt,** which, over time, may lead to congestive heart failure, often complicated by bacterial endocarditis. Unruptured aneurysms of a sinus of Valsalva extending into the right heart may cause tricuspid stenosis/incompetence, right ventricular outflow tract obstruction, or complete heart block. This lesion is commonly associated with other cardiac defects, particularly ventricular septal defect (usually of the perimembranous type), coarctation of the aorta, and aortic valve prolapse.

Diagnostic Keys

There are usually no physical manifestations of this anomaly prior to rupture unless the aneurysm distorts the aortic leaflets to such an extent that aortic insufficiency results. Once rupture occurs, on average between the second and fourth decades of life, about one-third of afflicted patients experience a sudden onset of chest pain followed by dyspnea and palpitations. A characteristic parasternal continuous murmur, often associated with a thrill, is also found. In nearly one-half of these patients, however, aneurysmal rupture is associated with a more gradual onset of symptoms. Over the ensuing weeks and months after rupture, cardiac failure progresses, becoming intolerable within 1 to 2 years. Electrocardiography and chest radiography reveal cardiac hypertrophy and pulmonary congestion. Two-dimensional echocardiography with Doppler, particularly transesophageal echocardiography, is usually diagnostic. Catheterization and cineangiography, specifically retrograde aortic root angiography, are useful in localizing the aneurysm's site of origin, identifying the cardiac chamber involved, estimating the degree of left-to-right shunting, and defining any associated cardiac defects.

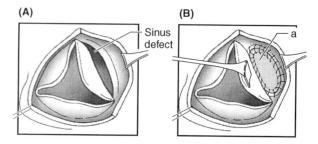

FIGURE 10–4.1. Operative repair of sinus of Valsalva aneurysm (right coronary sinus). *(A)* Through a median sternotomy and utilizing cardiopulmonary bypass, a transverse aortotomy is made just above the sinuses of Valsalva. The base of the aneurysm is exposed by retracting the aortic valve cusps. The aneurysm is withdrawn into the aorta from the chamber into which it extends and is excised across its base. *(B)* The resultant aortic defect is closed with a Dacron™ patch anchored with 4-0 Prolene™ sutures; direct suture closure of the defect may result in valve leaflet distortion and aortic insufficiency.

Operative Correction

Surgical correction of a ruptured sinus aneurysm should be performed promptly and involves closure of the defect in the sinus of Valsalva and repair of any associated lesions. Through a median sternotomy and utilizing cardiopulmonary bypass, a transverse aortotomy is made just above the sinuses of Valsalva (Fig. 10–4.1). The base of the aneurysm is exposed by retracting the aortic valve cusps. The aneurysm is withdrawn into the aorta from the chamber into which it extends and is excised across its base. The resultant aortic defect is closed with a Dacron™ patch anchored with 4-0 Prolene™ sutures; direct suture closure of the defect may result in valve leaflet distortion and aortic insufficiency. After this repair has been completed, along with repair of any associated defects, the aortotomy is closed, and the patient is weaned from cardiopulmonary bypass. Postoperative mortality after surgical repair of this anomaly is very low. Results and long-term prognosis after repair are generally excellent.

10.5 Double-Inlet Ventricle (Fig. 10.5)

Incidence: Comprises 2% to 3% of congenital heart defects

Pathophysiology: A single functional ventricle receives both systemic and pulmonary venous return via right- and left-sided atrioventricular valves or a single common valve, resulting in mixing of oxygenated and deoxygenated blood and, hence,

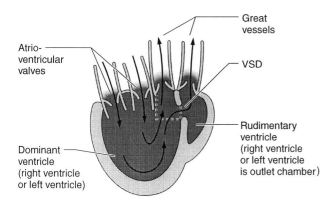

FIGURE 10–5. Schematic drawing of DIV.

TABLE 10–5.1. Anatomical Varinants of Double Inlet Ventricle

- Double inlet left ventricle w/left-sided rudimentary right ventricle & discordant ventriculoarterial connections
- Double inlet left ventricle w/right-sided rudimentary right ventricle & discordant ventriculoarterial connections
- Double inlet left ventricle w/right-sided rudimentary right ventricle & concordant ventriculoarterial connections
- Double inlet & double outlet left ventricle
- Double inlet and double outlet right ventricle
- Double inlet right ventricle w/left-sided rudimentary left ventricle & concordant ventriculoarterial connections
- Double inlet & double outlet from a solitary ventricle of indeterminate morphology

systemic arterial hypoxemia. This defect is also associated with excessive or inadequate pulmonary blood flow, depending on whether there is obstruction to pulmonary flow (e.g., pulmonary stenosis/atresia).

Clinical Features: The clinical presentation varies with alterations in pulmonary blood flow. Infants with increased pulmonary blood flow are not severely cyanotic but display signs and symptoms of pulmonary hypertension and congestive heart failure by early or mid-childhood. Infants with diminished pulmonary blood flow present with significant cyanosis during the early days or weeks of life. Electrocardiography and chest radiography typically reveal signs of pulmonary overcirculation and congestive heart failure. Echocardiography is diagnostic; a hallmark sign is the absence of an interventricular septum at the ventricular inlet.

Concepts of Correction: Initially, palliative procedures are performed to treat excessive or inadequate pulmonary blood flow and/or subaortic obstruction. These include pulmonary artery banding, systemic arterial/venous-to-pulmonary artery shunts (i.e., modified Blalock-Taussig, central, and modified Glenn shunts), resective widening of the left ventricular outflow tract, and the Damus-Kaye-Stansel procedure. Definitive surgical correction is effected by a Fontan-type operation.

Corrective Operation(s):

- *excessive pulmonary blood flow:* pulmonary artery banding
- *inadequate pulmonary blood flow:* modified Blalock-Taussig or central shunt (high PVR), modified Glenn shunt (normal PVR)
- *subaortic obstruction:* resection of the ventricular outflow tract muscle or Damus-Kaye-Stansel procedure
- *definitive repair—Fontan* operation.

Pathophysiology

Double-inlet ventricle (DIV) is a very rare congenital cardiac anomaly in which two separate atrioventricular valves or a single common atrioventricular valve empty into a single functional ventricle; the other ventricle is rudimentary and hypoplastic and communicates with the dominant chamber via a VSD. The atrioventricular valves are frequently morphologically indeterminate, neither mitral nor tricuspid, and are referred to as "left-sided" or "right-sided" corresponding to the atria they drain. DIV presents in several forms with variation in the types of functioning and hypoplastic ventricles (right or left), malformations of the atrioventricular valves, and ventriculoarterial connections (i.e., condordant/discordant, single-outlet/double-outlet) (Table 10–5.1). The most common anatomic pattern is double-inlet left ventricle with a left-sided rudimentary right ventricle and discordant ventriculoarterial connection. In this pattern, both atria (i.e., both systemic and pulmonary venous return) drain into a dominant right-sided "left ventricle," which, in turn, empties into the pulmonary artery. The left ventricle communicates with a rudimentary left-sided "right ventricle" via the bulboventricular foramen (VSD), from which the aorta arises. At least 30% of cases of DIV are associated with other cardiac anomalies including atrioventricular valve malformations (i.e., stenosis, insufficiency), pulmonary valve stenosis/atresia, coarctation of the aorta/interrupted aortic arch, and subaortic stenosis. Subvalvar pulmonary stenosis is particularly common; it results from infundibular narrowing or a restrictive VSD leading to an outflow chamber from which the pulmonary trunk arises. The two most common physiologic manifestations of this syndrome are (1) **cyanosis** from the mixing of oxygenated and deoxygenated blood prior to ejection into the aorta and (2) **excessive pulmonary blood flow,** resulting in pulmonary hypertension and congestive heart failure. The overall 1- and 5-year survival of untreated patients with DIV has been estimated to be 57% and 45%, respectively. Poor prognostic indicators include severe acidosis and low cardiac output on presentation, as well as systemic outflow obstruction.

It is also important to note that the morphology of the atrioventricular node and conduction system is abnormal in DIV; the atrioventricular node can lie anywhere around the perimeter of the right-sided atrioventricular valve.

Diagnostic Keys

The clinical presentation of DIV varies with the perturbations of pulmonary blood flow. Infants with increased pulmonary blood flow are not severely cyanotic, but suffer the sequelae of pulmonary hypertension and congestive heart failure by early or mid-childhood. Conversely, infants with decreased pulmonary blood flow secondary to pulmonary stenosis or atresia suffer from significant cyanosis during the early days or weeks of life. Electrocardiography and chest radiography reveal signs of pulmonary overcirculation and congestive heart failure. Two-dimensional echocardiography is diagnostic for DIV, with a hallmark sign being the absence of the interventricular septum at the inlet, between the atrioventricular valves. Cardiac catheterization and cineangiography are not essential for diagnosis, but they may add useful information including the pressure gradients across the ventricular outlets and systemic and pulmonary arterial anatomy.

Operative Correction

Most patients with DIV morphology are tracked toward a Fontan-type procedure (see Tricuspid Atresia section in Chapter 9). Initially, however, these patients may require a palliative procedure to treat one of three conditions: (1) excessive pulmonary blood flow, (2) inadequate pulmonary blood flow, or (3) subaortic obstruction. Patients with unrestricted pulmonary blood flow may require **pulmonary artery banding** (see Tricuspid Atresia section in Chapter 10) to attenuate pulmonary blood flow and prevent the development and sequelae of pulmonary hypertension (e.g., ventricular failure). Patients with inadequate pulmonary blood flow (e.g., pulmonary valvar stenosis/atresia, subvalvar pulmonary stenosis) and cyanosis may require a systemic-to-pulmonary artery shunt to augment blood flow to the lungs. This shunt may be in the form of a **modified Blalock-Taussig shunt** (subclavian artery-to-pulmonary artery; see Pulmonary Atresia with Intact Ventricular Septum section in Chapter 7), a central (GoreTex)™ **shunt**, or a **modified Glenn shunt** (bidirectional cavopulmonary anastomosis; see Tricuspid Atresia section in Chapter 9). A systemic arterial-to-pulmonary artery shunt (i.e., modified Blalock-Taussig or central shunt) is generally preferred for patients with an elevated pulmonary vascular resistance. For patients in whom pulmonary vascular resistance is not elevated, a systemic venous-to-pulmonary artery shunt (i.e., modified Glenn shunt) is preferred for several reasons: (1) since the modified Glenn shunt augments pulmonary blood flow at lower pressures than arterial shunts, pulmonary overcirculation and subsequent pulmonary vascular occlusive disease is avoided; and (2) systemic ventricular volume loading is reduced.

Subaortic obstruction develops in most patients with double-inlet left ventricle with discordant ventriculoarterial connection, resulting from restriction of the bulboventricular foramen. This condition can be treated with **resection** of obstructive ventricular outflow tract muscle (see Left Ventricular Outflow Tract Obstruction section in Chapter 7) or the **Damus-Kaye-Stansel procedure** (see *D*-Transposition of the Great Arteries section in Chapter 9) and modified Glenn shunt. In the Damus-Kaye-Stansel procedure, the main pulmonary artery is transected just proximal to its bifurcation. The proximal cut end of the main pulmonary artery is anastomosed end to side to the proximal ascending aorta, directing left ventricular blood to the aorta. The VSD is closed through a right ventriculotomy, and a valved conduit is placed between the right ventricle and the distal pulmonary artery bifurcation, directing right ventricular blood to the pulmonary artery.

Modifications of the Fontan procedure are now considered the definitive procedures of choice for most cases of DIV. The optimal age for repair is generally considered to be between 2 and 4 years of age. Optimal conditions for a successful Fontan repair include a normal pulmonary vascular resistance and pulmonary artery pressures (mean pulmonary artery pressure <15 mm Hg), adequate pulmonary artery caliber, and normal left ventricular function (ejection fraction >60%). Contraindications for this procedure include small or stenotic pulmonary arteries and an elevated pulmonary vascular resistance. Patients with high pulmonary vascular resistances and/or diminished ventricular function may require preliminary procedures including a modified Glenn shunt, atrioventricular valve repair/replacement, pulmonary artery reconstruction, and/or a Damus-Kaye-Stansel procedure, to optimize conditions for a successful, definitive Fontan procedure. The Fontan operation and its variants serve to direct systemic venous return to the pulmonary artery, bypassing the right ventricle. At Stanford, we prefer an extracardiac inferior vena cava-to-pulmonary artery connection. In this variation, the inferior vena cava is transected at its right atrial junction, and a GoreTex™ tube graft is interposed end to end between the inferior vena cava and the inferior surface of the right pulmonary artery. This operation, in conjunction with a previously performed bidirectional Glenn shunt, establishes a total cavopulmonary connection.

The results of the Fontan operation for DIV are similar to those achieved when this operation is performed for other congenital anomalies (i.e., tricuspid atresia). Operative mortality is reported to be less than 10%, with the primary preoperative risk factors being pulmonary vascular resistance and ventricular function. Ten-year survival rates have been reported to range between 60% and 80%. Satisfactory long-term results have been achieved, especially for patients who have a morphologic left ventricle as the

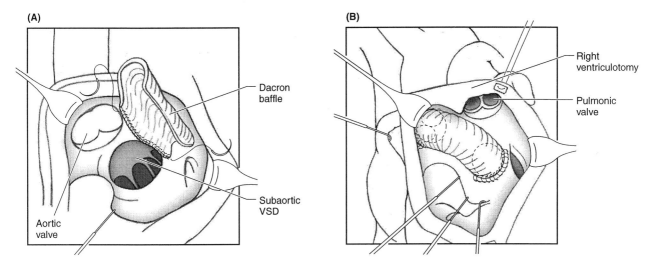

FIGURE 10–6.2.   Intraventricular tunnel repair of DORV with subaortic VSD. *(A)* The right ventricular chamber is accessed through a transverse ventriculotomy under cardiopulmonary bypass. *(B)* A tunnel tailored from a Dacron™ tube graft is placed between the subaortic VSD and the subaortic infundibulum using a continuous 4-0 or 5-0 Prolene™ suture line. The ventriculotomy should be closed with an autologous pericardial patch using a continuous Prolene™ suture, to avoid any narrowing of the right ventricular outflow tract.

relationships, coronary artery anatomy, VSD anatomy, and hemodynamic measurements.

Operative Correction

The variability of DORV configurations has resulted in variegated approaches to operative correction. Early palliative operations are performed for significant cyanosis or congestive heart failure and most commonly consist of a **systemic-to-pulmonary artery shunt** and **pulmonary artery banding**, respectively. Other palliative interventions may be appropriate for associated cardiac anomalies (e.g., patent ductus arteriosus, coarctation of the aorta). Although these palliative procedures are often very effective, early definitive correction for all types of DORV is now preferred to avoid the development of long-term complications.

In general, simple DORV with a subaortic VSD and without pulmonary stenosis should be repaired as early as possible and before 6 months of age to avoid the complications stemming from chronic pulmonary overcirculation. This form of DORV is corrected with an **intraventricular tunnel repair** whereby a tunnel is created within the right ventricle that conducts left ventricular blood emerging from the VSD directly to the aorta. The right ventricular outflow tract passes around this baffle. In this operation, the right ventricular chamber is accessed through a transverse ventriculotomy under cardiopulmonary bypass. Once the anatomy has been defined, a tunnel tailored from a Dacron™ tube graft is placed between the VSD and the subaortic infundibulum using a continuous 4-0 or 5-0 Prolene™ suture line (Fig. 10–6.2). The intraventricular tunnel may cause obstruction of the right ventricular outflow tract, necessitating augmentation of the right ventricular outflow tract with a right ventricular outflow patch or extracardiac right-ventricle-to-pulmonary artery conduit (see Pulmonary Stenosis with Intact Ventricular Septum section in Chapter 7 and Truncus Arteriosus section in Chapter 9). Regardless, the ventriculotomy should be closed with an autologous pericardial patch using a continuous Prolene™ suture to avoid any narrowing of the right ventricular outflow tract.

The indications for repair of DORV with a subaortic VSD and significant pulmonary stenosis resemble those for the tetralogy of Fallot; the repair may be deferred until 6 months to 2 years of age or until significant symptoms develop. The repair can be effected in a manner similar to that for tetralogy of Fallot (see Tetralogy of Fallot section in Chapter 9), substituting construction of an intraventricular tunnel for the VSD repair.

As with DORV with a subaortic VSD, DORV with a subpulmonic VSD (Taussig-Bing anomaly) can also be

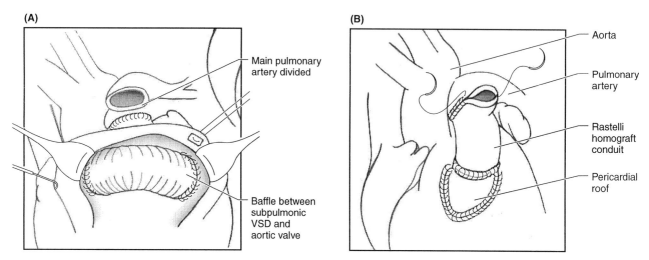

FIGURE 10–6.3. Intraventricular tunnel/Rastelli repair for DORV with a subpulmonic ventricular septal defect (Taussig-Bing anomaly). *(A)* An intraventricular tunnel between the subpulmonic VSD and the aortic infundibulum is created *(B)* If the tunnel lies across the pulmonary valve, a Rastelli procedure can be concomitantly performed whereby the main pulmonary artery is divided, oversewn proximally, and placed in continuity with the right ventriculotomy using a pulmonary or aortic homograft. An autologous pericardial hood is used to augment the ventricular anastomosis.

corrected using the intraventricular tunnel approach. In some cases, however, the pulmonic and tricuspid valves are in such close proximity that the intraventricular tunnel lies across the pulmonary valve, potentially obstructing the right ventricular outflow tract (Fig. 10–6.3). In this situation, a **Rastelli procedure** can be concomitantly performed whereby the main pulmonary artery is divided, oversewn proximally, and placed in continuity with the right ventriculotomy using a pulmonary or aortic homograft (see *D*-Transposition of the Great Arteries section in Chapter 9). Other alternative approaches to correction (in the absence of left ventricular outflow tract obstruction) include the **Jatene arterial switch operation** and VSD closure (see *D*-Transposition of the Great Arteries section in Chapter 9) and **reparation a l'étage ventriculare.** In the latter repair, the main pulmonary trunk is translocated (Lecompte maneuver) and anastomosed directly to the right ventriculotomy. DORV with a doubly committed VSD is corrected with an intraventricular tunnel repair. Surgical correction of DORV with a noncommitted VSD has been varied; however, the best results appear to be associated with an intraventricular tunnel repair combined with right ventricular outflow tract augmentation.

Morbidity and mortality associated with DORV correction vary with the clinical scenario and anatomic complexity; however, the overall operative risk ranges between 5%

and 10%, with variable long-term prognoses. Early deaths are generally due to low cardiac output and right ventricular failure. Morbidity consists of arrhythmias, recurrent VSD, aortic insufficiency, and conduit failure.

10.7 Anomalies of the Coronary Arteries (Fig. 10.7)

Incidence: Comprise <1% of congenital cardiac defects

Pathophysiology: The anomalous origin of the left coronary artery on the main pulmonary artery (ALCAPA) leads to reversal of left coronary arterial flow. This anomalous circuit results in coronary steal, myocardial ischemia, left ventricular dysfunction, and congestive heart failure. Coronary arteriovenous fistulae (CAVF) between the left or right coronary arteries and the right heart chambers or pulmonary artery also create a coronary steal phenomenon and myocardial ischemia.

Clinical Features: Signs and symptoms are often mild to absent in infancy but may include those of congestive heart failure and angina. Flow murmur (CAVF) may occasionally be detected. Electrocardiography may reveal signs of myocardial ischemia and left ventricular hypertrophy (ALCAPA). Chest radiograph may reveal signs of congestive heart failure (i.e., cardiomegaly, increased pulmonary vascularity). Cardiac catheterization with angiography is diagnostic, revealing abnormal coronary blood flow/fistulae and is necessary for planning surgical correction.

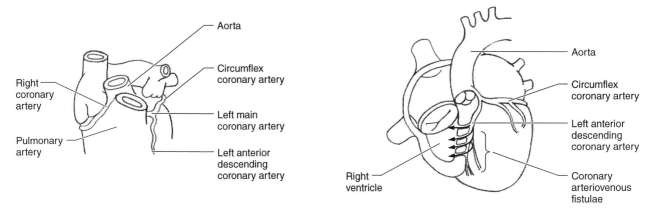

FIGURE 10–7. Schematic drawing of the coronary arteries.

Concept of Correction: For ALCAPA, correction involves the construction of a two-coronary system by establishing direct continuity between the left coronary ostium and the ascending aorta. For CAVF, operative correction is based on coronary fistula ligation.

Corrective Operation(s):

ALCAPA

- Coronary reimplantation
- Takeuchi procedure

CAVF

- Coronary fistula ligation (external or transcardiac chamber approach)
- Coronary artery aneurysmorraphy

General Considerations

Anomalous Left Coronary Artery from the Pulmonary Artery ALCAPA is a rare congenital cardiac defect in which the left main coronary ostium originates from the proximal main pulmonary artery or, less frequently, from the proximal right main pulmonary artery. The branching pattern of the left coronary artery remains normal, and the right coronary artery ostia is located in its normal aortic position. In utero, the PDA results in similar aortic and pulmonary artery pressures, allowing satisfactory antegrade perfusion of the anomalous left coronary artery. However, as the ductus closes and as the pulmonary vascular resistance and pulmonary artery pressure fall after birth, left coronary artery perfusion pressure declines. The right coronary arterial flow then predominates at normal aortic pressures and supplies blood to the entire myocardium and intracoronary collaterals, which, in turn, feed the left coronary artery. Consequently blood flow in the left coronary artery reverses and drains into the pulmonary artery. This anomalous coronary circuit results in a significant coronary steal, leading to myocardial ischemia, left ventricular dilatation, and congestive heart failure in infancy. Functional mitral regurgitation often results from left ventricular dilation and papillary muscle dysfunction.

Coronary Arteriovenous Fistula CAVF is a rare congenital anomaly defined as the presence of one or more communication(s) between a coronary artery and the lumen of any one of the four cardiac chambers, coronary sinus and tributaries thereof, superior vena cava, pulmonary artery, or pulmonary veins. Most commonly, however, isolated CAVFs from either the left or right coronary arteries terminate in the right heart chambers or pulmonary artery. Such fistulae lead to myocardial ischemia by creating a coronary steal and imposing an additional volume load on the left ventricle.

Diagnostic Keys

Anomalous Left Coronary Artery from the Pulmonary Artery Since relatively high postnatal pulmonary artery pressures limit left coronary artery runoff, myocardial ischemia and symptoms thereof are limited and are rarely severe enough to warrant intervention before 2 months of age. Symptoms, however, may be recognized within 1 to 2 weeks of birth. These symptoms include circumoral pallor and cyanosis, poor feeding, sweating, dyspnea, tachycardia, and discomfort, many of which probably stem from angina. When symptoms do not present in infancy, clinical evidence of congestive heart failure and ischemia may not become obvious until 20 years of age. Physical examination commonly reveals a precordial lift in association with gross cardiomegaly. Signs of congestive heart failure including hepatomegaly and pulmonary rales may also be present. As one would expect, the electrocardiogram frequently is suggestive of this diagnosis, with signs consistent with anterolateral infarction and left ventricular hypertrophy; cardiac enzymes may also be elevated. Chest radiography reveals cardiomegaly and interstitial pulmonary edema. Echocardiography usually shows a dilated, hypokinetic left ventricle. Definitive diagnosis, however, requires cardiac catheterization and cineangiography to demonstrate the anomalous left coronary ostium and retrograde left coronary artery blood flow.

Coronary Arteriovenous Fistula   Signs and symptoms stemming from CAVF depend on the volume of flow through the fistula and are usually absent to mild in the infant. Most patients are diagnosed and treated late in life after 20 years of age. In fact, detection of this anomaly often results from a continuous murmur found on routine physical examination or mild signs of cardiomegaly and pulmonary congestion on chest films. Symptoms are generally nonspecific and include effort dyspnea and fatigue and congestive heart failure signs; angina and myocardial infarction are rare. Electrocardiography is often normal but may occasionally suggest right or left ventricular overload depending on the fistula runoff. Chest radiography may likewise be normal or show signs of cardiomegaly and pulmonary congestion. Echocardiography may detect the arteriovenous fistula in conjunction with chamber dilation; however, cardiac catheterization with selected coronary cineangiography is necessary for definitive diagnosis and planning of surgical repair.

Operative Correction

Anomalous Left Coronary Artery from the Pulmonary Artery   The diagnosis of ALCAPA in infancy or adulthood is an indication for early surgical correction to prevent sequelae of myocardial ischemia. Currently, the optimal operation is the construction of a two-coronary system, which, simply put, entails the creation of direct continuity between the left coronary ostium and the ascending aorta. This is achieved with **coronary reimplantation** or the **Takeuchi procedure**, in which a transpulmonary artery tunnel/baffle is created from the aorta to the anomalous origin of the left coronary artery.

Coronary reimplantation is performed through a median sternotomy, using cardiopulmonary bypass. After both coronary ostia are clearly identified, the anomalous left coronary ostium is excised as a button from the main pulmonary artery. After adequately mobilizing the left coronary artery, the ostial button is anastomosed to a leftward and posteriorly placed aortotomy using a continuous 7-0 Prolene™ suture. The defect in the pulmonary artery is closed with an autologous pericardial patch, and the patient is weaned from cardiopulmonary bypass. Care must be taken that the coronary anastomosis is tension free.

The Takeuchi procedure is also performed through a median sternotomy under cardiopulmonary bypass. A short transverse incision is made in the main pulmonary artery and extended to create a hinged flap; this will serve as the baffle (Fig. 10–7.1). The ascending aorta is incised transversely at the same level of the pulmonary arteriotomy, and an aortopulmonary window is created using a continuous

7-0 Prolene™ suture. The hinged flap is then sutured to the posterior wall of the pulmonary artery, creating a tunnel that directs aortic blood flow from the aortopulmonary window to the anomalous origin of the left coronary artery. The aortotomy is closed, and the pulmonary artery is repaired with an autologous pericardial patch. The patient is then weaned from cardiopulmonary bypass.

The mortality associated with correction of ALCAPA varies widely with the spectrum of clinical presentations. Follow-up data are somewhat lacking; however, it is assumed that most patients who recover from this operation generally have a good long-term prognosis.

Coronary Arteriovenous Fistula   Since some CAVFs increase in size with age and predispose to heart failure, accelerated atherosclerotic changes, coronary aneurysmal dilation, and bacterial endocarditis, surgical closure of all but the smallest of fistulae is generally recommended. Simple **suture ligation** without cardiopulmonary bypass constitutes adequate therapy if the fistula arises from the distal aspect of the feeding coronary artery. However, if an important area of myocardium is supplied by the coronary artery distal to the fistula origin or if a large coronary artery aneurysm is present, fistula closure via a **transcardiac chamber approach** or **coronary aneurysmorrhaphy** with cardiopulmonary bypass will be required. The precise location and character of the fistula are determined preoperatively.

Simple suture ligation of distally placed coronary artery fistulae may be performed through a median sternotomy. If the fistula can be clearly identified on the surface of the heart, it can be suture ligated directly without cardiopulmonmary bypass. (Fig. 10–7.2). If the fistula location is not obvious on the surface, the involved cardiac chamber can be opened under cardiopulmonary bypass. This fistula can then be suture ligated under direct vision. Obliteration of a palpable thrill at the fistulae confirms accurate suture placement.

More proximally placed fistulae should be approached from within the affected cardiac chamber under cardiopulmonary bypass. The fistula openings are oversewn from within the chamber, and the fistula itself is excised. If the fistulae is associated with a coronary artery aneurysm, the anterior wall of the aneurysm is excised followed by exposure and direct suture closure of the underlying fistula (Fig. 10–7.3). The coronary artery is then repaired primarily with a continuous Prolene™ suture.

The mortality associated with closure of congenital CAVFs approaches zero. Postoperative complications are rare, and the long-term prognosis is generally excellent.

10.8 Hypoplastic Left Heart Syndrome (Fig. 10–8)

Incidence: Comprises 7% to 10% of cardiac defects in neonates diagnosed with congenital heart disease

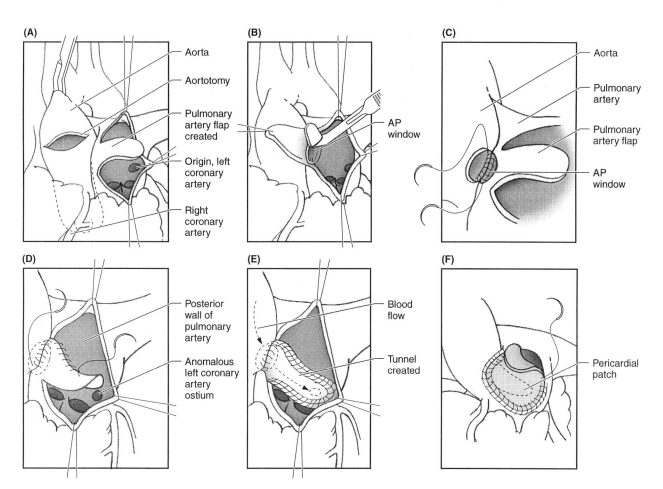

(A) Aorta
Aortotomy
Pulmonary artery flap created
Origin, left coronary artery
Right coronary artery

(B) AP window

(C) Aorta
Pulmonary artery
Pulmonary artery flap
AP window

(D) Posterior wall of pulmonary artery
Anomalous left coronary artery ostium

(E) Blood flow
Tunnel created

(F) Pericardial patch

FIGURE 10–7.1. Takeuchi procedure for ALCAPA. *(A)* After cardiopulmonary bypass has been established, a flap from the anterior wall of the main pulmonary artery is created *(B, C)* An AP window is constructed between the ascending aorta and main pulmonary artery using a continuous 7-0 Prolene™ suture. *(D, E)* The flap is sutured across the posterior wall of the pulmonary artery with a continuous 7-0 Prolene™ suture, creating a tunnel connecting the AP window to the anomalous left coronary artery ostium. *(F)* The pulmonary arteriotomy is closed with an autologous pericardial patch.

Pathophysiology: Hypoplastic left heart syndrome (HLHS) is characterized by marked hypoplasia or absence of the left ventricle, and severe aortic hypoplasia places the work of the pulmonary and systemic perfusion solely on the right ventricle. Pulmonary venous return enters the right atrium via an interatrial communication. Systemic perfusion is dependent on a PDA. Cyanosis, congestive heart failure, and systemic hypoperfusion results as pulmonary vascular resistance decreases and pulmonary blood flow increases at the expense of systemic blood flow.

Clinical Features: Neonates with HLHS typically present with tachypnea and mild cyanosis in the first 24 to 48 hours of life. A single S2, left parasternal systolic murmur, and right ventricular lift are noted on physical exam. Electrocardiography reveals right atrial enlargement and right ventricular hypertrophy. Chest radiography reveals cardiomegaly and increased pulmonary vascular markings. Echocardiography is diagnostic, revealing a hypoplastic/absent left ventricle and/or atretic ascending aorta.

Concepts of Correction: Surgical options include (1) a staged procedure to reconstruct the atretic aortic arch and create a Fontan-type circulation, eventually relieving the right ventricle of the pulmonary circulation. and (2) total cardiac replacement.

Corrective Operation(s):

• Norwood procedure

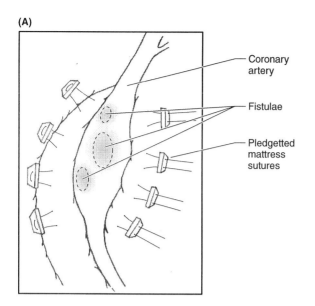

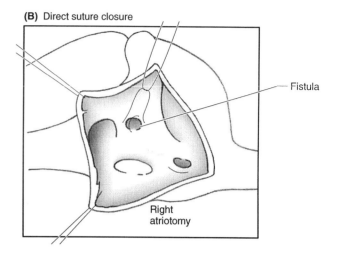

FIGURE 10–7.2.   Suture ligation of CAVF. Without cardiopulmonary bypass, double-pledgetted 6-0 or 7-0 Prolene™ sutures are passed beneath the coronary artery at the fistula sites.

Stage I: construction of neoaorta and modified Blalock-Taussig shunt

Stage II: revision of the Blalock-Taussig shunt to a Glenn shunt (hemi-Fontan procedure)

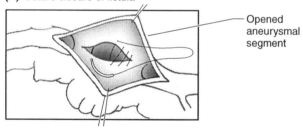

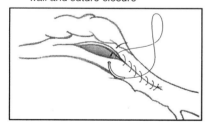

FIGURE 10–7.3.   CAVF closure with aneurysmorraphy. (A) Under cardiopulmonary bypass, the anterior aneurysm wall is excised followed by direct suture closure of the underlying fistula. (B) The coronary artery is then closed primarily, completing the aneurysmorraphy.

Stage III: completion of the Fontan procedure

• orthotopic cardiac transplantation

General Considerations

HLHS represents a spectrum of left-sided cardiac malformations based on a markedly hypoplastic or absent left ventricle and atretic ascending aorta (2 to 3 mm in diameter). Other associated malformations include hypoplasia of the aortic arch, aortic valve, and mitral valve. HLHS occurs in 7% to 10% of newborns diagnosed with congenital heart

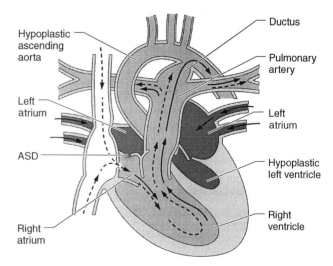

FIGURE 10–8.   Schematic drawing of HLHS. (■)——▸, Oxygenated; (□)----▸, Deoxygenated; (▨)----▸, mixed.

disease and accounts for 25% of cardiac deaths occurring within the first week of life.

Since the left ventricle is essentially nonfunctional in HLHS, the right ventricle supports both the pulmonary and systemic circulations. The right atrium receives systemic venous return as well as pulmonary venous return by way of an interatrial communication (i.e., patent foramen ovale, ASD). The admixture of systemic and pulmonary venous return is delivered into the right ventricle and pumped into the main pulmonary artery. Systemic flow is delivered into the aorta via a typically large PDA. Retrograde flow into the aortic arch and ascending aorta provides coronary and cerebral perfusion; antegrade flow into the descending aorta provides lower body systemic perfusion. Therefore, systemic oxygenation is critically dependent on the interatrial communication, and systemic perfusion is dependent on ductal patency and the balance between pulmonary and systemic blood flow. The relative ratio of pulmonary to systemic blood flow, in turn, is directly related to the pulmonary and systemic vascular resistances. In the immediate postnatal period, pulmonary vascular resistance is nearly equivalent to systemic vascular resistance, which generally results in a proper balance between pulmonary and systemic perfusion. However, as pulmonary vascular resistance decreases and as the ductus arteriosus closes after birth, pulmonary blood flow increases at the expense of systemic flow, resulting in congestive heart failure, renal insufficiency, and metabolic acidosis. The size of the interatrial communication is an extremely important determinant of pulmonary blood flow as the pulmonary vascular resistance falls. Furthermore, approximately 50% of patients with HLHS have some degree of tricuspid regurgitation.

Preoperative medical management of these infants is extremely important and is predicated on ensuring adequate systemic perfusion and oxygenation. The two major goals are the maintenance of ductal patency and maintaining an adequate balance between pulmonary and systemic blood flow ($Q_p/Q_s = 1$). Ductal patency can be reliably maintained with a continuous infusion of prostaglandin E1. Most neonates with HLHS diagnosed in the first few days of life have normal lungs and a Q_p/Q_s of approximately unity and do not require mechanical ventilation. Care must be taken to avoid significantly reducing the pulmonary vascular resistance, which would result in increased pulmonary blood flow at the expense of systemic perfusion and oxygenation. Consequently, high inspired oxygen concentrations are to be avoided. In fact, the addition of carbon dioxide to inspired gases is quite effective in raising pulmonary vascular resistance and, hence, treating systemic hypoperfusion and pulmonary overcirculation in these patients. Inotropes are generally avoided, since catecholamine-mediated increases in systemic vascular resistance lead to excessive pulmonary blood flow. Emergency operation for HLHS is rarely required except in cases of an intact interatrial septum not amenable to balloon septostomy. In these cases, oxygenated blood is not delivered to the right ventricle, resulting in severe hypoxemia and metabolic acidosis.

Diagnostic Keys

Neonates with HLHS typically present with tachypnea and mild cyanosis in the first 24 to 48 hours of life. A single S2, a left parasternal systolic murmur (ductal flow), and right ventricular lift are usually apparent on physical examination. Signs of right atrial enlargement and right ventricular hypertrophy are observed on electrocardiography. Chest radiography typically reveals cardiomegaly and increased pulmonary vascular markings; a reticular pattern suggestive of pulmonary venous obstruction may be observed if the interatrial communication is excessively restrictive. Two-dimensional echocardiography is diagnostic of HLHS, displaying the characteristic diminutive ascending aorta. The size of the ascending aorta, ductus arteriosus, and interatrial communication, in addition to the degree of tricuspid regurgitation, are important parameters to glean from echocardiographic examination. Cardiac catheterization is rarely required in the diagnosis of HLHS.

Operative Correction

The Norwood Procedure Surgical treatment of HLHS is directed toward **orthotopic cardiac transplantation** or the **staged Norwood procedure.** The Norwood procedure is a staged reconstruction leading up to a Fontan-type circulation. The mortality for neonates with HLHS is approximately 40% during the waiting period for an acceptable donor allograft. Improvements in the operative mortality for the Norwood procedure have resulted in most cardiac centers recommending the first stage of the procedure, since operative mortality is generally less than the combined mortality associated with waiting for and performing cardiac replacement. Moreover, this decision does not prohibit later crossover to transplantation if an appropriate donor organ becomes available.

High pulmonary vascular resistances encountered in the early neonatal period prohibit a single-stage Fontan procedure. The Norwood procedure comprises three stages designed to accommodate the changes in pulmonary vascular resistances until a Fontan-type circulation can be constructed. The first stage is directed toward maintaining balanced pulmonary and systemic hemodynamics and facilitating normal development of the pulmonary vasculature and the right ventricle. Through a median sternotomy on hypothermic cardiopulmonary bypass, the septum primum is excised through a right atriotomy to maximize the size of the interatrial communication. The main pulmonary artery is then transected just proximal to the origin of the right pulmonary artery, and the distal main pulmonary artery is closed with a patch to minimize stenosis (Fig. 10–8.1). The ductus arteriosus is ligated and divided at its entrance into

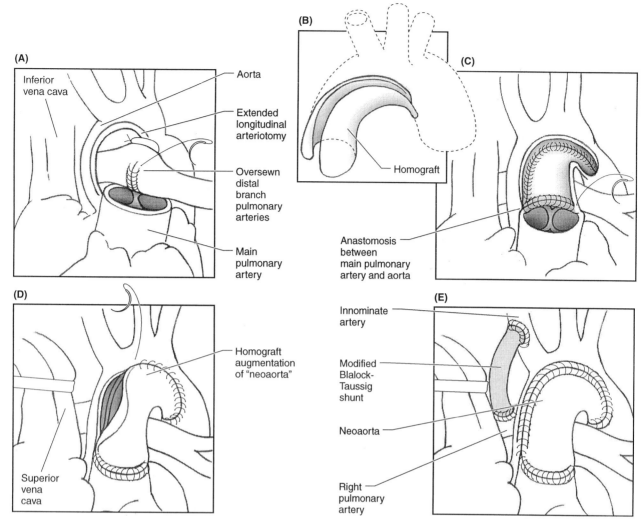

FIGURE 10–8.1. Norwood stage I for HLHS. Through a median sternotomy on hypothermic cardiopulmonary bypass, the septum primum is excised through a right atriotomy to maximize the size of the interatrial communication. *(A)* The main pulmonary artery is then transected just proximal to the origin of the right pulmonary artery, and the distal main pulmonary artery is closed with a patch to minimize stenosis. The ductus arteriosus is ligated and divided at its entrance into the thoracic aorta. An aortotomy is then performed extending from the inferior aspect of the aortic arch through the lateral aspect of the ascending aorta to the level of the transected pulmonary trunk. *(B–D)* The entire aortic arch complex is then augmented, creating a "neoaorta" comprising the proximal end of the transected main pulmonary artery anastomosed to the ascending aorta and arch. A cryopreserved homograft wall is used to reconstruct the aortic wall. *(E)* Finally, a systemic-to-pulmonary artery Blalock-Taussig shunt is constructed to provide pulmonary blood flow.

the thoracic aorta. A aortotomy is then performed extending from the inferior aspect of the aortic arch through the lateral aspect of the ascending aorta to the level of the transected pulmonary trunk. The entire aortic arch complex is then augmented, creating a "neoaorta" comprising the proximal end of the transected main pulmonary artery anastomosed to the ascending aorta and arch. A cryopreserved homograft wall is used to reconstruct the aortic wall. Finally, a systemic-to-pulmonary artery Blalock-Taussig shunt is constructed to provide pulmonary blood flow.

As the pulmonary vascular resistance falls in the weeks after completion of the first stage, excessive pulmonary blood flow from the systemic-to-pulmonary artery shunt may lead to right ventricular volume overload and congestive heart failure. Therefore, the **second stage** of the Fontan procedure is intended to reduce the volume load on the single ventricle. It consists of the first stage of the Fontan procedure (**hemi-Fontan**) and is performed at about 6 months of age. In this operation, the previous systemic-to-pulmonary artery shunt is occluded, and a bidirectional cavopulmonary Glenn shunt is performed, whereby the superior vena cava is divided and the cephalad end is anastomosed end to side to the superior aspect of the right pulmonary artery with a continuous 6-0 or 7-0 Prolene™ suture; the cardiac end of the superior vena cava is oversewn (Fig. 10–8.2).

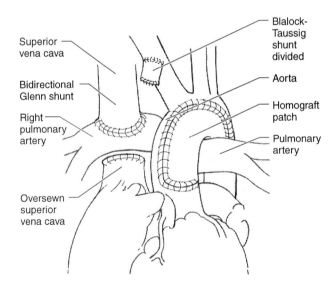

FIGURE 10–8.2. Norwood stage II for HLHS. The previous systemic-to-pulmonary artery shunt is divided, and a bidirectional cavopulmonary Glenn shunt is performed, whereby the superior vena cava is transected. Then the cephalad end is anastomosed end to side to the superior aspect of the right pulmonary artery with a continuous 6-0 or 7-0 Prolene™ suture, and the cardiac end of the superior vena cava is oversewn.

Alternatively, the cardiac end of the superior vena cava is anastomosed end-to-side to the inferior aspect of the right pulmonary artery, and its orifice is occluded from within the right atrium with a temporary patch of autologous pericardium or GoreTex.™ This step is intended to facilitate the third stage of the Norwood reconstruction in which the Fontan procedure is completed.

The third stage of the Norwood procedure, performed about 6 months to 1 year after the second stage hemi-Fontan, consists of the completion of the Fontan procedure. This consists of establishing continuity from the inferior vena cava to the confluence of the pulmonary arteries and the superior vena cava. The two most popular methods of achieving this are construction of a lateral atrial tunnel or an extracardiac interposition graft (see Tricuspid Atresia section in Chapter 9).

Orthotopic Cardiac Transplantation

The current technique for orthotopic cardiac transplantation has remained essentially unchanged from its initial description by Shumway and Lower in 1960.[1]

• *Donor Operation.* After the chest is entered through a median sternotomy, a retractor is placed and the pericardium is opened (Fig. 10–8.3). The heart is inspected and palpated for contusions, perforations, thrills, and coronary atherosclerosis. If the heart is deemed satisfactory, its final acceptance is immediately communicated to the recipient team. The aorta and pulmonary artery are dissected superiorly to the level of the arch and bifurcation, respectively, to ensure adequate length for implantation. The superior vena cava is then mobilized superiorly to the origin of the azygous vein and encircled with two ligatures. An adequate length of the inferior vena cava is dissected free from its pericardial reflection and is surrounded with an umbilical tape. The aorta is then encircled with an umbilical tape, and a 14-gauge cardioplegia perfusion cannula is inserted into its ascending segment. Intravenous heparin is administered at a dose of 300 U/kg and allowed to circulate for 3 to 5 minutes.

Excision of the heart commences with ligation of the superior and inferior venae cavae. The ascending aorta is then clamped distal to the perfusion cannula at the level of the innominate artery, and a hyperkalemic cardioplegic solution at 2 to 4°C is rapidly infused into the aortic root at a pressure of 150 mm Hg with the concurrent application of topical cold saline into the pericardial well. The inferior vena cava is divided, decompressing the right heart, which is now filling with cardioplegia. When the heart is fully arrested, cooled, and perfused with cardioplegia, it is elevated from the pericardial well, and each of the pulmonary veins is divided at their pericardial reflections. The pulmonary artery and aorta are divided at the level of the bifurcation and innominate artery, respectively. The explanted heart is placed in two sterile plastic bags with a cold saline interface.

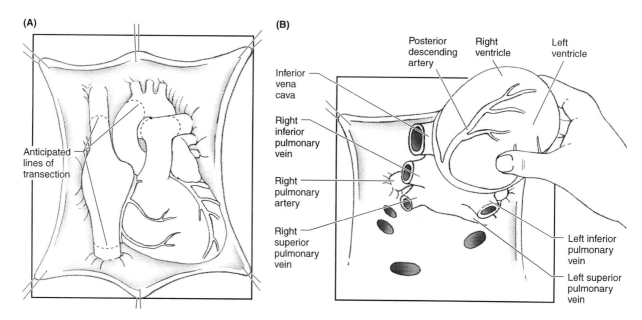

FIGURE 10–8.3.   Orthotopic cardiac transplantation (donor operation). *(A)* Lines of great vessel transection. *(B)* Excision of the donor heart beginning inferiorly commencing with division of the inferior vena cava and pulmonary veins, followed by transection of the superior vena cava, pulmonary arteries, and aorta. RPA = right pulmonary artery; RV = right ventricle; LV = left ventricle; PDA = posterior descending artery. (Reproduced with permission. Brown ME, et al.: Cardiac donor evaluation, retrieval, and matching to recipient. In: Smith JA et al (eds): *The Stanford Manual of Cardiopulmonary Transplantation*, Armonk, Futura Publishing, 1996, pp. 26–27.)

This is, in turn, placed within an air-tight container filled with ice-cold saline and transported in a standard ice-filled cooler.

• *Recipient Operation.* After anesthesia is induced and arterial and venous lines are placed, the supine patient's chest and groin areas are prepped and draped (Fig. 10–8.4). Central venous access via the left internal jugular vein is usually obtained, sparing the right side for future endomyocardial biopsies. After a median sternotomy is performed and the pericardium is opened, the patient undergoes routine cannulation of the aorta and both venae cavae. The arterial cannula is inserted in the most distal aspect of the ascending aorta. The venous cannulae are both placed laterally in the high right atrium near the superior vena caval junction. Following institution of cardiopulmonary bypass with moderate hypothermia (28 to 30°C) and snugging of caval snares, the ascending aorta is cross-clamped, and 50 to 100 mL of cardioplegic solution is rapidly infused into the aortic root, causing diastolic arrest. The aorta and pulmonary artery are separated and divided at the level of the semilunar valve commissures. The atria are then transected at the level of their atrioventricular grooves, ex-

cluding the atrial appendages, leaving two recipient atrial cuffs.

The donor heart is placed in a bowl of cold saline, and the left atrium is opened by connecting the pulmonary veins, fashioning the donor atrial cuff. The aorta and pulmonary artery are completely separated from each other. Under continuous application of topical cold saline into the pericardial well, implantation begins with direct anastomosis of the donor and recipient left atrial cuffs. The donor right atrium is then opened with an incision extending from the inferior vena cava orifice superiorly in a curvilinear fashion into the base of the right atrial appendage. Through this incision, an intact tricuspid valve and fossa ovalis are inspected and ensured. The right atrial cuff anastomosis is then performed followed by an end-to-end anastomosis of the donor and recipient pulmonary arteries. Systemic rewarming is initiated at this time, and caval snares are released, permitting blood to enter the heart and lungs and displacing any air trapped in the left-sided chambers. The end-to-end aortic anastomosis follows this maneuver. Just before completing the aortic anastomosis, additional attempts are made to vent any residual air by agitating the heart. Topical cold saline is

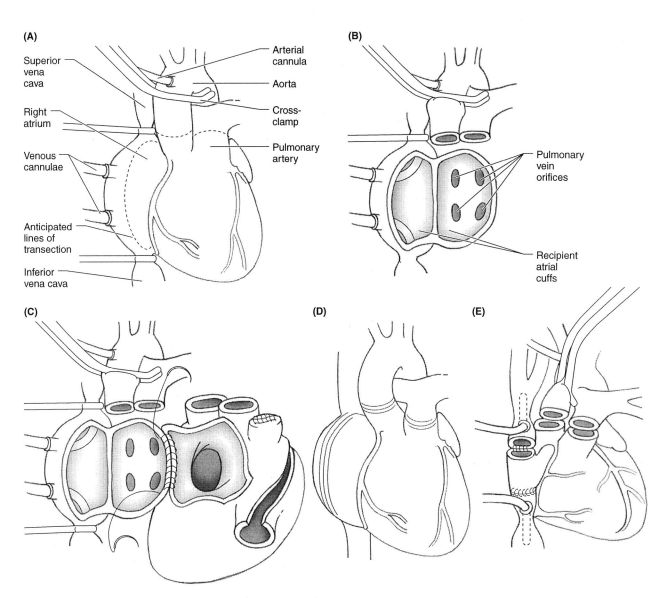

(A)

Superior vena cava

Arterial cannula

Aorta

Cross-clamp

Right atrium

Venous cannulae

Pulmonary artery

Anticipated lines of transection

Inferior vena cava

(B)

Pulmonary vein orifices

Recipient atrial cuffs

(C)

(D)

(E)

FIGURE 10–8.4. Orthotopic cardiac transplantation (recipient operation). *(A)* The aorta is cross-clamped and the caval snares are tightened as cardiopulmonary bypass is commenced. *(B)* Recipient right and left atrial cuffs and great arteries. *(C)* The left atrial cuff anastomosis is commenced at the left superior pulmonary vein. The right atrial cuffs are anastomosed in a similar fashion. *(D)* The operation is completed with the end-to-end aortic and pulmonary arterial anastomoses. Separation from cardiopulmonary bypass then begins. *(E)* Alternatively, the superior and inferior vena cava can be anastomosed end-to-end, instead of the right atrial cuff anastomosis. (Reproduced with permission. Yuh DD, et al.: Cardiac transplantation. In: Niederhuber JE: *Fundamentals of Surgery,* Stamford, Appleton & Lange, 1998, p. 665.)

then discontinued, 200 mg lidocaine is infused into the by-pass circuit, the aortic cross-clamp is removed, and a needle vent is placed in the ascending aorta. Although spontaneous defibrillation usually occurs at this time, electrical defibrillation is effected as necessary. Still under cardiopulmonary bypass, all suture lines are inspected for hemostasis before bypass is weaned. The superior vena cava cannula is drawn back into the right atrium, and the inferior vena caval cannula is removed just prior to discontinuation of bypass. An isoproterenol infusion (0.005 to 0.01 μg/kg/min) is titrated to achieve a heart rate of 90 to 110 bpm to maximize cardiac output chronotropically and inotropically and to lower pulmonary vascular resistance. Temporary atrial pacing wires are placed on the donor right atrium. The pericardium is left open. The right pleural space is opened, and chest tubes are placed in the right chest and the mediastinum. The sternum and overlying fascia and skin are closed in the usual fashion.

In recipients who have already undergone stage I of the Norwood operation, the donor aorta is anatomosed end to end to the recipient neoaorta, and the donor main pulmonary artery is anastomosed end to side to a longitudinal arteriotomy made in the recipient pulmonary artery bifurcation (Fig. 10–8.5). The right and left atrial cuff anastomoses are performed in the standard fashion. If a prior palliative operation has not yet been performed, the aortic arch is procured with the donor heart and is included in the transplant. Therefore, the recipient operation includes an end-to-end anastomosis between the proximal descending aorta of the donor to the recipient descending aorta below the level of the ductus arteriosus. The recipient arch vessels are anastomosed to the donor arch in the form of a Carrel patch. For recipients with anomalous pulmonary venous connections, procurement of extra lengths of the donor superior vena cava and innominate vein allows for direct end-to-end caval anastomoses.

In the Norwood staged reconstruction, operative mortality ranges between 20% and 50% for the first stage and generally lower mortalities for each of the second and third stages. Cardiac transplantation is associated with a lower operative mortality of 20%; however, 20% to 40% of neonates on waiting lists do not receive donor hearts. Moreover, cardiac transplantation is associated with lifelong immunosuppression and its associated risks.

10.9 Ebstein's Anomaly (Fig. 10–9)

Incidence: Comprises less than 1% of congenital cardiac defects

Pathophysiology: Downward displacement of the posterior and septal leaflets of the tricuspid valve and "atrialization" of the right ventricle leads to diminished right ventricular output and congestive heart failure, stemming from tricuspid insufficiency and/or right ventricular dysfunction. High right atrial pressures from tricuspid insufficiency and high pulmonary vascular resistances during the early postnatal period result in right-to-left shunting across an interatrial communication (i.e., ASD, patent foramen ovale) leading to varying degrees of cyanosis. An increased incidence of accessory

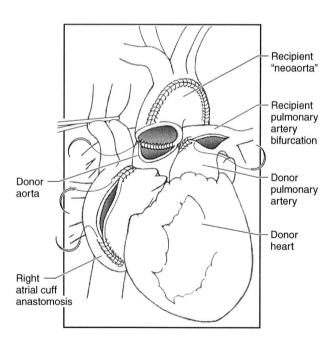

FIGURE 10–8.5.   Orthotopic cardiac transplantation after Norwood stage I. The donor aorta is anatomosed end to end to the recipient neoaorta, and the donor main pulmonary artery is anastomosed end to side to a longitudinal arteriotomy made in the recipient pulmonary artery bifurcation. The right and left atrial cuff anastomoses are performed in the standard fashion.

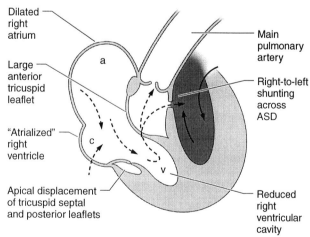

FIGURE 10–9.   Schematic drawing of Ebstein's anomaly. (■)——➤, Oxygenated; (□)---➤, Deoxygenated; (▨)===➤, mixed.

conduction pathways leads to paroxysmal supraventricular arrhythmias.

Clinical Features: Infants present with varying degrees of congestive heart failure and cyanosis. Paroxysmal supraventricular arrhythmias may also be noted. Electrocardiography reveals right atrial enlargement and Wolff-Parkinson-White patterns. Chest radiography reveals cardiomegaly from right atrial dilation and decreased lung markings. Echocardiography is diagnostic, revealing a downwardly displaced tricuspid valve, a small atrialized right ventricle, a dilated right atrium, and an atrial septal defect.

Concepts of Correction: Operative correction is predicated on repair or replacement of the tricuspid valve and closure of the atrial septal defect.

Corrective Operation(s):

- Danielson repair
- Carpentier repair
- Starnes procedure

General Considerations

Originally described by Wilhelm Ebstein in 1866, Ebstein's anomaly is a rare congenital cardiac lesion defined by malformation and downward displacement of the posterior and septal leaflets of the tricuspid valve toward the cardiac apex. The anterior septal leaflet is usually normal or enlarged to some degree. The malformed leaflet origins are inferiorly displaced into the right ventricle below the annulus fibrosus, creating a thin-walled "atrialized" portion of the right ventricle. A patent foramen ovale or secundum ASD is usually associated with this anomaly. The main physiologic disturbance associated with this defect is inadequate right ventricular output stemming from tricuspid insufficiency and right ventricular dysfunction. Increased pulmonary vascular resistance in the early neonatal period and tricuspid insufficiency result in high right atrial pressures and gross dilation, **right-to-left shunting** across the ASD, and significant cyanosis. Accessory conduction pathways, resulting in an increased incidence of paroxysmal supraventricular tachycardia or paroxysmal atrial fibrillation, are also associated with Ebstein's anomaly.

Overall survival in patients with Ebstein's anomaly is limited, with only about 50% to 70% of these patients surviving to 2 years of age. Death usually results from severe congestive heart failure, hypoxia, and cardiac arrhythmias.

Diagnostic Keys

Signs and symptoms of Ebstein's anomaly depend on the degree of tricuspid insufficiency, the size of the ASD, and the degree of right ventricular dysfunction. The early development of cyanosis and congestive heart failure is seen in many infants with severe tricuspid insufficiency and right-to-left shunting. Older patients with this anomaly usually present with dyspnea and cyanosis. Arrhythmias are also associated with this anomaly; 10% to 20% of these patients

have **Wolff-Parkinson-White syndrome.** Physical examination generally reveals a systolic flow murmur from tricuspid insufficiency, cyanosis, and clubbing. Electrocardiography and chest radiography usually reveal cardiomegaly due primarily to an markedly dilated right atrium and decreased pulmonary vascularity; they may show Wolff-Parkinson-White patterns. Two-dimensional echocardiography with Doppler is diagnostic, revealing a downwardly displaced tricuspid valve, small atrialized right ventricle, enlarged right atrium, and delayed closure of the tricuspid valve compared with the mitral valve. Cardiac catheterization with angiography is rarely required for the diagnosis.

Operative Correction

Indications for surgical correction of Ebstein's anomaly include New York Heart Association class III or IV status, moderate to severe cyanosis, paradoxical emboli, right ventricular outflow tract obstruction, and intractable arrhythmias. Medical management alone is only appropriate for mildly symptomatic children; these children will eventually need definitive surgical correction as their symptomatology

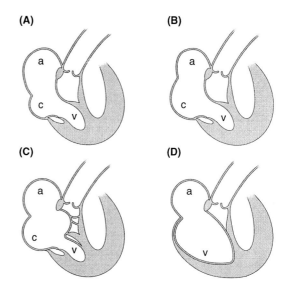

FIGURE 10–9.1. Four anatomic types of Ebstein's anomaly. *(A)* Small, contractile atrialized chamber (c) with mobile anterior leaflet. *(B)* Large, noncontractile atrialized chamber with a mobile anterior leaflet. *(C)* Resctricted motion of the anterior leaflet. *(D)* "Tricuspid sac" leaflet tissue forms a continuous sac adherent to the dilated right ventricle. a = atrium; v = ventricle. (Reproduced with permission from Carpentier A, Chuvaud S, Mace L, et al. A new reconstructive operation for Ebstein's anomaly of the tricuspid valve. *J Thorac Cardiovasc Surg,* 96:92, 1988.)

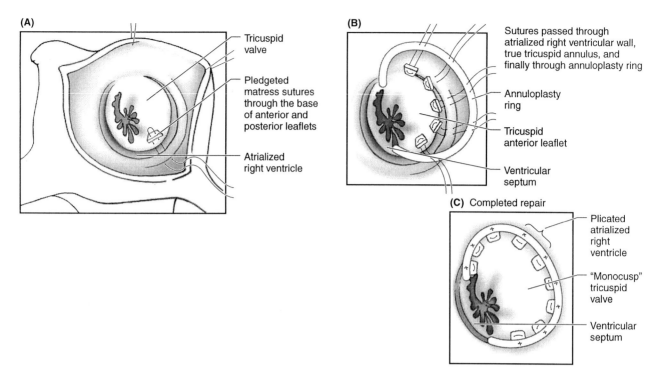

FIGURE 10–9.2. Danielson repair of Ebstein's anomaly. Through a median sternotomy on cardiopulmonary bypass, a right atriotomy is created, extending from the atrial appendage to the inferior vena cava. *(A)* The ASD is closed in the standard fashion with an autologous pericardial or prosthetic patch. A series of pledgeted mattress sutures is placed in the atrialized portion of the right ventricle in such a way as to plicate the aneurysmal free wall and to draw the downwardly displaced posterior leaflet toward the tricuspid annulus. *(B)* A posterior annuloplasty is then performed using one or more pledgeted mattress sutures to narrow the diameter of the tricuspid annulus. *(C)* The annulus is narrowed until there is satisfactory apposition between the previously displaced leaflets and the enlarged anterior leaflet, creating a monocusp valve. The atriotomy is then closed after excising redundant atrial wall, thereby effectively performing an atrioplasty.

and disability increase over time. Due to the wide anatomic variability of Ebstein's anomaly, a variety of techniques for surgical correction have been described. The most common approach involves repair or replacement of the tricuspid valve and ASD closure. Valvar repair is preferred to prosthetic replacement in young children, if feasible, due to the limited lifespan of tissue valves and the need to replace mechanical valves as the child grows.

The classic technique of tricuspid valve repair in Ebstein's anomaly is based on the construction of a monocusp valve, using the enlarged anterior leaflet of the tricuspid valve. The **Danielson repair** involves plication of the free wall of the atrialized portion of the right ventricle from the apex toward the base, posterior tricuspid annuloplasty, right

reduction atrioplasty, and ASD closure (see Fig. 10–9.2). The plication serves to draw the downwardly displaced tricuspid valve leaflets into the same plane as the tricuspid valve annulus and the enlarged anterior leaflet. The annuloplasty reduces the dilation of the tricuspid valve, bringing the enlarged anterior leaflet in closer apposition with the previously displaced leaflets, forming a monocusp valve. The atrioplasty reduces the right atrial dilation, and the ASD closure eliminates the right-to-left shunting. Furthermore, electrophysiologic mapping and division of accessory conduction pathways is performed, in the setting of ventricular pre-excitation. Tricuspid valve replacement is performed when the tricuspid valve is not reparable and is technically similar to adult tricuspid valve replacement.

Through a median sternotomy on cardiopulmonary bypass, a right atriotomy is created, extending from the atrial appendage to the inferior vena cava (Fig. 10–9.1). The ASD is closed in the standard fashion with an autologous pericardial or prosthetic patch (see Atrial Septal Defect (Ostium Secundum) section in Chapter 8). A series of pledgeted mattress sutures are placed in the atrialized portion of the right ventricle in such a way as to plicate the aneurysmal free wall and to draw the downwardly displaced posterior leaflet toward the tricuspid annulus. A posterior annuloplasty is then performed using one or more pledgeted mattress sutures to narrow the diameter of the tricuspid annulus. The annulus is narrowed until there is satisfactory apposition between the previously displaced leaflets and the enlarged anterior leaflet. The atriotomy is then closed after excising redundant atrial wall, thereby effectively performing an atrioplasty. The patient is then weaned from cardiopulmonary bypass.

The **Carpentier repair** is a modification of the Danielson repair in which the plication is performed in a circumferential manner, preserving the apex-to-base dimensions of the right ventricle (Fig. 10–9.3). As with the Danielson repair, the tricuspid valve is approached through a right atriotomy. The enlarged anterior leaflet is detached from the annulus, and the fused chordae tendinae are fenestrated to lengthen them. The atrialized portion of the right ventricle is then plicated in a vertical plane using a series of pledgeted mattress sutures; this plication also narrows the tricuspid annulus. The detached anterior leaflet is then reoriented and reattached to the annulus with a continuous suture. This repair is reinforced by attaching a Carpentier tricuspid annuloplasty ring to the annulus using circumferential mattress sutures. The ASD and atriotomy are then closed as in the Danielson repair.

Neonates with severe congestive heart failure and cyanosis may be treated by oversewing the tricuspid valve and performing a systemic-to-pulmonary artery shunt **(Starnes procedure)**. These patients are hence converted to a single ventricle configuration and are tracked toward an eventual modified Fontan procedure. In cases of Wolff-Parkinson-White syndrome, accessory pathways are also interrupted.

Overall early hospital mortality after surgical correction of Ebstein's anomaly is about 5%, usually from acute cardiac failure. Late deaths are uncommon after tricuspid valve repair or replacement and ASD closure, with most surviving patients achieving a significantly improved functional status.

10.10 Vascular Rings and Sling (Fig. 10–10.1)

Incidence: Comprises less than 1% of congenital heart defects

Pathophysiology: Maldevelopment of the embryonic aortic arches produces vascular rings/slings that may partially or completely encircle the trachea and/or esophagus, producing compressive symptoms.

Clinical Features: Tracheoesophageal compressive symptoms include respiratory distress, recurrent pulmonary infections, and dysphagia. The electrocardiogram is usually normal. Chest radiography may reveal signs of tracheal compression or pneumonia. Barium enema is usually diagnostic in detecting both tracheal and esophageal compression. Angiography is used for diagnostic confirmation and operative planning.

Concepts of Correction: Division of the vascular ring or sling to alleviate compression on the trachea or esophagus

Corrective Operations:

- double aortic arch: Division of the nondominant arch, usually the anterior (left) arch and ligamentum

- right aortic arch/ligamentum arteriosum: Division of the ligamentum

- left aortic arch (aberrant right subclavian artery): Division of the right subclavian artery at its origin with or without reanastomosis

- left aortic arch (anomalous innominate artery): Anterior aortic suspension

- pulmonary artery sling: Division and translocation of the left pulmonary artery or tracheal resection

General Considerations

The mediastinal great vessels are embryologically derived from a symmetrical array of paired (right and left) dorsal aortae and six pairs of branchial arches that are apparent by the fourth or fifth week of intrauterine life (Fig. 10–10.1). These vascular structures subsequently resorb and coalesce in an ordered sequence to form the aorta, include the aortic arch vessels. Most of the six pairs of branchial arches contribute to a particular arterial structure. The first and second arch pairs persist to form minor facial arteries: the maxillary, hyoid, and stapedial arteries. The third arch forms the common, internal (first portion), and external carotid arteries. The left fourth branchial arch forms a segment of the aortic arch extending from the left common carotid and left subclavian arteries, constituting the distal aortic arch and aortic isthmus. The right fourth arch forms the proximal right subclavian artery; the distal portion is contributed by the right dorsal aorta. The fifth arch is transient. The right sixth arch forms the proximal segment of the right pulmonary artery whereas its left pair persists as the ductus arteriosus. Perturbations of this developmental sequence leads to the vascular malformations known as rings or slings.

Vascular rings are a group of rare congenital anomalies of the aortic arch that commonly result in complete or partial encirclement and compression of the trachea and/or esophagus. Vascular sling is a condition whereby the left pulmonary artery originates from the right pulmonary artery and courses between the trachea and esophagus. These malformations can be grouped into four categories: (1) double

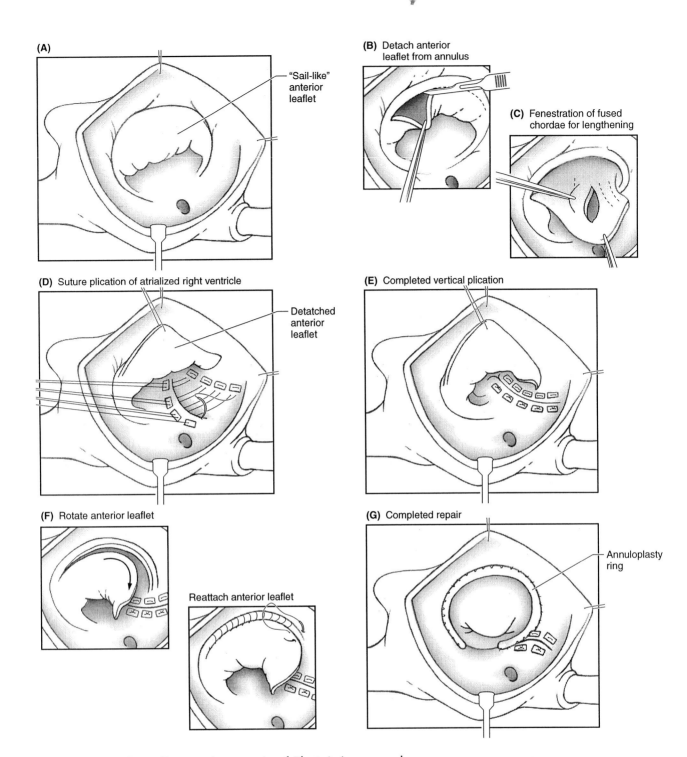

(A)

"Sail-like" anterior leaflet

(B) Detach anterior leaflet from annulus

(C) Fenestration of fused chordae for lengthening

(D) Suture plication of atrialized right ventricle

Detatched anterior leaflet

(E) Completed vertical plication

(F) Rotate anterior leaflet

Reattach anterior leaflet

(G) Completed repair

Annuloplasty ring

FIGURE 10–9.3. Carpentier repair of Ebstein's anomaly *(A–C)* Through a right atriotomy, the enlarged anterior tricuspid leaflet is detached from the annulus, and the fused chordae tendinae are fenestrated to lengthen them. *(D, E)* The atrialized portion of the right ventricle is then plicated in a vertical plane using a series of pledgeted mattress sutures; this plication also narrows the tricuspid annulus. *(F)* The detached anterior leaflet is then reoriented and reattached to the annulus with a continuous suture. *(G)* The repair is completed by attaching a reinforcing Carpentier tricuspid annuloplasty ring to the annulus using circumferential mattress sutures. Finally, the ASD closure and atrioplasty are performed as in the Danielson repair.

(A)

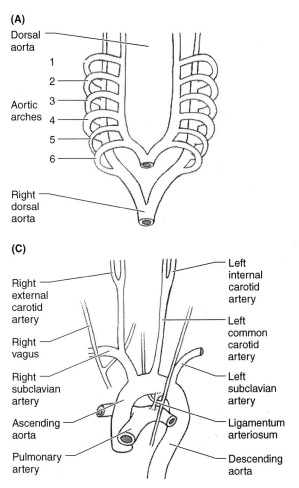

(B)

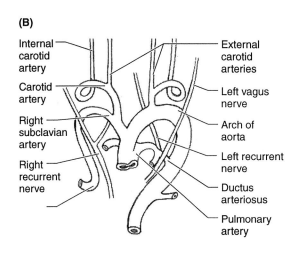

(C)

FIGURE 10–10.1. Embryological development of the branchial (aortic) arches. *(A)* Original aortic arch system with symmetric paired (right and left) dorsal aortae and six pairs of branchial arches. *(B)* Normal arch arterial pattern following an ordered sequence of resorption and fusion of the branchial arches and dorsal aortae. Derivations: first and second arch: minor facial arteries; third arch: carotid arteries; fourth arch (left): distal aortic arch and isthmus, (right): proximal right subclavian artery; fifth arch: resorbed; sixth arch (right): proximal right pulmonary artery (left): ductus arterious. *(C)* Normal adult pattern of mediastinal great vessels including arch vessels. (Reproduced with permission. Sadler TW: Cardiovascular system. In: Sadler TW: *Langman's Medical Embryology*, 5th ed. Baltimore, Williams & Wilkins, 1985, p. 198.)

aortic arch, (2) right aortic arch with left ligamentum arteriosum, (3) left aortic arch with anomalous arch vessels, and (4) pulmonary artery sling.

Double aortic arch (Fig. 10–10.2) is the most common type of vascular ring and results from a persistence of the right fourth arch. Morphologically, two arches arise from the ascending aorta, pass anteriorly and posteriorly to the trachea and esophagus, and rejoin the descending aorta,

completing the ring. The posterior (right) arch gives rise to the right common carotid and subclavian arteries; the anterior (left) arch gives rise to the left common carotid and subclavian arteries. The anterior arch is usually the smaller of the two arches.

Right aortic arch with left ligamentum arteriosum (Fig. 10–10.3) follows the double aortic arch in frequency. Persistence of the right fourth arch and deletion of the left

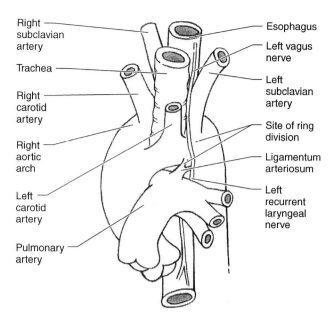

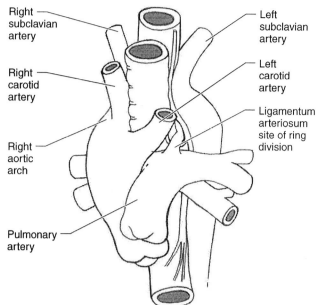

FIGURE 10–10.2. Double aortic arch, right arch dominant. Note the persistent right dorsal aorta. The trachea and esophagus are encircled between the two aortic arches. Repair consists of (1) division of the ring where the lesser (left) arch inserts into the descending aorta and (2) division of the ligamentum arteriosum. (Reproduced with permission. Mainwaring RD: Tracheoesophageal compressive syndromes of vascular origin. In Baue AE, et al. (eds): *Glenn's Cardiovascular and Thoracic Surgery*, 6th ed. Stamford, Appleton & Lange, 1996, p. 1096.)

FIGURE 10–10.3. Right aortic arch with retroesophageal left subclavian artery. The ring is divided at the (left) ligamentum arteriosum. (Reproduced with permission. Mainwaring RD: Tracheoesophageal compressive syndromes of vascular origin. In Baue AE, et al. (eds): *Glenn's Cardiovascular and Thoracic Surgery*, 6th ed. Stamford, Appleton & Lange, 1996, p. 1096.)

arch results in an anomalous retroesophageal left subclavian artery. The ligamentum arteriosum connects the descending aorta to the left pulmonary artery, forming a complete ring. When the left arch involutes between the subclavian artery and the descending aorta, a right aortic arch with "mirror-image" left innominate artery results.

Left aortic arch with an aberrant right subclavian artery (Fig. 10–10.4) results from regression of the right fourth arch between the subclavian and carotid arteries. The right subclavian artery branches from the descending aorta, passing posterior to the esophagus and often compressing it; this results in an incomplete ring. Left aortic arch with an anomalous innominate artery may cause anterior tracheal compression as the innominate artery passes anteriorly and upward toward the right apex.

Pulmonary artery sling (Fig. 10–10.5) results when the left pulmonary artery originates from the right pulmonary artery and passes between the trachea and esophagus, resulting in posterior tracheal compression. Pulmonary

artery slings are commonly associated with other intracardiac and tracheobronchial anomalies.

Diagnostic Keys

The diagnosis of a vascular ring or sling should be suspected in all neonates displaying symptoms of airway obstruction and/or dysphagia without an obvious etiology. Severe compressive symptoms (e.g., respiratory distress) may present shortly after birth. Dysphagia is usually more prominent in older children and young adults. Recurrent respiratory tract infections are also associated with this defect. Physical examination reveals sequelae of respiratory distress including tachypnea, stridor, wheezing, cyanosis, and intercostal retractions. Electrocardiography is usually normal; however, chest radiographic signs of tracheal compression or pneumonia may be seen. A barium swallow is usually diagnostic in detecting both tracheal and esophageal compression. Demonstration of posterior esophageal compression is diagnostic of a vascular ring. Anterior compression of the esophagus with posterior encroachment of the trachea is associated with a pulmonary artery sling. Computed tomography or magnetic resonance imaging studies with three-dimensional reconstructions are extremely

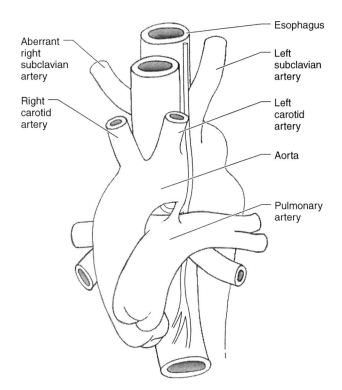

FIGURE 10–10.4. Left aortic arch with aberrant right subclavian artery. The course of the abnormal right subclavian artery crosses the midline behind the esophagus, often compressing it. (Reproduced with permission. Mainwaring RD: Tracheosophageal compressive syndromes of vascular origin. In Baue AE, et al. (eds): *Glenn's Cardiovascular and Thoracic Surgery*, 6th ed. Stamford, Appleton & Lange, 1996, p. 1097.)

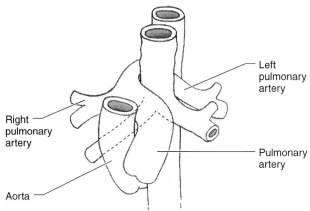

FIGURE 10–10.5. Pulmonary artery sling. The left pulmonary artery originates from the right pulmonary artery instead of the main pulmonary artery and passes between the trachea and esophagus, resulting in posterior tracheal compression. (Reproduced with permission. Mainwaring RD: Tracheoesophageal compressive syndromes of vascular origin. In Baue AE, et al. (eds): *Glenn's Cardiovascular and Thoracic Surgery*, 6th ed. Stamford, Appleton & Lange, 1996. p. 1098.)

accurate in demonstrating the anatomic configuration of the ring or sling. Fiberoptic bronchoscopy should be used to look for tracheomalacia or other tracheobronchial malformations, particularly in the cases of pulmonary artery slings. Echocardiography can identify abnormal arch anatomy and associated intracardiac defects but has limited utility in defining the anatomy of these lesions clearly. Angiography is usually performed for diagnostic confirmation and surgical planning.

Operative Correction

Patients diagnosed with vascular rings or slings who experience tracheal and/or esophageal compressive symptoms should undergo operative correction. Elective repair may be warranted in all cases of complete rings (i.e., double aortic arch and right aortic arch/left ligamentum arteriosum) to prevent progressive airway injury over time. Patients with asymptomatic incomplete rings may be managed expec-

tantly. Most arch anomalies may be approached through a left posterolateral thoracotomy in the fourth intercostal space. Median sternotomy may be necessary if any concomitant intracardiac repair is required.

The overall goal of operative repair is to divide the compressive vascular ring, relieve tracheoesophageal compression, and maintain normal perfusion of the aortic arch. In most cases, operative correction is performed through a left posterolateral thoracotomy at the fourth intercostal space without cardiopulmonary bypass.

Double aortic arch repair involves division of the smaller of the two arches at its narrowest point; in most cases, this will be the left (anterior) aortic arch. Through a left posterolateral thoracotomy, the left lung is retracted anteriorly, and the double arch is identifed through the mediastinal pleura (Fig. 10–10.6). The pleura overlying the arch to be divided is incised and reflected. Identification of the arch and arch vessels is facilitated by test occlusion and measurement of distal arterial pressures. If the left (anterior) arch is to be divided, it is divided between the left common carotid and descending aorta. If the right (posterior) arch is to be divided, it is divided between the right common carotid and the descending aorta. The segment to be divided is controlled with vascular clamps and transected at its narrowest point. The cut ends are then oversewn with a continuous Prolene™ suture line. The ligamentum arteriosum is also divided. The operation is concluded by reapproximating the incised

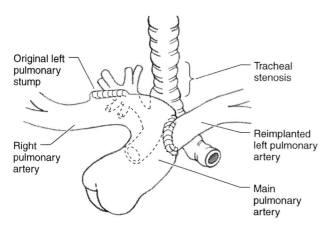

FIGURE 10–10.6. Traditional repair of a pulmonary artery sling. This repair involves division of the left pulmonary artery at its origin from the right pulmonary artery and its translocation anterior to the trachea with anastomosis to the main pulmonary artery. (Reproduced with permission. Castaneda AR, et al: Vascular rings, slings, and tracheal anomalies. In: *Cardiac Surgery of the Neonate and Infant*, Philadelphia, W.B. Saunders, 1994, p. 405.)

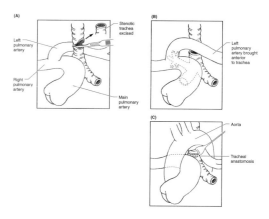

FIGURE 10–10.7. Modified pulmonary artery sling repair. *(A, B)* Because of the high incidence of tracheomalacia at the site of the vascular sling, an alternative approach is to perform a segmental resection of the stenotic trachea and anterior translocation of the left pulmonary artery. *(C)* This is followed by a primary anastomosis of the trachea posterior to the left pulmonary artery. (Reproduced with permission. Castaneda AR, et al: Vascular rings, slings, and tracheal anomalies. In: *Cardiac Surgery of the Neonate and Infant*, Philadelphia, W.B. Saunders, 1994, p. 406.)

mediastinal pleura, placing a thoracostomy tube, and closing the thoracotomy in routine fashion.

Right aortic arch/left ligamentum arteriosum correction simply involves division of the ligamentum arteriosum.

The technique of left aortic arch repairs is contingent on the vascular aberrancy. An aberrant right subclavian artery can be corrected with transection at its origin or transection and reimplantation, depending on the extent of collateral blood supply to the right arm. A compressive anomalous innominate artery may be corrected by anterior suspension of the aorta by tacking it to the posterior table of the sternum to relieve anterior tracheal compression.

Traditional repair of a pulmonary artery sling involves division of the left pulmonary artery at its origin from the right pulmonary artery and its translocation anterior to the trachea with anastomosis to the main pulmonary artery (Fig. 10–10.7). Because of the high incidence of tracheomalacia at the site of the vascular sling, an alternative approach is to perform a segmental tracheal resection with primary anastomosis of the trachea posterior to the left pulmonary artery (Fig. 10–10.7). Both procedures are performed via a median sternotomy or left thoracotomy under cardiopulmonary bypass.

Meticulous attention to postoperative respiratory care, including pulmonary toilet is essential. The effects of tracheal edema and tracheomalacia due to prolonged tracheal compression warrants cautious extubation. Operative correction of vascular rings and slings is associated with a low operative mortality and good long-term relief of compressive symptoms. Most morbidity and mortality is associated with the degree of tracheal maldevelopment.

Reference

1. LOWER RR, SHUMNAY NE. Studies on the orthotopic homotransplantation of the canine heart. *Surgical Forum* 1960;11:18.

PART 3

Postoperative Management in the Neonatal/Pediatric Intensive Care Unit

CHAPTER 11

Postoperative Care of the Neonate/Infant After Cardiac Surgery

Nancy A. Pike, RN, MN, FNP and Daniel A. Falco, MD

Introduction

The postoperative management of neonates/infants following cardiac surgery requires a technically skilled and knowledgeable multidisciplinary team in the intensive care unit (ICU). The trend toward earlier surgical correction versus palliation in the neonate and low birth weight infant has led to greater postoperative challenges, partly because of a significantly decreased threshold for human error. Longer cardiopulmonary bypass (CBP) times, myocardial/renal dysfunction, and the potential for profound bleeding diathesis may occur. The "single ventricle" requires an additional level of ICU expertise in balancing the pulmonary to systemic flow ratio in the postoperative period. Successful postoperative management of neonates and infants with congenital heart disease (CHD) depends on the combination of early preoperative stabilization, excellent surgical intervention, and an experienced ICU team.

This chapter was designed only as a brief overview of the postoperative management of those afflicted with CHD. Single ventricle physiology, pulmonary hypertension, mechanical ventilation, hemostasis and coagulation, electrolyte abnormalities, the surgical stress response, and nutritional support are covered.

Postoperative Management

The initiation of postoperative ICU management begins with a "report" from the operating room. The details of the surgical repair must include the anatomy, intraoperative hemodynamics, and an honest evaluation of the quality of the repair (i.e., any residual intracardiac shunts and/or stenosis, quality of repaired valvular function), including surgical arrhythmias, heart block, and overall ventricular function.

Intraoperative assessment by transesophageal echocardiography (TEE) and direct saturation and pressure measurements provide most of the needed information. With this knowledge at hand, the ICU team can anticipate further potential problems and develop a patient-specific plan of care.

Prompt evaluation of the initial postoperative chest x-ray can rule out any immediate problems such as a hydropneumothorax, a misplaced endotrachial tube, and/or an intravascular line.

The initial neonatal/infant assessment plan is thus based on the postoperative surgical physiology (i.e., an in-series versus an in-parallel circulation) or anatomy (i.e., single, one and one-half, or biventricular repair). Integration of the history, physical examination, noninvasive and invasive data, and biochemical data remains essential in the evaluation of the adequacy of oxygen delivery and end-organ function.

Noninvasive Monitoring

Noninvasive monitoring includes pulse oximetry, central and peripheral temperatures, and surface electrocardiographic (ECG) monitoring.

Pulse oximetry remains a vital noninvasive assessment of arterial oxygen saturation. Noninvasive monitoring is highly sensitive, and any dramatic changes should not be assumed to be inaccuracies or artifacts.

An increase in core temperature and decrease in peripheral temperature suggests inadequate cardiac output. These temperatures should be monitored for the first 48 to 72 hours after surgery.

The ECG provides heart rate and rhythm changes that remain critical for optimal cardiac output in the neonate, since neonatal stroke volume remains quite limited. Arrhythmias of junctional ectopic tachycardia (JET) and heart block can significantly alter cardiac output in the neonate. Bipolar atrial and ventricular temporary epicardial pacing wires are frequently placed. The epicardial wires can be utilized to diagnose the arrhythmia (an atrial ECG) and provide a more specific intervention to treat the arrhythmia (see Chap. 12).

Invasive Monitoring

Invasive monitoring in infants remains challenging and is not without the risks of infection and/or thrombosis. Central venous monitoring can be accomplished by either the percutaneous or direct transthoracic routes. If pulmonary arterial or left atrial pressures are necessary, the direct transthoracic approach is used.

The left atrial line can provide information relating to relevant mitral valve function, pulmonary shunting, and systemic ventricular function. Meticulous surveillance for air in the left and right atrial lines in infants with an atrial communication remains essential for the prevention of direct or paradoxical air emboli, respectively. A direct pulmonary artery line is usually placed in those at risk for pulmonary hypertension (PHTN), necessitating aggressive medical management including the possible use of nitric oxide (see section on PHTN, below).

Cardiac output measurements to assess cardiac function and oxygen delivery are not routinely performed in infants with CHD. Mixed venous oxygen saturation trends or $S\dot{V}O_2$ monitoring can provide assistance in assessing the adequacy of peripheral oxygen delivery. When such delivery is inadequate, metabolic and lactic acidosis occurs, requiring sodium bicarbonate administration and an alteration in the heart rate, preload, contractility, and afterload.

Serum lactate levels can also be utilized to assess adequacy of oxygen delivery. The lactate level is normally elevated by 6 to 10 mmol/L after circulatory arrest or deep hypothermia but should decrease to less than 2.0 mmol/L with adequate oxygenation and improved tissue perfusion. Most neonates require some inotropic support after cardiac surgery. Multiple pharmacologic agents may be utilized depending on the extent of the surgical repair and myocardial reserve. Escalation of inotropic agents may be needed in the first 10 to 24 postoperative hours due to myocardial edema and decreased ventricular function. Dopamine, epinephrine, calcium, and amrinone are commonly used agents. Physical assessment of cardiac function should be routinely practiced by assessing the distal extremity temperature, color, and capillary refill.

Left ventricular (LV) dysfunction is less common than right ventricular (RV) dysfunction in the neonate/infant, perhaps because the RV is more commonly abnormal. LV dysfunction would most likely be seen in correction of left-sided or septal lesions, i.e., multiple ventricular septal defects (VSDs), anomalous origin/course of the coronary arteries, or inadequate myocardial "protection." Optimizing heart rate and stroke volume can improve cardiac output. Cardiac pacing can be utilized to optimize heart rate. Stroke volume can be manipulated by augmenting preload (left arterial pressure [LAP] 8 to 10 mm Hg), and contractility can be managed with the use of inotropic/afterload support and/or calcium supplementation.

Mechanical ventilation needs to be carefully managed in order to optimize the cardiorespiratory system (see mechanical ventilation section below). Echocardiographic data can be utilized to assess LV function and rule out pericardial effusion and/or cardiac tamponade. When medical management of LV dysfunction fails, mechanical support from a left ventricular assist device (LVAD) or extracorporeal membrane oxygenation (ECMO) may need to be utilized as a lifesaving measure.

RV dysfunction is commonly seen in the hypertrophied ventricle that must bear a volume load following a period of pressure loading (i.e., tetralogy of Fallot with pulmonary insufficiency). The RV remains a "volume-loaded ventricle," and thus optimizing preload (right arterial pressure [RAP] < 15 mm Hg) remains critical. Alterations of afterload (pulmonary hypertension) may need to be addressed. Leaving the sternum open remains helpful in those with situs solitus, as the RV remains an anterior structure, easily compressed by the confines of the thorax. An "open" chest allows an increase in diastolic volume and reduces the effects of positive pressure ventilation.

Urinary output is an indirect indicator of end-organ function. Neonates can often have a 24 to 48 hour period of oliguria after a long CPB with or without circulatory arrest. Infants usually have a prompt diuresis of 1 ml/kg/hr or greater in the initial postoperative period usually due to an osmotic diuresis caused by hyperglycemia, stress response, intraoperative volume, a mannitol "pump prime," and diuretic administration.[1,2] After the initial 6 to 8 hours, urine output will decrease significantly, and diffuse lung and soft tissue edema may occur due to capillary leaking associated with endothelial damage by exposure to CPB. An assessment of the infant's volume status and optimizing cardiac function should always be evaluated with decreased urine output. Dopamine at 3 to 5 mcq/kg/min can also be utilized to improve renal blood flow and possibly increase urine output. Diuretic therapy is usually started on the first postoperative day with a test dose of furosemide (1 mg/kg). Neonates may take longer to excrete excess fluid due to lower glomerular filtration rate (GFR) in the immature kidney.[3] This also causes a decreased rate of drug metabolism and excretion. The use of a continuous furosemide infusion instead of intermittent bolus therapy allows for fewer fluctuations in electrolyte balance and undesirable hemodynamic instability with bolus administration.[4,5]

Single Ventricle Physiology

The postoperative management of the neonate with single ventricle physiology after first stage palliation is similar to the preoperative stabilization with an open ductus arteriosus. First-stage palliation varies depending on anatomy and consists of either a pulmonary artery band (nonrestricted pulmonary blood flow), or a Blalock-Taussig (BT) or central shunt (ductal dependent lesions or restricted pulmonary blood flow). Rarely is the circulation perfectly balanced. A Q_p/Q_s of 1:1 is vital for a successful outcome in children with single ventricles.

The goal of postoperative management is the maintenance of the pulmonary and systemic blood flow in order to achieve a Q_p/Q_s of 1:1, thus avoiding coronary or mesenteric insufficiency. The pulmonary vascular resistance (PVR) will normally drop by the fifth to seventh days of life. Timing of surgery is usually based on a drop in PVR by observing an increase in oxygen saturation and pulmonary overcirculation noted on clinical assessment and chest x-ray. Manipulating the PVR with ventilatory adjustments is usually attempted first. Overcirculation requires rapid intervention due to inadequate tissue perfusion producing a metabolic acidosis and low cardiac output state or shock. A 3.0–4.0-mm GoreTex tube is commonly utilized as a conduit to augment pulmonary blood flow. A 3.0-mm shunt is frequently too large for the premature or low birth weight infant. With pulmonary overcirculation (systemic arterial oxygen saturations > 85%), measures to increase the PVR by sedation and paralysis, hypoventilation, and supplemental nitrogen can be used to increase the PVR. Selectively decreasing the systemic vascular resistance (SVR) by reducing α-agonists and stimulating β-agonists can sometimes be helpful. Hemoconcentration (Hct > 40 g/dl) can help by increasing the viscosity of the blood through the small shunt. Inhaled CO_2 administered through the ventilator can also be utilized to produce hypercarbia and a resulting respiratory acidosis. The potential advantage to inhaled CO_2 is that respiratory acidosis can be induced without the use of severe hypoventilation, which may produce atelectasis. As a last resort, partial occlusion of the shunt with a titanium clip may be required if medical management fails to reduce overcirculation. The clip can usually be removed 1 to 3 days postoperatively once hemodynamic stability has been achieved.

With a decrease in the pulmonary circulation (systemic oxygen saturations < 70%), ventilator adjustments are needed to decrease PVR. A chest x-ray should be obtained, to assess first endotracheal tube (ETT) placement and the presence of a pleural effusion or pulmonary parenchymal disease. The neonate should be auscultated daily for the presence of a continuous shunt murmur at the right or left upper sternal boarder. All patients with modified BT shunts (GoreTex) are placed on aspirin (10 mg/kg/dose) daily to reduce the risk of platelet aggregation and subsequent shunt thrombosis. The neonate may also have an anatomic source for pulmonary undercirculation. Too small a shunt or narrowing at the proximal or distal anastomotic site are the most frequent causes. This produces a resistance to flow relative to the fourth power along with hyperviscosity in a linear fashion.

The assessment of low cardiac output in the neonate with clinical signs of tachycardia, hypotension, oliguria, and metabolic acidosis needs to be critically evaluated. A decrease in ventricular output (primary pump or low output failure), excessive maldistribution of blood flows with an elevated Q_p/Q_s (high output failure), or atrioventricular (AV) valve failure producing a (backwards) failure may be present. Coronary ischemia must be ruled out in those children with aortic atresia/mitral atresia or stenosis. The cause for low cardiac output in the single ventricle neonate can be determined by using the same approach as noted above, i.e., invasive/noninvasive monitoring, clinical exam, and laboratory data to decide on the most appropriate treatment.

Pulmonary Hypertension

In the fetus, pulmonary and systemic pressures are equal, due to the ductus arteriosus. After birth, the ductus arteriosus normally closes at around 24 to 72 hours of age. The pulmonary arterial pressure decreases to half the systemic arterial pressure and continues to decrease over the next 3 to 6 months when the PVR reaches adult levels. Ventilation and oxygenation are utilized at birth to decrease PVR. The clinical conditions of respiratory distress syndrome, meconium aspiration, congenital diaphragmatic hernia, sepsis, PHTN, and congenital heart defects with large communications at the ventricular or great vessel level can alter the natural progression in the reduction of PVR. The mechanism for a delay in reduction of PVR in the presence of increased blood flow is unclear. Endothelial injury secondary to increased pulmonary blood flow or pressure may contribute to PVR changes and the development of PHTN probably due to an alteration in the balance of endothelin-1 versus nitric oxide synthetase.[6]

Neonates with preoperative increased pulmonary blood flow and pressure are at risk for PHTN postoperatively. Congenital heart defects at risk for PHTN crisis postoperatively are large VSD, complete AV canal, truncus arteriosus, large patent ductus arteriosus or aortopulmonary window, D-transposition of the great arteries, and total anomalous venous return.

PHTN is demonstrated by an increase in pulmonary artery pressure, increased right heart pressure, RV dysfunction, decreased cardiac output, and decreased oxygen delivery producing a metabolic acidosis. Infants at risk for PHTN should be identified on arrival to the ICU and preventive therapy should be initiated. Stimulation such as hypoxia, hypothermia, hypoglycemia, pain, and tracheal stimulation should be avoided. Appropriate sedation and analgesia should be initiated with continuous infusions of opioids (fentanyl) and benzodiazepine (midazolam). Studies have suggested that suppressing the intraoperative stress response by administration of high-dose narcotics can reduce postoperative complications in the pulmonary circulation and thus potentially the mortality.[7,8] Neuromuscular blockade with pancuronium or vecuronium can be added for infants who are sensitive to changes in pattern of ventilation or changes in partial pressure of arterial CO_2 ($PaCO_2$). This will allow more control of PVR through mechanical ventilation and minimize rapid changes due to coughing or straining.

Ventilatory strategies include increasing alveolar and arterial oxygen by increasing Fraction of inspired oxygen (FIO_2) and positive pressure ventilation, alkalinization with bicarbonate administration, decreasing $PaCO_2$ with a low ventilator rate (15–20 bpm), high tidal volume (15 to 20 ml/kg), and decreasing mean airway pressure with low positive end-expiratory pressure (PEEP; <4 cm H_2O) and ventilatory rate. The goal in reducing PVR is to achieve a pH > 7.50 while maintaining normal serum bicarbonate levels, increasing partial pressure of arterial O_2 (PaO_2) and PAO_2, decreasing $PaCO_2$ (to 25 to 30 mm Hg), and minimizing intrathoracic pressures. The postoperative chest x-ray should be evaluated to assess for pneumothoraces and pleural effusions, which can increase intrathoracic pressures and PVR. High-frequency ventilation is a nonconventional mode of mechanical ventilation that can be utilized to maintain oxygenation and gas exchange by attempting to reduce the peak and mean airway pressures when conventional ventilation fails.

Cardiovascular strategies to decrease pulmonary artery pressures and improve RV function involve increasing preload (RA 10 to 12 mm Hg) and contractility. Increasing contractility with inotropic support such as dopamine and epinephrine has limited effectiveness due to the insensitivity of the RV to inotropes and not treating the primary problem of reducing RV afterload. Amrinone (phosphodiesterase inhibitor) can be utilized to reduce RV afterload by decreasing the PVR and SVR while increasing cardiac output. A variety of other vasodilators have been used to reduce PVR and treat postoperative pulmonary hypertension such as sodium nitroprusside, nitroglycerin, prostaglandin E_1 (PGE_1), and prostacyclin (PGI_2) but not without systemic vasodilating effects.

The only true selective pulmonary vasodilator that can be utilized when medical management fails is inhaled nitric oxide (NO). NO is an endothelium-derived relaxing factor administered as an inhaled gas that causes rapid pulmonary vasodilation with no systemic effects. NO is commonly used in a last attempt to reduce PVR prior to the initiation of ECMO in the unstable neonate not able to be weaned from

CPB. NO should be administered under institutional protocols because administration errors may produce potentially lethal methemoglobin formation. NO is usually started at 5 ppm and increased to 20 or 80 ppm, while observing for responses, which include a reduction in PA pressures (transthoracic line), increase in PaO_2, or increase in oxygen saturation. The postoperative administration of NO can also be utilized as a diagnostic tool to rule out PHTN versus a structural abnormality requiring surgical intervention.

Mechanical Ventilation

The removal of CO_2 and the replenishment of oxygen to the bloodstream should be treated independently. Minute ventilation is the product of tidal volume (TV) and respiratory rate (RR). Adequate minute ventilation is assessed via the measurement of the $PaCO_2$. A normal spontaneous tidal volume is approximately 3 to 5 ml/kg. A normal mechanical ventilator tidal volume is approximately 6 to 12 ml/kg. The normal respiratory rate remains dependent on a patient's age (Table 11–1). With inadequate ventilation (i.e., $PaCO_2$ higher or lower than desired), one can manipulate either the TV or RR. Deciding which to change is patient dependent. To assess whether or not a given tidal volume is optimal, one must evaluate the patient's chest wall movement, auscultate both lung fields, and assess the degree of lung expansion on chest x-ray.

Oxygenation of the blood depends on multiple factors, including the delivery of oxygen to the lungs, the ability of the lung to transfer oxygen into the bloodstream (diffusion capacity), and the degree of intracardiac and/or intrapulmonary shunting of blood from the right side to the left side of the heart. One can quantify/monitor the amount of shunt via multiple mechanisms: calculating the alveolar to arterial O_2 gradient (A-a gradient), the oxygenation index (OI), or the shunt flow (Q_s/Q_t).

Adequate oxygenation is assessed through the measurement of the PaO_2. Determining optimal oxygenation is dependent on the patient's cardiac anatomy and the type of repair. In ductal dependent cardiac lesions (i.e., tetralogy of Fallot with PA and single ventricle defects), increasing PaO_2 will increase blood flow to the lungs at the expense of critically limiting the systemic blood supply. To optimize

TABLE 11–1. Range of Normal Respiratory Rates for Age

Newborn	30–50
6 months	20–40
1–2 years	20–30
2–6 years	15–25
>6 years	13–20

Source: From Blumer J., *A Practice Guide to Pediatric Intensive Care.* 3rd ed. St. Louis: Mosby-Year Book; 1990.

oxygenation, one can change the F_{IO_2} or alter the amount of lung that is available for oxygen exchange through the manipulation of the mean airway pressure. Deciding which to change is patient dependent. One must always keep in mind that changes in the mean airway pressure can have serious consequences on cardiac output. The latter is especially true in right-sided versus left-sided lesions, particularly when the pulmonary valve remains incompetent.

Respiratory Care for Infants Returning Extubated to the ICU

The evaluation of an extubated infant returning to the pediatric ICU after cardiac surgery includes assessing the adequacy of the airway and breathing. This includes a visual assessment of the level of sedation and the work of breathing, listening for noisy breathing or stridor, and auscultation of the lung fields.

The infant's level of sedation includes knowing the amount of sedation/analgesia an infant received during surgery and determining the stimulation required to arouse the infant. If the infant is under sedation, the crying can produce PHTN, and struggling places an added stress upon the heart. Oversedation can lead to apnea and depressed cardiac output and can cause the posterior oropharynx to become floppy and obstruct breathing.

The assessment of the work of breathing includes determining the RR (Table 11–1), evaluating the infant for grunting, flaring, or retractions, and ascertaining the adequacy of chest wall movement. Keep in mind that a fatiguing infant will have a decreasing respiratory rate, spells of apnea, and decreased level of consciousness. A restless infant must always be assessed for hypoxemia and not assumed to be undersedated.

Noisy breathing or stridor is a symptom of upper airway narrowing or obstruction. Resistance in a tube is proportional to the length and radius of the tube. Infants have a small diameter airway to begin with, and even a small amount of swelling in the upper airway can significantly increase the resistance and make breathing more difficult. When auscultating an infant's lungs, one must ensure adequate air exchange in both lung fields and listen for wheezes/crackles. Mucus plugging and pneumothoraces are not infrequent complications following cardiac surgery. Tracheobronchomalacia may be a concomitant finding in those infants with vascular ring, pulmonary sling, or abnormal distal pulmonary arterial arborization. Recurrent laryngeal nerve palsy should be suspected if the findings are new following a left thorocotomy or arch reconstruction.

If ventilation is determined to be inadequate, one needs to determine the cause. If swelling in the airway is the reason, one can optimize the position of the infant's head, consider a trial of nebulized racemic epinephrine (if not contraindicated), attempt heliox, or administer steroids. Nasal

trumpets in the infant are difficult to keep patent because of their small size. If the patient has a family history of asthma or wheezing, consider nebulized albuterol. If the infant is oversedated, consider a small dose of naloxone HCl (1 to 5 mcq/kg) or flumazenil. Nasal continuous positive airway pressure (nasal CPAP) should be considered before reintubating the trachea. If nasal CPAP is used, remember that it often fills the stomach with air and a nasogastric tube should be placed to decompress the stomach.

If oxygenation is determined to be inadequate, one must determine etiology. A thorough physical exam should exclude most significant cases of pnuemothorax or pleural effusion. The postoperative chest x-ray should always be reviewed to eliminate these causes. The chest x-ray will also help to determine the presence of atelectasis, pulmonary edema, or other lung pathology not recognized preoperatively. Persistent intracardiac shunts should be considered, and an echocardiogram should be obtained if other reasons for arterial oxygen desaturations are not found. Treatment depends on the etiology and severity of the pathology.

One can increase the F_{IO_2} through a variety of oxygen-delivery devices including blow-by oxygen, nasal cannula, face mask, or oxygen tents; all of these deliver a varying quantity of oxygen. If a proper workup is not undertaken to determine the etiology of the arterial oxygen desaturation, simply delivering a higher F_{IO_2} can delay the treatment of the underlying pathology.

Respiratory Care for Infants Returning Intubated to the ICU

The initial evaluation of an intubated infant returning to the pediatric ICU after cardiac surgery includes assessing the adequacy of the airway and breathing. This includes an assessment of the level of sedation and the work of breathing, ensuring that the ETT is properly sized and positioned, auscultation of the lung fields, and making certain the mechanical ventilator is properly set up.

Evaluating an infant's level of sedation includes knowing the amount of sedation/analgesia an infant received during surgery and determining the stimulation required to arouse the infant. If the infant is undersedated, the crying and struggling can produce PHTN, which places an added stress on the heart. Furthermore, it is very difficult for a mechanical ventilator to synchronize its breaths with a struggling infant. Oversedation can lead to depressed cardiac output.

The assessment of the work of breathing includes determining the patient's RR (Table 11–1), assessing the infant for flaring or retractions, and ascertaining the adequacy of chest wall movement. Patients returning intubated to the pediatric ICU should not be working hard to breath; the mechanical ventilator should provide most of the work of breathing.

TABLE 11–2.   Endotracheal Tube Sizes[a]

Age Group	Size	Oral Length (cm)	Suction Catheter
Newborn		11–12	
<1.0 kg	2.5		—
1–2 kg	3.0		6
>2 kg	3.5		8
1–6 months	3.5	12–13	8
1 year	4.0	13	8–10
2–3 years	4.5	15	8–10
4–5 years	5.0	16	10
6–7 years	5.5	18	10
8–9 years	6.0	20	10
10–11 years	6.5	22	10
12–13 years	7.0	22	10
14–15 years	7.5	24	10

[a]External diameter of a *cuffed* tube is equivalent to an uncuffed tube of 1/2 size larger, i.e., 5.0 cuffed = 5.5 uncuffed.
Source: From Blumer J., *A Practice Guide to Pediatric Intensive Care.* 3rd ed. St. Louis: Mosby-Year Book; 1990.

Ensuring the proper placement of an ETT begins with noting the size of the tube and the depth of its insertion. The appropriate size of an infant's uncuffed ETT depends on age (Table 11–2). A half size smaller or larger is generally acceptable, but proper assessment includes determining the amount of leak around the ETT. This is ascertained by using a self-inflating anesthesia bag connected to a manometer and the ETT. The pressure in the ETT is slowly increased while the practitioner auscultates the anterior neck and notes the pressure at which a leak of air is first heard. All infants and neonates should have a leak at pressures between 10 and 30 mm Hg. A leak beginning below 10 mm Hg indicates that the ETT is too small and that a significant amount of ventilation may be lost around the tube. If no leak is heard at a pressure > 35 mm Hg, the tube may be too large for the airway, which can lead to irritation of the tracheal mucosa. This can produce swelling or damage to the upper airway. Factors to consider when deciding to change an improperly sized ETT are the amount of time an infant is expected to be intubated, the level of difficulty in ventilating or oxygenating the patient, and the stability of the patient.

The optimal depth of insertion of an ETT is approximately 1 cm above the carina. The depth of insertion of an orotracheal tube should be roughly three times the inner diameter, in millimeters, of the ETT. Confirming the depth of the ETT by chest x-ray is an important part of the initial assessment.

When auscultating an intubated infant's lungs, one must ensure adequate air exchange in both lung fields and listen for wheezes/crackles. Unequal breath sounds can be a sign of a right main stem intubation, mucus plugging, and/or pneumothoraces, which are not infrequent complications following cardiac surgery. Poor or no breath sounds may be a sign of an obstructed or dislodged ETT, pneumothorax, or equipment failure. Wheezes may be a sign of bronchospasm or pulmonary edema.

Ensuring that the mechanical ventilator has been properly set up includes determining the mode of ventilation, the FIO_2, the RR of the mechanical ventilator, PEEP, pressure support (PS), and the inspiratory time (I-time).

The monitoring of the intubated patient for adequacy of ventilation and oxygenation includes arterial blood gas (ABG) measurements, noninvasive CO_2 monitors, and continuous pulse oximetry. ABGs are considered the gold standard for determining the sufficiency of ventilation and oxygenation. Because of the expense and quantity of blood required for regular ABGs, noninvasive measurements of $PaCO_2$ and oxygenation are often employed.

The two means of following CO_2 noninvasively are the end-tidal and transcutaneous monitors. If calibrated properly and checked for accuracy with an ABG, these can be helpful in following trends without having to obtain regular ABGs. If there is a significant change in either of these CO_2 monitors, one should first check to ensure that the patient is still receiving adequate ventilation and then check an ABG.

Noninvasive measurements of O_2 saturation include the continuous pulse oximeter. This measures the percentage of hemoglobin that is saturated with oxygen. Oxygen saturation and partial pressure of O_2 are related. When O_2 saturations are <90%, a small change in O_2 saturation can mean large PaO_2 changes.

The decision of when to wean an infant from mechanical ventilation is made in concert with the cardiac surgery team, is multifactorial, and is beyond the scope of this chapter. Once the decision has been made to wean the patient to extubation, several factors need to be considered. The physician should ensure that no invasive procedure is scheduled for later in the day that will require significant sedation. Air leak should once again be evaluated, and a trial of steroids should be considered 6 to 8 hours before attempting extubation in any patient without an air leak at >30 cm H_2O. The amount of secretions should be determined. If secretions are excessive and thin, one can consider a trial of glycopyrrolate. If secretions are excessive and thick, one should consider waiting to extubate the infant pending a workup for pneumonia, realizing that it is difficult for infants to cough up secretions on their own. Frequently, a nasopharyngeal swab may elucidate an infectious element such as adenovirus or respiratory syncytial virus (RSV). The level of consciousness should be addressed, and analgesic/sedation drugs should be decreased 1 to 2 hours prior to extubation if possible. Feeds should be held 4 hours prior to extubation to ensure an empty stomach if reintubation is necessary.

How to wean an infant from mechanical ventilation is as much style as science. One usually decreases the mechanical ventilator's minute ventilation by alternately decreasing the TV and RR. The rate of ventilator weaning is dependent on how well the patient tolerates it, which is determined by monitoring the $PaCO_2$.

One can consider extubation once mechanical ventilation and supplemental oxygen delivery are minimized. A minimal mechanical breath TV is usually 5 to 7 ml/kg. A minimized RR depends on age. It is not unusual to extubate a neonate from a mechanical RR of 12 to 20. Patients should not be requiring more than 40% FIO_2 with minimal PEEP (no greater than 5 cm H_2O).

The respiratory care of the neonate returning from cardiac surgery is a complex endeavor. Ensuring adequate ventilation and oxygenation are vital components of a successful postoperative course.

Hemostasis and Coagulation

Healthy neonates and infants up to 6 months of age have low levels of coagulation factors compared with adults. These factors reach adult levels by 6 months to 1 year of age. Coagulation factor levels are approximately 30% to 40% lower in newborns with CHD than in neonates without structural abnormalities.[9] The inhibitors of coagulation, proteins C and S and antithrombin III (AT-III), are all depressed in the neonatal period.[10] One can postulate that these low levels can be caused by impaired hepatic synthesis secondary to liver hypoperfusion. Infants at the highest risk are those with cyanotic or ductal dependent lesions, left-sided obstructive lesions, and poor cardiac output. Platelet abnormalities such as thrombocytopenia occur in one-third of children with cyanotic CHD.[11] Newborns placed on PGE[1] infusions preoperatively to maintain patency in ductal dependent lesions can have decreased platelet function by preventing activation.

The major hemostatic abnormality associated with CPB is platelet dysfunction.[12] There is a 50% to 70% reduction in circulating platelets in infants compared with adults due to hemodilution associated with high CPB priming volumes versus extracellular fluid ratios. CPB is also associated with the reduction in plasma concentrations of coagulation factors. This is also related to hemodilution. The CPB priming volume is two to three times the circulating blood volume of the neonate. The general practice for priming the CPB circuit is with whole blood or fresh frozen plasma (FFP) instead of packed red blood cells. A unit of whole blood should also be available for separation from CPB. Fresh whole blood is a more balanced product, containing red blood cells, platelets, and coagulation factors. The availability of whole blood and the timing of surgery in the neonate require cooperation from the transfusion services.

Prior to initiation of CPB, heparin is utilized to produce systemic anticoagulation. Heparin is believed to have a more prolonged effect in infants due to the decreased metabolic capability of the infant and the exposure to more profound levels of hypothermia, which also reduces heparin metabolism. Prior to CPB removal, modified ultrafiltration can be initiated in the bypass circuitry to remove excess fluid from the circulation. Protamine is utilized to neutralize heparin and restore clotting activity after CPB. Systemic hypotension from protamine administration is not as pronounced in neonates as seen in adults. The protamine dose requirement in neonates is higher than in older children due to a more pronounced heparin effect, as stated above.

Management of postoperative bleeding in the neonate can be extremely challenging. The differentiation of medical versus surgical bleeding can be difficult. Bleeding >10% of circulating blood volume per hour or >3 to 5 ml/kg in 3 consecutive hours, despite adequate heparin reversal and factor replacement, usually requires surgical reexploration. It remains critically important during periods of component replacement that adequate ionized calcium levels be obtained due to chelation of calcium with the citrated preservative in FFP, cryoprecipitate, and even albumin. Infants and neonates have a multifactorial coagulation defect with a severe reduction in factor activity and platelet number and function compared with adult patients. Restoration of normothermia and the use of fresh whole blood (<48 hours old) after CPB has been associated with a significant reduction in postoperative bleeding compared with component therapy in neonates.[13] Optimal hematocrit levels are individually based on patient age, preoperative hematocrit, surgical correction versus palliation, and postoperative myocardial function. Neonates undergoing palliation or with moderate to severe myocardial dysfunction usually benefit from hematocrits levels around 40% to assist with oxygen-carrying capacity in the postoperative period. Neonates with physiologic correction and good myocardial function postoperatively can tolerate lower hematocrit levels of around 30% to 35%. Similarly, a neonate with a biventricular repair can tolerate a lower Hct than those neonates with a single ventricle repair.

Pharmacologic agents utilized to improve hemostasis following CPB are antifibrinolytic drugs such as epsilon aminocaproic acid and transexamic acid. Aprotinin is a serine protease inhibitor that binds to and inactivates various enzymes involved in coagulation. These drugs have been shown to have some benefit in decreasing bleeding in adults, with varying results in children.[14,15] Further investigation in infants and the pediatric use of pharmacologic agents following CPB will need to be evaluated.

Children can sometimes have a reaction to heparin both preoperatively and postoperatively. Heparin-induced thrombocytopenia (HIT) is a rare complication of heparin therapy in the preoperative or postoperative period. The incidence of HIT in children is presumably less than that in adults (0.5% to 5%). HIT is an idiosyncratic, antibody-mediated reaction that occurs within 6 to 12 days of heparin administration. The clinical signs are thrombocytopenia and thrombosis with increasing heparin requirements.

Electrolyte Abnormalities

Electrolyte abnormalities are common in the initial postoperative period. The severity of the abnormalities depends on the intraoperative stability of the infant. Initial fluids utilized are 10% dextrose with one-quarter normal saline at two-thirds maintenance for neonates and 5% dextrose with one-quarter normal saline at two-thirds maintenance for older children. Once oliguria has resolved or an improvement in urine output is seen, then potassium can be added to the solution. The dextrose concentration can be increased as needed after the glucose has stabilized post CPB.

Hypokalemia is treated with intravenous potassium chloride supplimentation (0.5 mEq/kg) over 1 hour via a central venous line. The goal is to maintain a normal serum K^+ level (3.5 to 4.5 mEq/L). Very few hemodynamic effects are seen in infants with hypokalemia, but the effects of hyperkalemia can produce significant mortality and morbidity. Hyperkalemia should be verified by repeating the test to confirm the value and then removing all potassium in the intravenous fluids. The ECG monitor should be inspected for the peaked T wave commonly seen with hyperkalemia. Glucose (2 to 4 ml/kg of 25% dextrose) and insulin (0.1 to 0.3 U/kg of regular insulin) can be administered to reduce K^+ acutely along with sodium polystyrene sulfonate (1 g/kg) every 6 hours rectally or via a nasogastric tube and diuretics (furosemide 1 to 2 mg/kg IV). Calcium chloride (10% 10 to 20 mg/kg IV) and sodium bicarbonate (1 to 2 mEq/kg IV) can be used to generate an alkalemia and redistribute K^+ into the cells. If hyperkalemia and oliguria is present intraoperatively, a peritoneal dialysis catheter is usually placed and allowed to drain by gravity unless it is needed for dialysis when the above treatments have failed.

Hypocalcemia is seen in neonates due to decreased myocardial storage in the immature heart, difficulty buffering the changes in ionized serum calcium when giving citrated blood products, dilution on CPB, and respiratory alkalosis. Hypocalcemia is also associated with DiGeorge anomaly, which is a congenital parathyroid insufficiency, or thymic hypoplasia/aplasia. This is seen in conotruncal defects and aortic arch anomalies such as tetralogy of Fallot, interrupted aortic arch (type B), truncus arteriosus, right-sided aortic arch, aberrant right subclavian artery, and some high ventricular septal defects. These infants require frequent intravenous calcium chloride supplementation and ultimately may need a continuous calcium infusion until conversion to oral supplementation. Calcium chloride (10% 10 to 20 mg/kg IV) is administered to achieve a normal serum ionized Ca^{2+} level (1.10 to 1.30 mmol/L). Calcium is an excellent positive inotrope in the neonate with postoperative systolic dysfunction. Hypercalcemia is very rare and is usually related to excessive calcium supplementation.

Surgical Stress Response

The metabolic response to the stress of surgery and critical illness is the secretion of the counterregulatory hormones (cortisol, glucagon, catecholamines, growth hormones) and the inhibiting of insulin secretion, which may facilitate postoperative catabolism and substrate mobilization from energy stores.[18,19] The infant is poorly equipped to respond to the severe catabolic processes that accompany surgery and critical illness, partly because of a modest reserve of carbohydrates, fat, and protein in a state of enormous utilization to support growth, thermoregulation, and organ maturation. The neonatal hormonal and metabolic manifestations of the stress response during cardiac surgery and in the postoperative period can be suppressed by high-dose opioid administration.[1] The brief duration of the infant stress response can be managed by a continuous intervenous narcotic infusion alone or in combination with local anesthetics during the initial 24-hour postoperative period. Some research has demonstrated that the postoperative stress response can be affected by the route of opioid administration. Epidural administration has been shown to decrease cortisol, norepinephrine, and vasopressin responses more than parenteral administration.[16,17] The anesthetic control of the stress response intraoperatively and in the first 24 postoperative hours can decrease catabolism and improves postoperative mortality and morbidity.[20]

Nutritional Support

Nutritional requirements after cardiac surgery are greatly affected by the patient's presurgical status and age, as well as the nature of the stress response to surgery and CPB. Nutritional support initially after cardiac surgery is usually 5% to 10% dextrose with electrolytes. Surgical procedure (palliation or complete repair), age, and postoperative stability are factors affecting timing of initiation of nutritional support. Feedings are usually started once bowel sounds have resumed and the infant is stabilized after surgery. The use of enteral, parenteral, or a combination of both forms of nutrition are evaluated per individual. Enteral feedings in infants with significant diastolic runoff, i.e., patent ductus arteriosus or AP window, are often withheld early in the postoperative period due to the fear of necrotizing enterocolitis. This diagnosis should be considered in any infant with postoperative abdominal distention, bloody stools, and pneumotosis intestinalis. Total parenteral nutrition (TPN) is an alternative to enteral feedings when gut absorption capacity and motility are severely disturbed in the postoperative period. Long-term complications are associated with the use of TPN in critically ill infants, including excessive CO_2 production and difficulty in weaning from mechanical ventilation, nosocomial infections, hepatic dysfunction, and hyperglycemia.

TABLE 11–3. An Approach to Feeding and Analgesia After Cardiac Surgery and Cardiopulmonary Bypass in Infants Based on Time Frame After Surgery and Clinical Condition

Postoperative Time Frame (hr)	Cardiorespiratory Status	Nutrition	Analgesia
<24	Unstable	5%–10% dextrose with electrolytes	1. Continuous IV fentanyl or sufentanil or 2. Epidural fentanyl and lidocaine
24–48	Unstable	TPN with or without continuous trophic NG feeding (1–2 ml/hr)	1. Continuous IV fentanyl or sufentanil or 2. Epidural fentanyl and lidocaine
24–48	Intubated and stable	Slowly advance continuous NG feeding	Wean continuous narcotic infusion
>48	Extubated and stable	Switch from continuous NG to bolus oral feeds	Discontinue narcotics
>48	Unstable (but no abdominal distention or GI hemorrhage	Advance continuous NG feeding and decrease TPN as tolerated	Switch from continuous fentanyl to intermittent morphine and diazepam

IV = intravenous; *TPN* = total parenteral nutrition; *NG* = nasogastric; *GI* = gastrointestinal.
Source: From Zuckerberg AL et al. Nutrition and metabolism in the critically ill child with heart disease. In: Nichols DG et al., eds. *Critical Heart Disease in Infants and Children.* St. Louis, MO: Mosby-Year Book, 1995.

A combination of TPN and small-volume enteral feedings (PO or NG) at 10 to 12 ml/kg/day is often utilized in neonates and low birth weight infants in an attempt to evaluate whether the infant is ready to transition to enteral feedings in the postoperative period (Table 11–3). The transpyloric route of enteral feedings can be utilized to decrease gastric distention, overcome delayed emptying, and minimize risk of aspiration if the infant is not able to feed by mouth. Reflux through the pylorus can be a complication of transpyloric and nasogastric feedings. Reflux issues can be medically treated with ranitidine and metoclopramide while nasogastric feedings are being used. The goal of transitioning the infant on TPN is to increase enteral feeds slowly while decreasing the TPN and maintaining a normal glucose.

Once on enteral feeds, the volume of feeds can be increased as tolerated, and the addition of supplementations or more calorie-rich formulas (24, 27, or 30 cal/oz) can be attempted if needed for catch-up growth. Many infants with CHD are fed via nasogastric tubes due to congestive heart failure and poor weight gain. These infants may require nasogastric feedings after surgical repair and assistance with oral stimulation to reintroduce feedings by mouth once they have recovered from surgery. Occasionally in infants with RV diastolic dysfunction, the lymphatic system is overwhelmed or direct surgical trauma to the thoracic duct leads to a chylothorax. This requires dietary or formula changes to low fat or no fat with the supplementation of intravenous lipids or oral medium-chain triglycerides (MCT oil). This is usually noted by the presentation of a new effusion on chest x-ray once formula or dietary fats are reintroduced after surgery. The fluid drained is usually milky or cloudy in color with a fluid triglyceride level greater than 110.

Conclusions

The postoperative care of neonates/infants after cardiac surgery is challenging for the multidisciplinary team. Initial stabilization after surgery requires intense observation and early interventions to combat the physiologic changes postoperatively. Knowledge of the postoperative anatomy/physiology, being able to anticipate sequelae, and initiating preventive interventions can only improve patient outcomes in this fragile population.

References

1. ANAND K, HANSEN D, HICKEY P. Hormonal-metabolic stress response in neonates undergoing cardiac surgery. *Anesthesiology* 1990;73:661–670.
2. BENZING G, FRANCIS P, KAPLAN S, et al. Glucose and insulin changes in infants and children undergoing hypothermic open heart surgery. *Am J Cardiol* 1983;52:133–136.
3. GUIGNARD J, TORRADO A, DA CUNHA O, et al. Glomerular filtration rate in the first 3 weeks of life. *J Pediatr* 1975;87:268–272.
4. LAHAV M, REGEV A, RA'ANANI P, et al. Intermittent administration of furosemide vs continuous preceded by a loading dose for congestive heart failure. *Chest* 1992;102:725–731.

5. SINGH NC, KISSOON N, AL MOFADA A, et al. Comparison of continuous versus intermittent furosemide administration in postoperative pediatric cardiac patients. *Crit Care Med* 1991;20:17–21.

6. LITTLE RC, LITTLE WC. Local control of peripheral circulation. In: *Physiology of the Heart and Circulation*. 4th ed. Chicago: Year Book Medical Publishers; 1989:267–283.

7. ANAND KJ, HICKEY PR. Halothane-morphine compared with high-dose sufentanil for anesthesia and postoperative analgesia in neonatal cardiac surgery. *N Engl J Med* 1992;326:1–9.

8. HICKEY PR, HANSEN DD, WESSEL DL, LANG P, JONAS RA, ELIXSON EM. Blunting of the stress response in the pulmonary circulation of infants by fentanyl. *Anesth Analg* 1985;64:1137–1142.

9. ANDREW M, PAES B, MILNER R, et al. Development of the human coagulation system in the full term infant. *Blood* 1987;70:165–172.

10. PETERS M, TEN CATE JW, KOO LH, BREEDERVELD C. Persistent antithrombin III deficiency: risk factor for thromboembolic complications in neonates small for gestational age. *J Pediatr* 1984;105:310–314.

11. ROSOVE MH, HOCKING WG, HARWIG SS, PERLOFF JK. Studies of beta-thromboglobulin, platelet factor 4, and fibrinopeptide A erythrocytosis due to cyanotic congenital heart disease. *Thromb Res* 1983;29:225–235.

12. CAMPBELL FW. The contribution of platelet dysfunction to postbypass bleeding. *J Cardiothorac Vasc Anesth* 1991;5:8–12.

13. MANNO CS, HEDBERG KW, KIM HC, et al. Comparison of the hemostatic effects of fresh whole blood, stored whole blood, and components after open heart surgery in children. *Blood* 1991;77:930–936.

14. ROYSTON D. High dose aprotinin therapy: a review of the first 5 years' experience. *J Cardiothorac Vasc Anesth* 1992;6:76–100.

15. ELLIOT MJ, ALLEN A. Aprotinin in paediatric cardiac surgery. *Perfusion* 1990;5(suppl):73–76.

16. HAKANSON E, RUTBERG H, JORFELDT L, MARTENSSON J. Effects of the extradural administration of morphine or bupivacaine on the metabolic response to upper abdominal surgery. *Br J Anaesth* 1985;57:394–399.

17. RUTBERG H, HAKANSON E, ANDERBERG B, JORFELDT L, MARTENSSON J, SCHILDT B. Effects of the extradural administration of morphine or bupivacaine on the endocrine response to upper abdominal surgery. *Br J Anaesth* 1984;56:233–238.

18. CUTHBERTSON DP. Second annual Jonathan E. Rhoads Lecture. The metabolic response to injury and its nutritional implications: retrospect and prospect. *J Parenter Enteral Nutr* 1979;3:108–129.

19. ELLIOT M, ALBERTI KGM. The hormonal and metabolic response to surgery and trauma. In Kleinberger G, ed. *New Aspects of Clinical Nutrition*. Basle: Karger; 1983:247–270.

20. ANAND KJ, SIPPELL WG, SCHOFIELD NM, AYNSLEY-GREEN A. Does halothane anesthesia decrease the metabolic and endocrine stress responses of newborn infants undergoing operation? *Br Med J (Clin Res Ed)* 1988;296:668–672.

21. BLUMER J. *A Practice Guide to Pediatric Intensive Care*. 3rd ed. St. Louis, MO: Mosby-Year Book; 1990.

22. ZUCKERBERG AL, et al. Nutrition and metabolism in the critically ill child with heart disease. In: Nichols DG et al., eds. *Critical Heart Disease in Infants and Children*. St. Louis, MO: Mosby-Year Book; 1995.

CHAPTER 12

Postoperative Arrhythmias

Anne M. Dubin, MD, and George Van Hare, MD

Introduction

Arrhythmias are commonly encountered in the postoperative cardiac patient and can be catastrophic. These patients start out with a predisposition to hemodynamic instability, owing largely to the effects of cardiopulmonary bypass. The early postoperative period following a palliative or definitive correction of a preexisting congenital heart defect often leads to a variety of problems including impairment of oxygenation and cardiac performance. Patients with certain cardiac defects are predisposed to the development of bradyarrhythmias and tachyarrhythmias due to associated electrophysiologic diagnoses.

Several congenital heart defects are commonly associated with an accessory pathway. These include Ebstein's anomaly of the tricuspid valve, L-transposition of the great arteries, and hypertrophic cardiomyopathy. However, the fact that accessory pathways are relatively common in the general population (0.30% prevalence, 1.6/1,000 live births) means that one will also see accessory pathways in the most common types of congenital heart disease, e.g., atrial septal defects (ASDs), ventricular septal defects (VSDs), and tetralogy of Fallot. In fact, as data from the Pediatric Radiofrequency Catheter Ablation Registry clearly show, accessory pathways are seen in all forms of congenital cardiac disease.[1]

Hemodynamic abnormalities commonly encountered in unrepaired patients may also predispose to arrhythmias. Patients with Ebstein's anomaly or other causes of severe tricuspid regurgitation may have atrial flutter, most likely due to right atrial wall stretch.[2] Likewise, patients with mitral stenosis may develop atrial fibrillation secondary to left atrial dilation. Finally, patients with left ventricular failure and those with pulmonary hypertension and/or suprasystemic right ventricular pressure may also have increased atrial pressures and may develop both atrial and ventricular arrhythmias.

Tachyarrhythmias

Sinus Tachycardia

The most common tachyarrhythmia seen in the immediate postoperative period is sinus tachycardia (Fig. 12–1). It may be difficult to distinguish sinus tachycardia from the various etiologies of tachyarrhythmias. A careful search for correctable causes of sinus tachycardia, including fever, dehydration, bleeding, pain, and anxiety, is important. One additional clue is the ventricular rate. For example, sinus rates above 250 beats per minute (bpm) are essentially not seen. Therefore, a tachyarrhythmia with a rate in excess of 250 bpm is not sinus tachycardia.

Junctional Ectopic Tachycardia

The rhythm that generates the most concern in the immediate postoperative period is junctional ectopic tachycardia (JET). The anatomic substrate for automatic JET is essentially unknown, but it is assumed to be due to a small focus of abnormal automaticity somewhere in the atrioventricular (AV) node or bundle of His. Experience with transcatheter ablation has suggested that the substrate is supraventricular, located adjacent to or within the compact AV node, since lesions created in the atrial septum have been successful in treating this arrhythmia.[3–6]

JET is most commonly encountered in the immediate postoperative period in children following cardiac surgery utilizing cardiopulmonary bypass, especially surgery involving the atrial and/or ventricular septum. Postoperative JET develops within several hours of discontinuation of bypass and may last for several days. If untreated, it is associated with a high mortality rate, as the high ventricular rate and AV dissociation may lead to hemodynamic decompensation.

JET is classically recognized as a narrow QRS tachycardia with AV dissociation and an atrial rate that is slower than

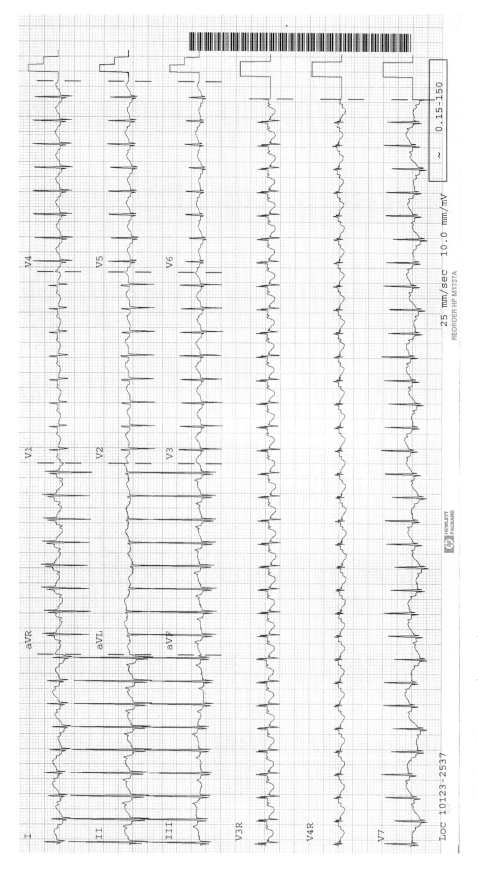

FIGURE 12–1.   Sinus tachycardia.

the ventricular rate (Fig. 12–2). The ectopic focus conducts down the His-Purkinje system giving the appearance of normal ventricular activation. Retrograde conduction from the junctional focus back to the atrium is usually absent. The atrium is activated by the normal sinus impulses at a much slower rate, leading to AV dissociation. This AV dissociation will allow for capture beats to be seen in the arrhythmia. Capture beats result from occasional antegrade conduction of a normal sinus impulse, causing the next QRS complex to occur slightly earlier than expected. Such capture beats, since they utilize the same His-Purkinje system as the junctional focus, will occur with an identical QRS morphology to that seen with the underlying JET. In some patients, 1:1 conduction from the junctional focus to the atrium is present: P waves will be superimposed on QRS complexes.

Atrioventricular Reentrant Tachycardial/Atrioventricular Nodal Reentrant Tachycardia

If a patient has a preexisting substrate for supraventricular tachycardia (SVT), such as the Wolff-Parkinson-White syndrome, which is not ablated preoperatively, incessant tachycardia may occur postoperatively. Atrioventricular reentrant tachycardia (AVRT) is also narrow complex, with rates usually between 200 and 300 bpm, depending on the age of the child (Fig. 12–3). AVRT can lead to significant hemodynamic instability and may be very difficult to treat.

Atrial Fibrillation and Atrial Flutter

Atrial fibrillation or flutter can also be seen in the immediate postoperative period. These arrhythmias may cause hemodynamic instability. Rapid AV conduction will lead to elevated ventricular rates, insufficient ventricular filling time, and the loss of the normal atrial contribution to stroke volume. Atrial fibrillation or flutter is strongly associated with reversible conditions such as postoperative pericarditis. Therefore, the occurrence of postoperative atrial fibrillation or flutter does not necessarily mandate long-term antiarrhythmic therapy.

Electrocardiographically, atrial fibrillation is recognized by the occurrence of a narrow-QRS tachycardia with irregular R-R intervals ("irregularly irregular") (Fig. 12–4). With slower ventricular rates, a chaotic baseline may be seen with no discernable P waves.

Atrial flutter may be difficult to recognize with rapid AV conduction. However, unlike atrial fibrillation, the regular atrial activity usually leads to regular R-R intervals such as one would observe with persistent 2:1 or 3:1 conduction (Fig. 12–5). With AV nodal blockade, the baseline will have a saw-toothed pattern (flutter waves).

In both atrial fibrillation and atrial flutter, atrial activity may be evaluated with the administration of adenosine.[7] It is unlikely that adenosine will terminate the arrhythmia, but it will provide a short episode of AV block during which

the atrial activity can be appreciated. An esophageal lead, or direct recording from epicardial atrial wires in the immediate postoperative period may also be helpful in determining atrial activity.

Ventricular Tachycardia

Ventricular arrhythmias are rare following cardiac surgery in children. Frequent premature ventricular contractions or the occurrence of ventricular tachycardia should raise the possibility of inadequate coronary perfusion, as occasionally seen after arterial switch procedures for transposition of the great vessels or tetralogy of Fallot repairs with inadvertent sacrifice of a major epicardial coronary artery. One may also observe ventricular ectopy in patients with very poor ventricular function following cardiopulmonary bypass, particularly in the setting of high-dose inotropes (e.g., isoproterenol, epinephrine). Finally, the use of halothane as an anesthetic agent has been associated with the occurrence of ventricular tachycardia and premature ventricular contractions.

Ventricular tachycardia may be recognized by the observation of a sustained tachycardia with abnormally wide QRS complexes (Fig. 12–6). The occurrence of AV dissociation with an atrial rate slower than the ventricular rate makes this diagnosis more likely. It should be noted, however, that ventriculoatrial conduction is often present in children, preventing the occurrence of AV dissociation.

Bradyarrhythmias

Atrioventricular Block

AV block is the bradyarrhythmia of most concern in the postoperative period. Cardiac surgery that involves the atrial or ventricular septum, particularly perimembranous VSD repairs, may lead to AV block resulting from damage to the bundle of His. Patients with certain types of heart defects are also predisposed to the development of AV block at surgery, as they are thought to have conducting systems that are more "fragile" than normal. These defects include complete AV canal and L-transposition of the great arteries. In the latter defect, also known as ventricular inversion or congenitally corrected transposition, there is a high rate of spontaneous complete AV block, even in the absence of cardiac surgery. Another mechanism of AV block is damage to the compact AV node on the atrial side of the AV junction. It is thought that traction or suction catheter damage to the compact AV node occurs, which leads to second- or third-degree AV block in the immediate postoperative period. In practice, for patients with second-degree AV block, it is important to differentiate between Wenckebach conduction (Mobitz type I) and non-Wenckebach conduction (Mobitz type II), since the former has a much better prognosis for recovery of conduction and will often be responsive to pharmacologic agents (e.g., atropine, catecholamines). It is usually true that

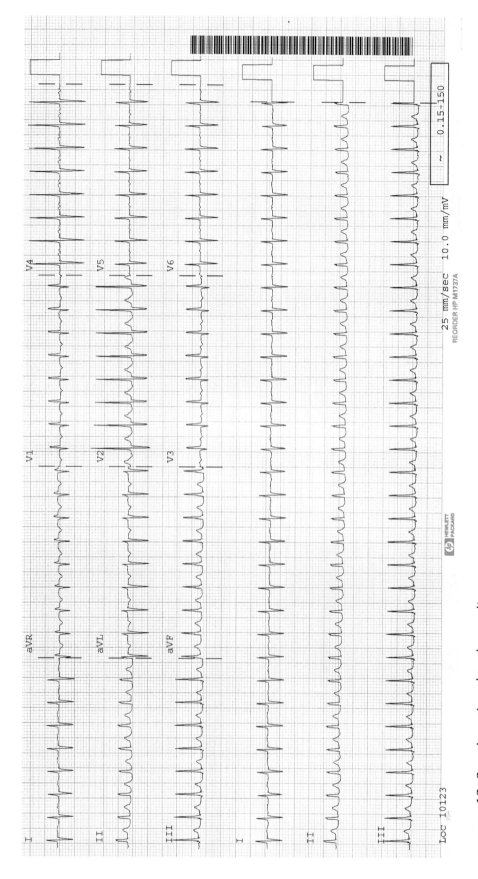

FIGURE 12–2. Junctional tachycardia.

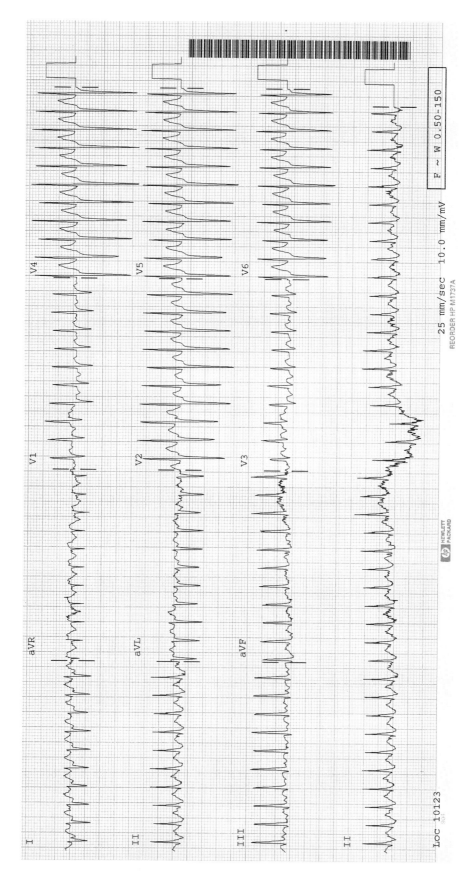

FIGURE 12–3. AV reentrant tachycardia.

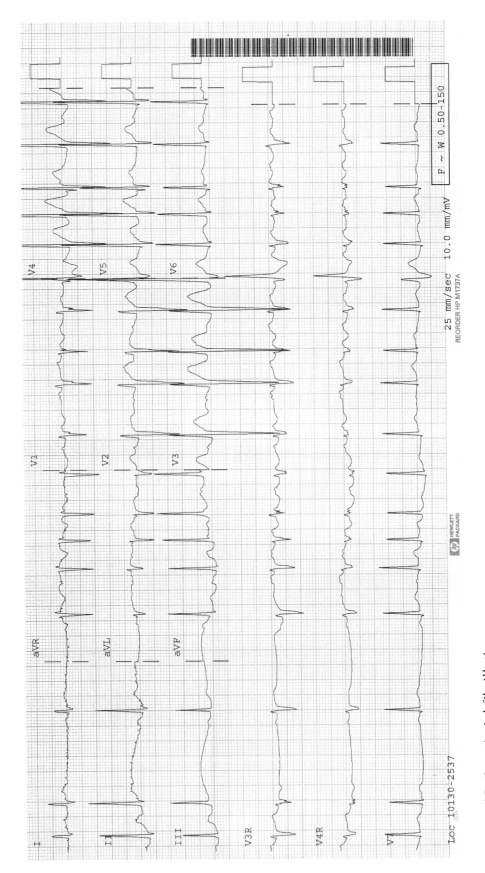

FIGURE 12–4. Atrial fibrillation.

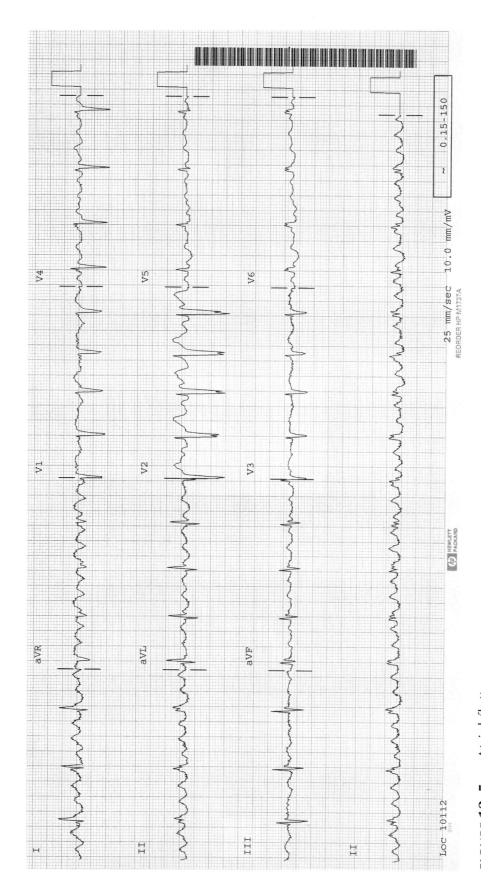

FIGURE 12–5. Atrial flutter.

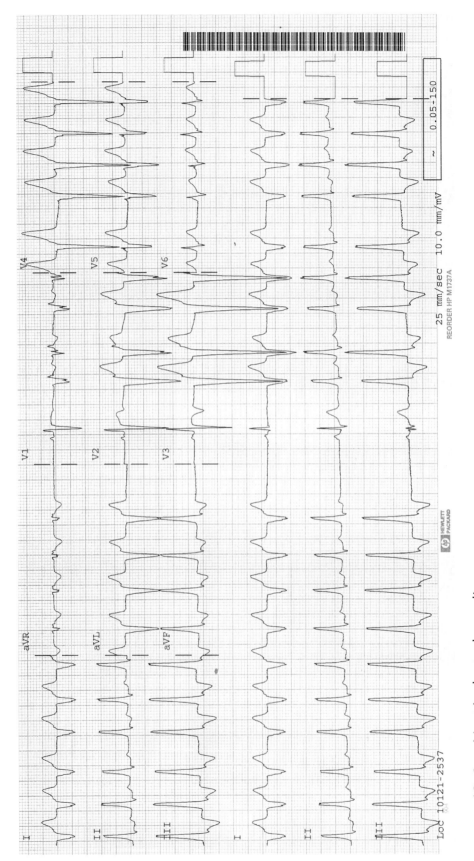

FIGURE 12–6.   Ventricular tachycardia.

Mobitz I conduction is most frequent in cases of injury to the compact AV node, whereas Mobitz II conduction is mainly seen with damage to the bundle of His and distal conducting system (Figs. 12–7 and 12–8).

Therapy

Direct-Current Cardioversion

Hemodynamically unstable patients who are known or suspected to be suffering from a reentrant tachycardia should undergo direct-current (DC) cardioversion as soon as possible. When such an arrhythmia is only suspected, a trial of cardioversion may allow for the firm diagnosis to be made. Automatic focus tachycardias and, of course, sinus tachycardia will not respond to cardioversion for longer than 1 or 2 seconds. Waiting and failing to perform cardioversion in a hemodynamically unstable patient may cause more harm than inappropriately attempting to cardiovert a patient without a reentrant tachycardia. Initially, cardioversion should always be attempted in a synchronized mode except if the rhythm is ventricular fibrillation. If the device cannot synchronize to the QRS complexes, cardioversion must proceed in an asynchronous mode. In this circumstance, there is some risk of delivering current on the vulnerable part of the T wave, which may precipitate ventricular fibrillation. The dose for routine DC cardioversion of tachycardias other than atrial or ventricular fibrillation is 1 to 2 J/kg. For atrial and ventricular fibrillation, initial attempts at 2 J/kg are reasonable; however, higher doses up to 6 J/kg may be required.

Medications

In both AV reentrant and AV nodal reentrant tachycardia, the most common forms of SVT, the AV node is part of the reentrant circuit. Therefore, pharmacologic agents that block the AV node generally comprise first-line therapy: digoxin, beta-blockers, and calcium channel blockers. In the immediate postoperative period, however, digoxin is not immediately effective, and beta-blockers and verapamil may precipitate hypotension due to their negative inotropic potential. Diltiazem, which has less negative inotropic potential than verapamil and can be titrated by continuous infusion, can be effective in this situation. Importantly, calcium channel blockers must never be used in small infants younger than 6 months, due to the propensity of verapamil to cause cardiac arrest in this age group.[8,9] One may also consider an esmolol infusion, as its action is short lived and can be stopped quickly. Other intravenous agents that may be effective include procainamide, which influences accessory pathway function, and intravenous amiodarone, which has a number of antiarrhythmic actions (see below).

For atrial fibrillation and atrial flutter with a rapid ventricular response, similar considerations apply. The initial goal is to slow AV conduction and thereby limit the ventricular rate, rather than to convert the rhythm; therefore an AV nodal blocking agent may be useful. Pharmacologic cardioversion is sometimes possible with procainamide or intravenous amiodarone; alternatively, these agents may potentiate subsequent DC cardioversion. It should be noted that class I antiarrhythmic agents (e.g., procainamide, quinidine) given to patients in atrial flutter may slow the atrial rate, which may, in turn, permit more rapid AV conduction and paradoxically increase the ventricular rate. Since this circumstance may lead to hemodynamic instability, patients receiving class I antiarrhythmic agents should also receive AV nodal blocking agents.

Most intravenous medications have been disappointing in the management of JET. Digoxin, propranolol, and procainamide are only occasionally effective. Intravenous propranolol and procainamide should be used cautiously in the immediate postoperative period because of their negative inotropic potential. Amiodarone, either orally or intravenously, is perhaps the most effective agent for the acute management of JET.[10–12] Bradycardia and asystole has occasionally been encountered with intravenous amiodarone loading; hence, backup ventricular pacing is advised when intravenous amiodarone is administered in the immediate postoperative period. Amiodarone has not been associated with significant decreases in ventricular function after the initial loading dose.

For the treatment of ventricular arrhythmias, lidocaine is the agent of first choice. When lidocaine is unsuccessful, one may consider the use of intravenous procainamide, which has proarrhythmic and negative inotropic effects. Intravenous amiodarone is also a reasonable choice for ventricular arrhythmias, particularly in patents who are critically ill, as it is extremely effective with minimal proarrhythmic effects. Amiodarone must be used with extreme care, however, as acute hypotension and/or bradycardia may be precipitated by the loading dose.

Cooling

In general, patients with JET who are febrile in the immediate postoperative period should be cooled to normothermia. Often, with mild cases of JET, this is all that is necessary. In more significant cases of JET, surface cooling to a central temperature of 34°C may be very effective in lowering tachycardia rates[13,14] and may permit atrial pacing (see below). Sedation or even paralysis may be necessary to permit this extent of cooling in older children. More aggressive surface cooling should be avoided, as this may result in significant elevations in systemic vascular resistance and detrimental hemodynamic consequences.

Radiofrequency Ablation

It would be quite rare to consider the use of radiofrequency (RF) ablation in the immediate postoperative period. However, should ablation be required as a last resort, standard

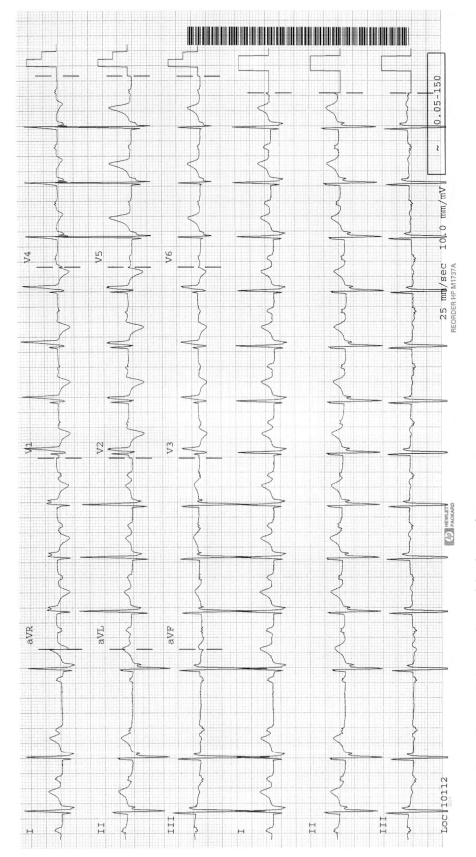

FIGURE 12–7. Second-degree heart block, Mobitz type I.

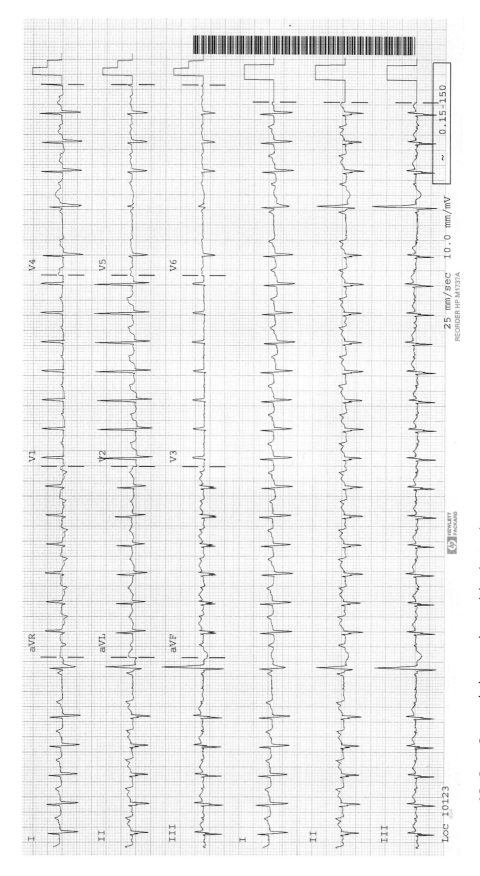

FIGURE 12–8. Second-degree heart block, Mobitz type II.

methods are employed, albeit at higher risk due to the likely hemodynamic instability in such patients. In the postoperative setting, RF ablation should be considered only as a last resort when other measures have failed.

Pacing

Multiple reports have demonstrated the effectiveness, safety, and convenience of atrial overdrive pacing for conversion of atrial flutter in adults and children by endocardial and transesophageal approaches.[15–17] Although sedation may be required, this technique can be performed at the bedside and is a means of providing atrial pacing if the patient manifests a bradyarrhythmia after conversion. Using intracardiac and transesophageal techniques in pediatric patients, Campbell et al.[17] successfully converted atrial flutter to sinus rhythm in 63% and 73% of patients, respectively. There were no complications using either technique.

Pacing may be considered in several circumstances of JET. First, pediatric patients most likely develop JET as a consequence of damage to the cardiac conducting system. As such, progression to complete AV block is possible and has been observed. Therefore, backup pacing with temporary epicardial pacing wires is reasonable. Second, the use of atrial pacing at a rate slightly above the JET rate may capture and overdrive the JET; the improvement in hemodynamics resulting from restoration of AV synchrony may permit discontinuation of catecholamines or substitution with a noncatecholamine inotrope (e.g., amrinone).

When treating bradyarrhythmias, pacing is the primary mode of therapy. Pharmacologic agents (e.g., atropine, isoproterenol) comprise short-term therapy for some forms of bradycardia, particularly sinus node dysfunction and Mobitz I (Wenckebach) second-degree AV block. However, transition to temporary and ultimately permanent pacing is often necessary. In most centers, temporary atrial and ventricular pacing wires are placed in patients undergoing intracardiac repairs that put them at risk for the development of AV block. These wires cannot be used in the long term, however, as patients usually develop exit block after 5 to 10 days. When patients develop persistent postoperative AV block, a permanent pacemaker is required. Permanent pacemakers may be placed by a transvenous approach for children of adequate size without anatomic obstructions or intracardiac shunting, or by an epicardial approach for infants of very small size or those with intracardiac shunting or lack of atrial and ventricular access (e.g., Fontan procedure). The timing for placement of a permanent pacing system is controversial. Certainly, AV block that persists beyond 10 days following surgery warrants pacemaker placement. An earlier decision to pace may well be appropriate based on other clinical factors, including the presence or absence of an underlying rhythm and the impression of the surgeon with respect to the degree of conducting system damage.

References

1. KUGLER JD, DANFORD DA, DEAL BI, et al. Radiofrequency catheter ablation for tachyarrhythmias in children and adolescents. *N Engl J Med* 1994;330:1481–1487.

2. SCHEIBLER GL, ADAMS P, ANDERSON RC, AMPLATZ K, LESTER RG. Clinical study of twenty three cases of Ebstein's anomaly of the tricuspid valve. *Circulation* 1959;19:165–187.

3. BHARATI S, MOSKOWITZ WB, SCHEINMAN M, ESTES NAD LEV M. Junctional tachycardias: anatomic substrate and its significance in ablative procedures. *J Am Coll Cardiol* 1991;18:179–186.

4. YOUNG ML, MEHTA MB, MARTINEZ RM, WOLFF GS, GELBAND H. Combined alphaadrenergic blockade and radiofrequency ablation to treat junctional ectopic tachycardia successfully without atrioventricular block. *Am J Cardiol* 1993;71:883–885.

5. VAN HARE GF, VELVIS H, LANGBERG II. Successful transcatheter ablation of congenital junctional ectopic tachycardia in a ten-month-old infant using radiofrequency energy. *PACE* 1990;13:730–735.

6. SCHEINMAN MM, GONZALEZ RP, COOPER MW, LESH MD, LEE RJ, EPSTEIN LM. Clinical and electrophysiologic features and role of catheter ablation techinques in adult patients with automatic atrioventricular junctional tachycardia. *Am J Cardiol* 1994;74:565–572.

7. CROSSON JE, ETHERIDGE SP, MILSTEIN S, HESSLEIN PS, DUNNIGAN A. Therapeutic and diagnostic utility of adenosine during tachycardia evaluation in children. *Am J Cardiol* 1994;74:155–160.

8. ABINADER E, BOROCHOWITZ Z, BERGER A. A hemodynamic complication of verapamil therapy in a neonate. *Helv Paediatr Acta* 1981;36:451–455.

9. GARSON A Jr. Medicolegal problems in the management of cardiac arrhythmias in children. *Pediatrics* 1987;79:84–88.

10. VILLAIN E, VETTER V, GARCIA IM, HERRE I, CIFARELLI A, GARSON AL. Evolving concepts in the management of congenital junctional ectopic tachycardia. A multicenter study. *Circulation* 1990;81:1544–1549.

11. PERRY IC, KNILANS TK, MARLOW D, DENFIELD SW, FENRICH AL, FRIEDMAN RA. Intravenous amiodarone for life-threatening tachyarrhythmias in children and young adults. *J Am Coll Cardiol* 1993;22:95–98.

12. RAJA P, HAWKER RE, CHAIKITPINYO A, et al. Amiodarone management of junctional ectopic tachycardia after cardiac surgery in children. *Br Heart J* 1994;72:261–265.

13. PFAMMATTER IP, PAUL T, ZIEMER G, KALLFELZ HC. Successful management of junctional tachycardia by hypothermia after cardiac operations in infants. *Ann Thorac Surg* 1995;60:556–560.

14. BASH SE, SHAH II, ALBERS WH, GEISS DM. Hypothermia

for the treatment of postsurgical greatly accelerated junctional ectopic tachycardia. *J Am Coll Cardiol* 1987;10:1095–1099.

15. BENSON DW, DUNNIGAN A, BENDITT DG, SCHNEIDER SP. Transesophageal cardiac pacing: history, application, technique. *Clin Prog Pacing Electrophysiol* 1984;2:360–372.

16. HENTHORN R, ROBERTS WS, KELLY K, LEIER CV. Conversion of atrial flutter: rapid atrial pacing as a bedside technique. *Pacing Clin Electrophysiol* 1980;3: 202–206.

17. CAMPBELL RM, DICK MD, JENKINS IM, et al. Atrial overdrive pacing for conversion of atrial flutter in children. *Pediatrics* 1985;75:730–736.

CHAPTER 13

Pediatric Cardiopulmonary Resuscitation

Frederick Tibayan, MD

Epidemiology

The precise etiology of cardiac arrest in children varies with the population studied. In contrast to adults, primary cardiac diseases are not the major cause of arrest. In a study of 119 outpatient pediatric arrests, sudden infant death accounted for 32% of cases, followed by drowning (22%) and respiratory disease (9%). Congenital heart disease and other cardiac causes made up only 7%. However, in studies including pediatric inpatients, cardiac diseases may constitute as much as 40% to 42% of the cardiac arrests.[1,2]

Pediatric arrests also differ from adult arrests in the initial rhythm. Adults usually present with the sudden onset of ventricular fibrillation, whereas in the majority of pediatric arrests, bradycardia degenerates into asystole.[3] Overall, asystolic arrests make up 68% to 78% of pulseless arrests in children. In contrast, ventricular fibrillation is found in 6% to 9% and pulseless electrical activity (PEA) in 4% to 10%.[1,4,5] The predominance of asystole has many explanations. First, the hypoxia and acidosis secondary to respiratory failure that underlies most pediatric arrests suppresses the atrioventricular (AV) node. This leads to bradycardia and eventually asystole. Second, there may be a higher incidence of unwitnessed arrests in children. These unwitnessed arrests have more time to degenerate into asystole. Congenital heart disease is a leading cause of ventricular arrhythmias, particularly ventricular fibrillation. Accordingly, in hospitals caring for children with unoperated and postoperative congenital heart abnormalities, ventricular fibrillation may be a more common presenting rhythm.

Once a child presents with pulseless arrest, the outcome is poor, and many survivors carry permanent neurologic deficits. In a metaanalysis of 734 cardiac arrests, overall survival was only 8.5%.[5] This contrasts with the 44% to 75% survival seen with pure respiratory arrests.[1,2] Most pediatric cardiac arrests represent prolonged respiratory arrests, so it is not surprising that cardiac arrest outcomes are worse. Analysis of survival by presenting rhythm suggests that patients with ventricular fibrillation may be a more treatable subgroup, with survival ranging from 17% to 26%. In contrast, only 2% to 4% of children with asystole survive to discharge.[6,7]

The higher overall mortality of pediatric cardiac arrests could arise from the greater frequency of asystole, which, in adults and children, is a lethal rhythm. O'Rourke[8] notes that most pediatric cardiac arrests arise from secondary causes and result from a preceding or precipitating period marked by disturbance of homeostasis. This is in contrast to the typical adult case, in which a primary cardiac disease (i.e., coronary artery disease) suddenly initiates the arrest. In the child, resuscitation must address the underlying cause and restore homeostasis in addition to treating the cardiac arrest. This complex backdrop to pediatric arrests contributes to poor survival rates.

Basic Life Support

Proper delivery of basic life support provides the foundation of any resuscitation. Particularly in the pediatric population, *prompt restoration of ventilation and oxygenation* is usually the only therapy needed. After determining responsiveness, the airway should be opened and rescue breathing initiated. If loss of central pulses is confirmed, chest compressions should be delivered to circulate blood to the vital organs. Basic life support should be continued until advanced life support can be begun. A complete discussion of basic life support techniques may be found in the guidelines published by the American Heart Association and the American Academy of Pediatrics.

Access

The timely establishment of reliable vascular access for the administration of fluid and resuscitative medications is fundamental to successful treatment of cardiopulmonary arrest.

The venous system is the preferred route for drug administration during resuscitation. Both central and peripheral infusion are acceptable, but if a peripheral vein is used, it should be flushed with at least 5 mL of saline to deliver the drug to the central circulation.

Intraosseous infusion is another safe and effective route of drug administration. When venous access is difficult to obtain in a small child, intraosseous (IO) access can be rapidly secured. It is considered equivalent to intravenous (IV) infusion, as the marrow is a large vascular compartment. Large volumes of fluid and virtually all medications may be infused by this route.

The endotracheal (ET) tube may be used for delivery of selected drugs, including epinephrine, atropine, naloxone, and lidocaine. Peak levels of some drugs such as epinephrine may be lower when delivered through the ET tube.[9] Therefore, the recommended dose for epinephrine is 10 times the IV/IO dose. Drugs delivered by this route should be diluted to a volume of 3 to 5 mL, instilled, and then flushed into the lower airways via suction catheter with 3 to 5 mL normal saline. Several positive pressure breaths should follow to aid in absorption of the drug.

Pharmacology

Epinephrine

Epinephrine is an endogenous catecholamine with alpha- and beta-adrenergic effects. Beta-adrenergic effects of epinephrine include increases in cardiac contractility, heart rate, oxygen requirements, and automaticity.[10] Intensity of ventricular fibrillation is also augmented, which may make the rhythm more amenable to electrical defibrillation.[11] Alpha-mediated vasoconstriction in dermal, renal, mucosal, and splanchnic vessels increases perfusion pressure to the brain and myocardium.[12] In treatment of cardiac arrest, the alpha-adrenergic vasoconstriction has been shown to be the most important pharmacological action of epinephrine. The resulting increase in aortic diastolic pressure is critical in a successful resuscitation.[13]

Indications   Because of the increased coronary and cerebral perfusion pressure associated with alpha-mediated vasoconstriction, epinephrine is indicated in essentially all forms of cardiac arrest, including asystole, pulseless ventricular tachycardia, ventricular fibrillation, and bradycardia, not responsive to adequate ventilation and oxygenation. In children with ventricular fibrillation, epinephrine may increase the vigor of fibrillation, making successful defibrillation more likely.[11]

Epinephrine infusion may also be indicated after restoration of spontaneous circulation. It may be used to support coronary perfusion, to augment systolic and diastolic blood pressure, or to increase cardiac inotropy and chronotropy.

Dosage   Recent animal data suggest that higher than previously recommended doses of epinephrine may result in greater coronary and cerebral perfusion pressure, as well as an increased rate of return to spontaneous circulation.[14] One clinical trial in the pediatric population showed improved survival and neurologic outcome using higher doses of epinephrine.[15] However, these results have not been supported by trials in adults.[16]

As the benefit of high-dose epinephrine is still controversial, the first IV or IO dose given for pulseless arrest remains **0.01 mg/kg,** or 0.1 mL/kg of the 1:10,000 solution. If the arrest persists, subsequent IV/IO doses may be increased to **0.1 mg/kg** (0.1 mL/kg of a 1:1000 solution). Epinephrine should be administered every 3 to 5 minutes during the resuscitation. Because epinephrine is now available in two different dilutions, special care must be taken to ensure that the correct dose is being given.

The tracheobronchial tree absorbs epinephrine. In studies of adults, ET administration resulted in blood levels one-tenth as high as with equal doses given IV.[9] Few data are available on ET administration in children. Nevertheless, extrapolating from the adult studies, the recommended ET dose is 10 times the IV dose, or 0.1 mg/kg. As with other drugs delivered through the ET tube, epinephrine should be diluted in 3 to 5 mL normal saline before instillation. Another method includes delivery of the drug through a suction catheter placed beyond the tip of the ET tube, followed by saline flush of 3 to 5 mL. Either way, several positive-pressure breaths should follow ET administration. Once IV or IO access is obtained, this should be used in favor of the ET route.

If epinephrine is given as an infusion, the predominant cardiovascular effects will depend on the dosage. At <0.3 μm/kg/min, beta-adrenergic effects predominate, whereas at larger doses, the alpha effects are more evident.

Adverse Effects   Epinephrine can lead to tachycardia and ectopy through its beta-adrenergic effects. Excessive vasocontriction can result in ischemia or necrosis of an extremity or the mesenteric or renal vascular beds. Tissue infiltration causes ischemia and ulceration. Finally, care must be taken that epinephrine is not mixed with sodium bicarbonate, as alkaline solutions inactivate catecholamines.

Atropine

Atropine is a belladonna alkaloid that blocks the muscarinic synapses of central and peripheral parasympathetic nerves. Its primary cardiovascular effects are to increase the rate of sinoatrial pacemakers and AV conduction. Atropine may also activate latent ectopic pacemakers. Atropine has little effect on contractility, systemic vascular resistance (SVR), or coronary perfusion pressure.[17]

Indications   Atropine is indicated in cases of symptomatic bradycardia (with or without AV block) that persists after adequate ventilation and oxygenation and administration of epinephrine.[18] In children, bradycardia usually results from hypoxemia. Thus, treatment must include support of ventilation and oxygenation prior to drug administration. Atropine is also used in the prevention or treatment of vagally induced bradycardia associated with intubation. Efficacy has not been demonstrated in cardiac arrest, but a vagolytic dose may be given to infants and children in cardiac arrest.

Dosage The recommended dose of atropine is **0.02 mg/kg,** with a minimum dose of 0.1 mg and a maximum single dose of 0.5 mg in a child and 1.0 mg in an adolescent. The dose may be repeated after 5 minutes, up to a maximum total dose of 1.0 mg in a child and 2.0 mg in an adolescent. At lower than recommended doses, paradoxical bradycardia may occur, due to central activation of vagal outflow.

Atropine may be given via the IO route at the same dosages as the IV route. Atropine is also absorbed by the tracheobronchial tree. No optimal ET dose is known, but administration of two to three times the IV dose is recommended. As with epinephrine, the drug should either be diluted in 3 to 5 mL saline or delivered beyond the tip of the tube via suction catheter and flushed with saline, followed by several positive pressure breaths.

Adverse Effects As noted previously, atropine may result in paradoxical bradycardia if given at low doses. More often, it can cause a sinus tachycardia, which is usually well tolerated in children. At very high doses, central nervous system effects, including hallucinations, delirium, and coma, have been observed. Use of atropine may block hypoxemia-induced bradycardia. Thus, continuous pulse oximetry should be used when giving atropine before intubation.

Adenosine

Adenosine is an endogenous purine used as the drug of choice in the treatment of supraventricular tachycardia (SVT). Adenosine leads to the activation of inhibitory G-proteins, which inhibit slow calcium channels and open potassium channels, causing hyperpolarization of pacemaker cells. The overall effect is to delay AV node conduction and slow the ventricular response to atrial tachycardia. Red blood cells quickly sequester adenosine, giving it a half-life of <10 seconds and a duration of action <2 minutes.

Indications Adenosine is the drug of choice for the treatment of SVT in the pediatric population.[19] It is effective in terminating SVT due to a reentrant pathway, the most common cause of SVT in children. Additionally, in tachycardia secondary to unrecognized atrial fibrillation or atrial flutter, transient slowing of the AV node may aid in the diagnosis of the underlying rhythm.

Dose Adenosine should first be given as a rapid IV bolus of **0.1 mg/kg** followed by a saline flush of 2 to 5 mL to avoid sequestration of the drug before reaching the heart. If no effect is observed, the dose may be doubled up to a maximum of 12 mg or 0.3 mg/kg.

Adenosine may be given IO, but not via the ET tube. Due to its short half-life, it is critical to administer it as fast as possible and follow the dose with a saline flush.

Adverse Effects The common side effects of adenosine are transient and generally resolve within a few minutes. The include chest pain, dyspnea, flushing, bradycardia, and irritability. Children with transplanted, denervated hearts are very sensitive to the effects of adenosine.[20] Adenosine should be used with caution and at lower doses in this population.

Lidocaine

Lidocaine is a class Ib antiarrhythmic with complex effects on myocardial electrical activity. First, by reducing the slope of phase 4 depolarization, it decreases automaticity and suppresses ventricular arrhythmias. Second, as a local anesthetic rapidly binding to and dissociating from sodium channels, lidocalne shortens the duration of phase 0 of the action potential.[21] Lidocaine has also been demonstrated to inhibit ventricular reentry.[22]

Indications Ventricular arrhythmias are uncommon in children with normal hearts, except in cases of drug intoxication or electrolyte imbalances. They are much more common in children with structural heart disease and myocarditis. In cases of metabolic disturbance or intoxication, the treatment is to address the underlying cause. If no such cause is identified or structural heart disease is suspected, lidocaine may be used in the treatment of wide complex tachycardia.[22] Lidocaine is also indicated as the first antiarrhythmic in a pulseless arrest that persists despite defibrillation and epinephrine.

Lidocaine delivered as an infusion may also be useful in the prevention or treatment of recurrent ventricular arrhythmias after resuscitation of infants and children. Finally, as it may suppress ectopy and raise the threshold for ventricular fibrillation, lidocaine infusion may be used prior to DC cardioversion in a stable patient provided that access and the drug are readily available.[23]

Dose When injected IV or IO, the recommended dose of lidocaine is **1 mg/kg.** Lidocaine may also be delivered via ET tube (also 1 mg/kg), with the drug diluted or flushed with 3 to 5 mL saline and followed by several positive pressure breaths.

Lidocaine infusion should be preceded by a loading dose of 1 mg/kg and then started at **20 to 50 μm/kg/min.** Note that higher serum concentrations (>6 μm/mL) are needed to suppress ventricular fibrillation than ectopy. However, as lidocaine is cleared by hepatic metabolism, children in low cardiac output states with decreased hepatic blood flow are more susceptible to lidocaine toxicity. In these cases, the infusion rate should be reduced to 20 μm/kg/min.

Adverse Effects   High serum levels of lidocaine may produce myocardial and circulatory depression. Central nervous system side effects, such as confusion, muscle twitching, and seizures, are also observed.

Calcium Chloride

Ionized calcium plays a central role in myocardial excitation-contraction coupling. In response to an influx of calcium, the sarcoplasmic reticulum releases intracellular calcium, which binds to troponin and tropomyosin. This interaction allows myosin and actin to form crossbridges and initiate contraction.

Calcium is also implicated in increasing ventricular contractility and automaticity in asystole. Conversely, hypocalcemia has been linked to impaired ventricular performance and attenuation of the hemodynamic response to catechol.[24]

The positive inotropic effects of calcium have been demonstrated in patients after cardiopulmonary bypass. Calcium chloride has previously been recommended for children in asystole or electromechanical dissociation. However, recent studies demonstrate that intracellular calcium accumulation may be deleterious for the cell. Calcium influx is the final common pathway for cell death and is a mediator for reperfusion injury. This injury is thought to occur through activation of intracellular enzymes such as nitric oxide synthase and phospholipases.[25] Moreover, studies demonstrate that calcium channel blockers increase myocardial blood flow and function after ischemia and also increase the threshold for ventricular fibrillation.[26] Finally, data have not supported improved outcome after using calcium in asystole or PEA.[27] These considerations resulted in new guidelines for the use of calcium therapy in pediatric arrest.[28]

Indications   The indications for calcium therapy are now limited to the following specific situations: hypocalcemia, hyperkalemia, hypermagnesemia, and calcium channel blocker overdose. Calcium is not recommended for either asystole or PEA.

Dose   Calcium chloride is prepared as a 10% solution, with 27.2 mg/mL elemental calcium. Calcium gluconate contains 9 mg/mL elemental calcium. Few data exist for the pediatric population, but the recommended dose derived from adult studies is **5 to 7 mg/kg** elemental calcium. This amounts to 0.2 to 0.25 mL/kg calcium chloride. The infusion should be given slowly to prevent bradycardia. In cases of documented hypocalcemia, the dose may be repeated as needed.

Adverse Effects   Calcium infused too quickly can cause bradycardia or asystole. Children on digoxin are especially susceptible to this effect. Locally, calcium can cause vein sclerosis or soft tissue necrosis in cases of infiltration.

Sodium Bicarbonate

The bicarbonate buffer system is critical in maintaining acid-base balance and in the excretion of volatile acids. Acidosis adversely affects the cardiopulmonary system in several ways: 1) diminishing spontaneous cardiac activity and contractility, 2) lowering the fibrillation threshold, 3) blunting the response to catechols in the heart and peripheral vessels, and 4) raising pulmonary vascular resistance. Overall, SVR and cardiac output can be reduced, with resulting hypotension. The increase in pulmonary vascular resistance can profoundly affect patients with significant right-to-left shunting, such as those with septal defects or patent ductus arteriosus.

Administration of bicarbonate promotes a reaction with hydrogen to form carbonic acid and eventually water and carbon dioxide:

$$H_2CO_3^- + H^+ \leftrightarrow H_2CO_3 \leftrightarrow H_2O + CO_2$$

The lungs then excrete the carbon dioxide, provided ventilation is adequate. This buffering capacity of bicarbonate minimizes the change in pH for a given amount of acid. Paradoxically, bicarbonate therapy may transiently worsen intracellular acidosis as the CO_2 produced diffuses into the cell more quickly than the hydrogen ions can egress.[28]

Indications   Bicarbonate therapy has failed to show benefit during CPR.[22,29] Consequently, indications for administration of sodium bicarbonate are limited. Definite indications are hyperkalemia and tricyclic antidepressant overdose, although bicarbonate may also be considered in prolonged arrests with documented severe acidosis. It must be stressed that the primary treatment of acidosis in pediatric arrest is the restoration of adequate ventilation and tissue perfusion.

Dose   The optimal dose of bicarbonate varies with every situation. The acuity and severity of acidosis dictates the proper amount of bicarbonate required. Initially, **1 mEq/kg IV/IO** may be tried. Further dosing may be based on arterial blood gases. However, these data may be misleading, as arterial blood gases tend to reflect ventilation rather than tissue perfusion and often do not correlate with venous gases in cardiac arrests.[30]

Sodium bicarbonate is available in two concentrations. Older infants and children may be given 8.4% sodium bicarbonate. The high osmolarity of this solution carries a greater risk of periventricular hemorrhage in neonates, who should be given 4.2% sodium bicarbonate.

Adverse Effects   After bicarbonate therapy, paradoxical intracellular acidosis may transiently occur through the rapid diffusion of CO_2 into the cells. Metabolic alkalosis may also occur if too much bicarbonate is given. Alkalosis causes leftward displacement of the oxyhemoglobin dissociation curve, decreasing delivery of oxygen to the tissues. It also lowers ionized calcium, forces an intracellular shift of potassium, and decreases the fibrillation threshold. Hypernatremia and hyperosmolarity can also follow bicarbonate therapy. Finally, bicarbonate causes the precipitation of calcium and slowly inactivates catechols, so the clinician must ensure that bicarbonate is not infused in the same line as these other medications.

Naloxone

Narcotic overdose depresses the central nervous system including the respiratory center. Narcosis may manifest through respiratory depression, sedation, or hypotension secondary to vasodilation or direct myocardial depression. Naloxone is a rapidly acting, essentially pure competitive narcotic receptor antagonist.[31]

Indications   Naloxone is the drug of choice for reversal of the respiratory and central nervous system effects of narcotic overdose.[32]

Dose   IV or endotracheal access is recommended in the treatment of narcotic overdose, but intramuscular and subcutaneous routes have also been used. The initial dose of naloxone in children under 5 years or 20 kg is **0.1 mg/kg IV.** For older or heavier children, 2 mg is standard. Naloxone has an onset of action of approximately 2 minutes. Naloxone is generally very safe, even at high doses, so the drug may be administered repeatedly at the same dose every 2 minutes until the desired effect is achieved. However, as the effect lasts only 45 minutes, the clinician should be vigilant for recurrent narcosis. In cases of prolonged narcosis, continuous infusion is a viable option beginning at 0.04 to 0.16 mg/kg/min and titrated to desired effect.

Adverse Effects   Naloxone is quite safe, even at high doses. However, abrupt reversal of opiate overdose may lead to tachycardia, nausea, vomiting, hypertension, tremulousness, seizure, and cardiac arrhythmias.[32]

Dopamine

Dopamine is an endogenous catechol and the precursor of norepinephrine. Dopamine's predominant actions vary with the dosage. At low doses (2 to 5 μm/kg/min), D_1 receptors in renal and splanchnic vascular beds cause dilation, increasing renal blood flow and thus glomerular filtration rate.[10] Between 5 and 10 μm/kg/min, beta-1 properties become apparent, mediated through direct receptor stimulation and promotion of norepinephrine release from cardiac sympathetic nerves. At this dose, augmentation of cardiac output occurs via increases in heart rate and contractility. Note that the indirect effects mediated by norepinephrine may be diminished or absent in infants, whose sympathetic innervation may be incomplete, and in patients after heart transplant. At higher doses (10 to 20 μm/kg/min),

alpha-1 mediated peripheral vasoconstriction causes increases in SVR.

Indications   Consider the use of dopamine in euvolemic patients with hypotension. Dopamine's beta-1 and alpha-1 properties make it especially useful in hypotensive, bradycardic patients, or in stabilization after cardiac arrest once a stable rhythm has been restored.

Dose   Dopamine is administered through an IV drip titrated to the desired response. If >20 μm/kg/min is required, another pressor agent should be added.

Adverse Effects   Dopamine's most serious side effects include tachycardia and other arrhythmias. Infiltration into the skin causes necrosis.

Dobutamine

Dobutamine, a synthetic analog of dopamine, has complex beta-1, beta-2, and alpha-1 agonist properties. Dobutamine does not have affinity for the dopaminergic receptor, and it does not facilitate norepinephrine release from cardiac sympathetic nerves. As alpha-mediated vasoconstriction is counterbalanced by beta-2 vasodilation, dobutamine's overall hemodynamic effects are increased cardiac output with a slight reduction in wedge pressure and SVR. Augmentation of cardiac output is largely due to improvement in stroke volume. In studies of the pediatric population, dobutamine increased contractility without significant change in heart rate except at high infusion rates.[33,34]

Indications   The hemodynamic profile of dobutamine makes useful in patients with poor cardiac output but high SVR, particularly in heart failure with pulmonary congestion. Dobutamine may be indicated after cardiac surgery in children with suspected or confirmed myocardial dysfunction.[30]

Dose   Dobutamine is delivered IV as a continuous drip. The initial dose is 2 μm/kg/min, titrated to effect. The smallest dose that obtains the desired response should be used.

Adverse Effects   Dobutamine can cause both hyper- and hypotension. Beta-1 stimulation can precipitate tachycardia and other dangerous arrhythmias. Tissue necrosis can result from extravasation.

Isoproterenol

Isoproternol is a synthetic catecholamine with essentially pure beta-agonist activity. Through its actions on the beta-1 receptor, isoproternol increases heart rate, speeds conduction through the AV node, and augments contractility. These actions tend to raise cardiac output as well as myocardial oxygen demand. Its actions on the beta-2 receptor, abundant in skeletal muscle, mediate peripheral vasodilation and thereby lower blood pressure.

Indications Since isoproterenol has a tendency to lower diastolic blood pressure and coronary perfusion, its utility in cardiac arrest is limited. Other pressor agents with alpha activity such as epinephrine may be preferable. However, isoproterenol's chronotropic effects make it indicated in the treatment of symptomatic bradycardia unresponsive to atropine and epinephrine.

Adverse Effects Because it can increase myocardial oxygen demand while decreasing coronary perfusion pressure, isoproterenol may precipitate cardiac ischemia. Isoproterenol may also result in dangerous tachyarrhythmias and hypokalemia.

Direct Current Defibrillation/Cardioversion

Defibrillation

Defibrillation aims to depolarize a critical mass of myocardium asynchronously, creating asystole, in the hope of allowing natural cardiac pacemakers to take over and restore organized contractions. Defibrillation is the only treatment for ventricular fibrillation and must be initiated without delay in patients with ventricular fibrillation. As fibrillating myocardium consumes the heart's energy stores, the chance of conversion to a natural rhythm diminishes with time, and conversion to asystole is more likely.[35]

The mass of myocardium depolarized is directly proportional to the amount of current delivered and indirectly proportional to the transthoracic impedance. A dose of **2 J/kg** is initially recommended, followed by second and third doses of 4 J/kg. After three unsuccessful attempts at defibrillation, chest compressions and ventilation with 100% oxygenation are resumed, and epinephrine administration is instituted. Defibrillation is repeated after each medication is given.

Synchronized Cardioversion

Synchronized cardioversion, like defibrillation, depolarizes the heart, creating a temporary asystole that allows the fastest pacemaker (usually the sinus node) to restore a viable rhythm. The shock is delivered during the QRS complex, avoiding the relative refractory period, to reduce the possibility of inducing ventricular fibrillation. Cardioversion is the treatment of choice for all supraventricular tachycardias (including atrial fibrillation and atrial flutter) associated with poor perfusion. Ideally, vascular access is secure, and the patient is intubated and sedated. However, cardioversion must not be delayed in an unstable patient.

Arrhythmias

Arrhythmias in infants and children may be dangerous as a result of decreased cardiac output or the tendency to deteriorate into a lethal arrhythmia. Cardiac output, and thus tissue perfusion, may be compromised by slow rates, fast rates that limit diastolic filling and stroke volume, or rates that generate no pulse at all. Thus, in the acute setting, arrhythmias may be grouped by pulse rate. Bradyarrhythmias are a common response to hypoxia in the pediatric population. The primary treatment is good ventilation and oxygenation through a secure airway. The tachyarrhythmias include sinus tachycardia, supraventricular tachycardia, and the less common atrial fibrillation and flutter. In the unstable patient with a tachyarrhythmia, immediate synchronized cardioversion is the treatment of choice. If no pulse is detected, the patient has a collapse rhythm or pulseless arrest. Pulseless ventricular tachycardia and ventricular fibrillation have a very different treatment protocol from asystole and PEA. Therefore the rhythm should be confirmed in more than one lead before instituting therapy for pulseless arrest.

Bradyarrhythmias

Bradycardia is defined as a heart rate <60 bpm. Bradycardia progressing to asystole is the most common presenting rhythm in pediatric cardiac arrest.[3] In most cases, the arrest is secondary to a respiratory process. This distinction is in stark contrast to adults, who typically have a primary cardiac arrest presenting as ventricular fibrillation. Children primarily augment cardiac output by increasing heart rate, and the development of bradycardia often signals imminent cardiopulmonary failure due to an inability to compensate for poor tissue perfusion. Etiologic factors include hypoxia, hypotension, and acidosis, which can depress AV node conduction and induce sinus bradycardia, sinus arrest with junctional or ventricular escape, or AV block. Excessive vagal tone (common after deep suctioning of the airway) and medications can also precipitate bradycardia. If the child is suffering from poor perfusion due to the bradycardia, exact diagnosis is usually not needed at the time, rather, treatment must be begun immediately after determining that the child has a slow heart rate and cardiopulmonary compromise.

Most pediatric arrests are primarily respiratory in origin. Children have a higher metabolic rate than adults, with greater oxygen consumption per kilogram body weight.[30] This predisposes them to hypoxemia and respiratory failure. Respiratory failure causes hypoxemia and acidosis, which slows AV conduction and leads to bradycardia.

The key intervention in the treatment of bradyarrhythmias in children is the establishment of **a secure airway** and adequate ventilation and oxygenation[22] (Fig. 13–1). Usually, these interventions are sufficient to restore normal sinus rhythm and achieve good survival and neurological outcome. Outcome is significantly worse if the bradycardia is allowed to deteriorate into asystole. Thus, the rapid delivery of 100% oxygen with effective ventilation cannot be overemphasized.

In cases of bradycardia that persists after effective oxygenation and ventilation, **epinephrine** may be used.

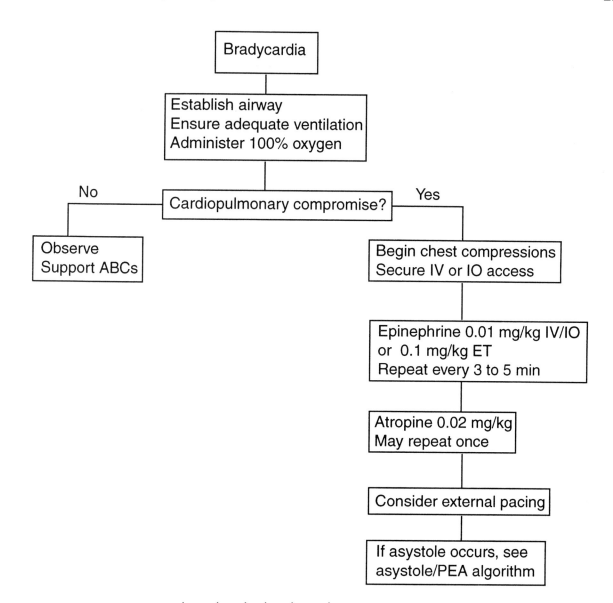

FIGURE 13–1. Treatment algorithm for bradycardia.

Epinephrine's alpha effects cause peripheral vasoconstriction, increasing coronary and cerebral perfusion. Beta stimulation increases contractility and heart rate through enhancement of both Sinoatrial node automaticity and conduction through the AV node. The initial IV dose is 0.01 mg/kg. Alternately, epinephrine can be given through the ET at 10 times the dose (0.1 mg/kg). Epinephrine should be repeated every 3 to 5 minutes until spontaneous circulation is restored.

Atropine may also be used for treatment of bradycardia. It is usually reserved for cases in which ventilation and oxygenation have been established and the patient has not responded to epinephrine. Vagolytic doses of atropine increase sinoatrial node automaticity and AV node conduction. It is especially useful in vagally mediated bradycardia during intubation and bradycardia with AV block. The dose

is 0.02 mg/kg, repeated in 5 minutes if necessary. A dose of at least 0.5 mg for a child and 1.0 mg for adolescents must be used to avoid paradoxical bradycardia.

Tachyarrhythmias

When the normal heart rate for the age of the child or infant is exceeded, a tachyarrhymia is present[36]. Tachyarrhythmias arise from three possible mechanisms: increased automaticity, reentry, and triggered activity. These arrhythmias can be classified according to width of the QRS complex, morphology of the P waves, and the relationship between the P waves and the QRS.[37]

Sinus Tachycardia Sinus tachycardia (ST) results from a higher than normal rate of sinoatrial node discharge. Usually, increased sympathetic output raises sinoatrial node

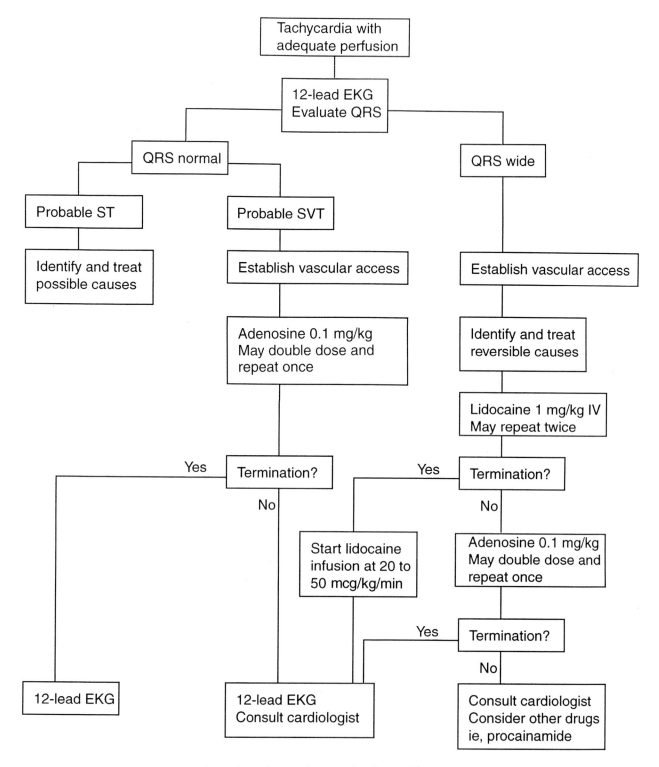

FIGURE 13–2. Treatment algorithm for tachyarrythmias with adequate perfusion.

automaticity. P waves and QRS complexes are normal, and each P wave is followed by a QRS. Infants and children augment their cardiac output primarily through increasing heart rate. Thus, ST should prompt a search for an underlying need for increased oxygen delivery, such as fever, sep-

sis, hypovolemia or hypoxia, intoxication, electrolyte imbalance, tamponade, or pneumothorax. Anxiety, pain, and a physiologic response to exercise may also cause ST. Treatment consists of addressing the cause of the tachycardia[22] (Fig. 13–2).

Supraventricular Tachycardia   SVT can often be distinguished from ST in several ways. First, it is often paroxysmal, with abrupt changes to and from normal sinus rhythm. Second, the P waves may be abnormal, or even absent. Third, SVT is usually faster than ST.[22] SVT originates from two mechanisms, reentry and automaticity. The more common mechanism is reentry, typically with an accessory pathway. In the case of Wolff-Parkinson-White syndrome, an accessory bypass tract connects the atria and ventricles. The ventricles are stimulated earlier by the impulse that was not delayed in the AV node. Thus the electrocardiogram shows a shorter PR interval and a widened QRS with a slurred upstroke (the delta wave). Increased automaticity also accounts for a small fraction of SVT.

Although most patients with SVT have normal heart structure (except for the possible bypass tract), several congenital heart defects are associated with SVT. Most notably, Ebstein's anomaly can be found in 10% to 25% of patients with WPW. Other abnormalities associated with Wolff-Parkinson-White syndrome include *L*-transposition of the great arteries, ventricular septal defect, and aortic stenosis.[38]

Treatment of SVT depends on the stability of the patient and the availability of vascular access (Fig. 13–2). In the pediatric patient in SVT with adequate perfusion, **adenosine** (0.1 mg/kg) is the treatment of choice. If unsuccessful, the dose may be doubled and repeated. Adenosine is highly effective in terminating SVT due to reentry with a bypass tract. In other cases of tachycardia, adenosine may slow the ventricular response enough to elucidate the diagnosis. Because of its very short onset of action, adenosine may also be used in the unstable child with readily available vascular access.

In hemodynamically unstable children without vascular access, **synchronized cardioversion** (0.5 to 1.0 J/kg) is recommended. In the ideal situation, patients should be intubated, oxygenated, and adequately ventilated with consideration given to sedation and analgesia prior to cardioversion. However, if shock is present, cardioversion should not be delayed.

Atrial Fibrillation and Atrial Flutter   Atrial flutter is a regular atrial tachycardia characterized by "sawtooth" P waves. Some evidence exists for automatic and triggered mechanisms, but most of the flutter is probably due to intra-atrial reentrant loops. Most newborns with atrial flutter have structurally normal hearts. In older children, this is not the case. In a study of 380 children from 12 months to 25 years of age, only 6% of patients had a normal heart, whereas almost 75% had previously undergone operations for congenital heart disease.[39,47] Abnormalities associated with a large right atrium, such as tricuspid atresia and Ebstein's anomaly, are most likely to lead to atrial flutter.

Atrial fibrillation is an irregular, chaotic rhythm with no discernible P waves. Multiple, reentrant atrial wave-fronts often reach a refractory AV node and then conduct impulses to the ventricles in an irregularly irregular pattern. This rhythm, rare in both infants and children, is almost always associated with an abnormal heart. In a retrospective study of 35 pediatric patients with atrial fibrillation, 17 had congenital heart disease (13 were postoperative patients), and only one had a normal heart.[40] Acutely, atrial fibrillation presents problems because the rapid ventricular rate may compromise stroke volume, leading to a drop in cardiac output. In turn, this may result in hypotension and pulmonary congestion.

The algorithm for treatment of atrial fibrillation or flutter in the hemodynamically unstable pediatric patient follows that of supraventricular tachycardias. Establishing access and giving medications to slow the ventricular rate should not delay synchronized cardioversion (0.5 to 1.0 J/kg) if the child has evidence of cardiovascular compromise. If the clinical condition permits, sedation and analgesia should be given prior to cardioversion.

Ventricular Tachycardia   Defined as three or more consecutive, rapid excitations originating from the ventricle, ventricular tachycardia can also be described as sustained (>30 seconds) or nonsustained, monomorphic or polymorphic. The QRS complex typically is wide, but (especially in infants) may appear almost normal. The rate may vary from just above normal for age to over 400 bpm.

The symptoms of ventricular tachycardia vary with the heart rate and the duration of the arrhythmia. Slower rates may be well tolerated, but very rapid ventricular tachycardia does not allow for diastolic filling and compromises cardiac output. Thus patients may present with hypotension and signs of poor perfusion, such as shortness of breath and loss of consciousness. The most feared consequence of ventricular tachycardia is deterioration into ventricular fibrillation, a rhythm incompatible with life.

The electrophysiologic mechanism of ventricular tachycardia is unclear. Evidence supports both automaticity and reentry hypotheses.[37] Ventricular tachycardia may be caused by hypoxemia, acidosis, electrolyte imbalances, temperature changes, trauma, and medications, particularly antiarrhythmics and tricyclic antidepressants. These etiologies may precipitate ventricular tachycardia in any child, but ventricular arrhythmias are exceedingly rare in infants and children with normal hearts. Two pediatric populations at markedly increased risk for developing ventricular arrhythmias are those with **long QT syndrome** and those with structural heart disease or myocarditis.

Long QT syndrome was initially characterized in 1957.[41] Since then, evidence has accumulated that this population has a tendency toward cardiac electrical instability and resulting syncope or sudden death. These patients usually but not always have a prolonged QT interval, and half display hereditary transmission. Congenital deafness may also be associated. The natural history of the long QT syndrome is not truly known, as most patients are symptomatic before presentation.[42]

Scarring in the ventricle may serve as a focus for arrhythmias. As surgical treatment for congenital heart disease became more common, clinicians noted a high incidence of sudden death in postoperative patients. This was especially true following repairs involving the ventricles, such as tetralogy of Fallot. In addition, children with unoperated congenital heart disease or otherwise structurally abnormal hearts are also at risk for ventricular arrhythmias. These cases are often associated with abnormal hemodynamics, such as aortic stenosis with a worsening transvalvar gradient.[43]

The treatment for ventricular tachycardia depends on the hemodynamic status of the patient (Fig. 13–3). In the stable patient with good perfusion, reversible causes may be sought, such as hypoxia, drug overdose, or electrolyte imbalance. Second, **lidocaine** (1 mg/kg IV) may be administered and repeated up to two times if necessary.[22] Conversion to sinus rhythm with lidocaine should prompt stabilization with a lidocaine drip of 20 to 50 μm/kg/min. In the presence of cardiopulmonary compromise, **synchronized cardioversion** 0.5 to 1.0 J/kg should be attempted and repeated as required. Lidocaine may be given as in the stable patient, but cardioversion must not be delayed. Again, underlying causes (i.e., hypothermia, profound acidosis, electrolyte imbalances) should be diagnosed and corrected. **Bretylium,** a class III antiarrhythmic, has not been proved effective in the pediatric population, but it may be used if cardioversion and lidocaine are unsuccessful.[28]

Ventricular Fibrillation and Pulseless Ventricular Tachycardia   In ventricular fibrillation, multiple waves of reentry result in disordered ventricular depolarizations with no cardiac output. The electrocardiogram appears irregular without discrete P, QRS, or T waves. This arrhythmia is rare in infants and children. In one study, ventricular fibrillation was the terminal rhythm in only 6% of patients under the age of 18 years.[3] However, in children with congenital heart disease, it is much more common. Like ventricular tachycardia, fibrillation is associated with structural heart disease and long QT syndrome. Hypoxia, hypothermia, electrolyte abnormalities, acidosis, and drug intoxication may rarely induce ventricular fibrillation in children with normal hearts. Unless rapidly treated, ventricular fibrillation is irreversible and incompatible with life.

The treatment for ventricular fibrillation and pulseless ventricular tachycardia is **immediate defibrillation**[22] (Fig. 13–4). Cardiopulmonary resuscitation should be delivered until the shocks are administered. The first recommended dose is 2 J/kg. If ventricular fibrillation persists, 4 J/kg should be delivered and repeated if necessary. Neither the administration of medication nor securing vascular access should delay defibrillation. Defibrillation attempts to depolarize the myocardium, giving spontaneous pacemakers an opportunity to regain control. If fibrillation continues too long, myocardial cells may not have sufficient energy stores to resume spontaneous activity.[44,45]

After three defibrillations, **epinephrine** (0.01 mg/kg IV/IO or 0.1 mg/kg ET) should be administered. Vasoconstriction due to alpha-1 stimulation raises aortic diastolic pressure and increases coronary and cerebral perfusion.[46] Epinephrine may also make ventricular fibrillation more amenable to successful defibrillation. In light of data that a higher dose may improve perfusion pressure and possibly contribute to a better neurologic outcome, epinephrine should be repeated every 3 to 5 minutes during resuscitation at 0.1 mg/kg regardless of route.

If arrhythmia persists despite epinephrine, **lidocaine** (1 mg/kg IV/IO) may be given to suppress ventricular reentry and ectopy. **Bretylium** (5 mg/kg IV first dose, 10 mg/kg second dose) may be considered, but it is unproved in infants and children. Sodium bicarbonate may be indicated in prolonged arrests with documented severe acidosis. Importantly, defibrillation at 4 J/kg should be repeated after each medication.

Asystole and Pulseless Electrical Activity   Asystole consists of the absence of electrical activity on electrocardiogram, associated with loss of central pulses. The rhythm should be confirmed in more than one lead before making the diagnosis. Since there is no depolarization, there is no ventricular contraction and no cardiac output. Asystole can present as an initial rhythm, or it may follow bradycardia or a ventricular arrhythmia. Hypoxia, hypothermia, hyper- and hypokalemia, drug intoxication, and profound acidosis can all cause asystole. These possible reversible causes should be promptly diagnosed and corrected[22] (Fig. 13–4). Once an airway is obtained with adequate oxygenation and ventilation, vascular access should be secured. **Epinephrine** to support coronary and cerebral perfusion should be administered and repeated every 3 to 5 minutes as in ventricular fibrillation (0.01 mg/kg IV/IO or 0.1 mg/kg ET first dose, 0.1 mg/kg second dose all routes). Defibrillation is not beneficial in asystole and may inhibit natural spontaneous cardiac pacemaker activity.

PEA is a term applied to organized activity on the electrocardiogram without detectable central pulses. Importantly, PEA is often secondary to treatable underlying causes that must be rapidly diagnosed to restore spontaneous circulation. Hypovolemia, hypoxia, hypothermia, hyperkalemia, tension pneumothorax, pulmonary embolism, tamponade, and drug intoxication may cause PEA. Treatment is similar to that of asystole. Again, defibrillation is not indicated, as organized electrical activity is already present. Support of blood pressure with epinephrine is appropriate. A fluid bolus of 10 to 20 ml/kg may be considered since hypovolemia is a common etiology of PEA.

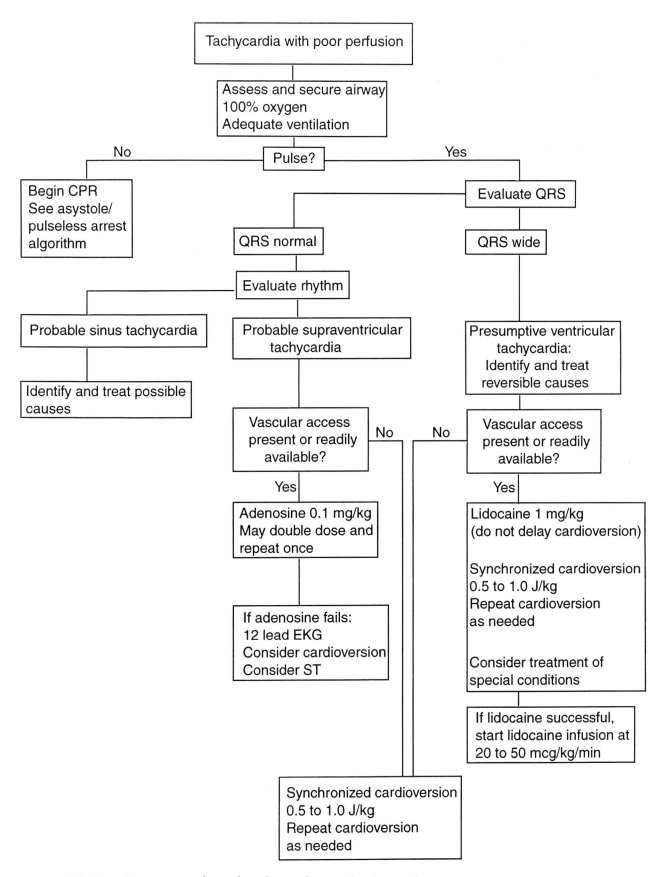

FIGURE 13–3. Treatment algorithm for tachyarrythmias with poor perfusion.

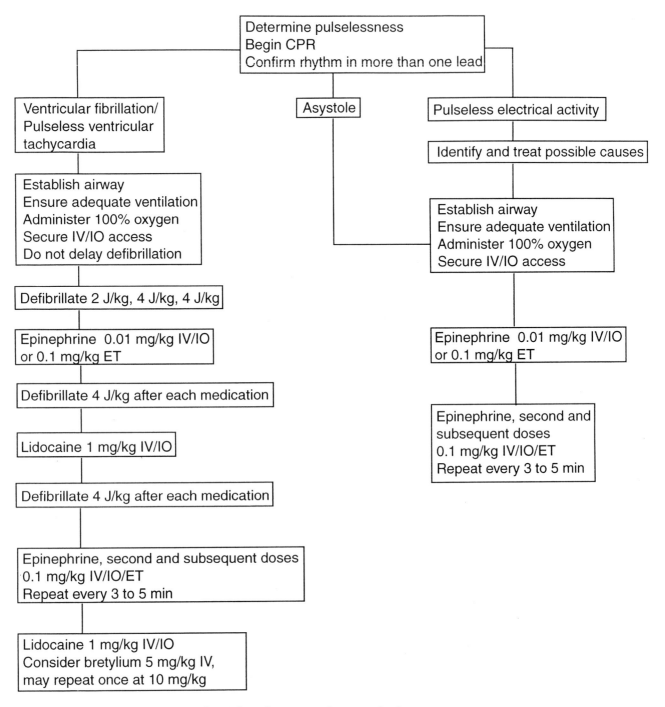

FIGURE 13–4.   Treatment algorithm for asystole or pulseless electrical activity.

Conclusions

Pediatric cardiac arrest is very different from adult cardiac arrests and is commonly the end result of a gradual decline from a secondary cause, such as respiratory failure. Support of airway, breathing, and circulation before deterioration into a collapse rhythm is critical, particularly in light of the poor outcome after cardiac arrest. Ventilation and

oxygenation are the primary treatments of bradycardia, with epinephrine and atropine being secondary measures to support blood pressure and stimulate automaticity and conduction. Synchronized cardioversion is the treatment of choice for unstable children with SVT. However, adenosine may be therapeutically and diagnostically useful in the patient with adequate perfusion. Children with congenital heart disease are at special risk for ventricular arrhythmias, which may have a better prognosis than other pulseless arrest rhythms. Ventricular fibrillation is first treated with electrical defibrillation, followed by epinephrine to improve cerebral and coronary blood flow. Asystole is the most lethal rhythm in children and adults. After securing adequate ventilation and oxygenation, reversible causes must be identified and treated. Epinephrine again serves to support the circulation. PEA is the least common collapse rhythm found in children, commonly resulting from reversible causes that must be diagnosed and treated. Although cardiac arrest carries a high mortality rate in the pediatric population, prompt and appropriate intervention may prove lifesaving.

References

1. GILLIS J, DICKSON D, RIEDER M, et al. Results of inpatient pediatric resuscitation. *Crit Care Med* 1986;14:469–471.

2. LEWIS JK, MINTER MG, ESHELMAN SJ, et al. Outcome of pediatric resuscitation. *Ann Emerg Med* 1983;12:297–299.

3. WALSH CR, KRONGRAD E. Terminal cardiac electrical activity in pediatric patients. *Am J Cardiol* 1983;51:557–561.

4. EISENBERG M, BERGNER L, HALLSTROM A. Epidemiology of cardiac arrest and resuscitation in children. *Ann Emerg Med* 1983;12:672–674.

5. HICKEY RW, COHEN DM, STRAUSBAUGH S, et al. Pediatric patients requiring CPR in the prehospital setting. *Ann Emerg Med* 1995;25:495–501.

6. COFFING CR, QUAN L, GRAVES JR, et al. Etiologies and outcomes of the pulseless, nonbreathing pediatric patient presenting with ventricular fibrillation. *Ann Emerg Med* 1992;21:1046. Abstract.

7. MOGAYZEL C, QUAN L, GRAVES JR, et al. Out-of-hospital ventricular fibrillation in children and adolescents: causes and outcomes. *Ann Emerg Med* 1995;25:484–491.

8. O'ROURKE PP. Outcome of children who are apneic and pulseless in the emergency room. *Crit Care Med* 1984;14:466–468.

9. RALSTON SH, TACKER WA, SHOWEN L, et al. Endotracheal versus intravenous epinephrine during electromechanical dissociation with CPR in dogs. *Ann Emerg Med* 1985;14:1044–1048.

10. HOFFMAN BB, LEFKOWITZ RJ. Catecholamines and sympathomimetic drugs. In: Gilman AG, Rall TW, Nies AS, Taylor P, eds. *The Pharmacologic Basis of Therapeutics*. 6th ed. New York: Pergamon Press; 1990:187–220.

11. OTTO CW, YAKAITIS RW. The role of epinephrine in CPR: a reappraisal. *Ann Emerg Med* 1984;13:840–843.

12. MICHAEL JR, GUERCI AD, KOEHLER RC, et al. Mechanisms by which epinephrine augments cerebral and myocardial perfusion during cardiopulmonary resuscitation in dogs. *Circulation* 1984;69:822–835.

13. OTTO CW, YAKAITIS RW, BLITT CD. The mechanism of action of epinephrine in resuscitation from asphyxial arrest. *Crit Care Med* 1981;9:321–324.

14. BROWN CG, WERMAN HA. Adrenergic agonist during cardiopulmonary resuscitation. *Resuscitation* 1990;19:1–16.

15. GOETTING MG, PARADIS NA. High-dose epinephrine improves outcome from pediatric cardiac arrest. *Ann Emerg Med* 1991;20:22–26.

16. BROWN CG, MARTIN DR, PEPE PE, et al. A comparison of standard-dose and high-dose epinephrine in cardiac arrest outside the hospital. *N Engl J Med* 1992;327:1051–1055.

17. BROWN JH. Atropine, scopolamine, and related antimuscarinic drugs. In Gilman AG, Rail TW, Nies AS, Taylor P, eds. *The Pharmacologic Basis of Therapeutics*. 6th ed. New York: Pergamon Press; 1990:187–220.

18. COON GA, CLINTON JE, RUIZ E. Use of atropine from brady-asytolic prehospital cardiac arrest. *Ann Emerg Med* 1981;10:462–467.

19. CLARKE B, TILL J, ROWLAND E, et al. Rapid and safe termination of supraventricular tachycardia in children by adenosine. *Lancet* 1987;1:299–301.

20. ELLENBOGEN KA, THAMES MD, DIMARCO JP, et al. Electrophysiological effects of adenosine in the transplanted human heart: evidence of supersensitivity. *Circulation* 1990;81:821–828.

21. BIGGER JT, HOFFMAN BF. Anti-arrhythmic drugs. In: Gilman AG, Rail TW, Nies AS, Taylor P, eds. *The Pharmacologic Basis of Therapeutics*. 6th ed. New York: Pergamon Press; 1990:840–873.

22. Cardiac rhythm disturbances. In: Chameides L, Hazinski MF, eds. *Pediatric Advanced Life Support*. Dallas, TX: American Heart Association; 1997:7-1 to 7-16.

23. SPEAR JF, MOORE EN, GERSTENBUTH G. Effect of lidocaine on the ventricular fibrillation threshold in the dog during acute ischemia and premature ventricular contractions. *Circulation* 1972;46:65–73.

24. SCHLEIEN CL, KULUZ JW. Cardiopulmonary resuscitation. In: Garson A, Bricker JT, Fisher DJ, Neish SR, eds. *The Science and Practice of Pediatric Cardiology*. 2nd ed. Baltimore, MD: Williams & Wilkins; 1998:2553–2583.

25. KATZ AM, REUTER H. Cellular calcium and cardiac cell death. *Am J Cardiol* 1979;44:188–190.

26. RESNEKOV L. Calcium antagonist drugs: myocardial preservation and reduced vulnerability to ventricular fibrillation during CPR. *Crit Care Med* 1981;9:360–361.

27. STUEVEN HA, THOMPSON B, APRAHAMIAN C, et al. The effectiveness of calcium chloride therapy in refractory electromechanical dissociation. *Ann Emerg Med* 1985;14:626–629.

28. Guidelines for cardiopulmonary resuscitation and emergency cardiac care: Emergency Cardiac Care Committee and Subcommittee, American Heart Association, VI: Pediatric advanced life support. *JAMA* 1992;268:2262–2274.

29. GAZMURI RJ, VON PLANTA M, WEIL MH, et al. Cardiac effects of cabon dioxide-consuming and carbon dioxide-generating buffers during cardiopulmonary resuscitation. *J Am Coll Cardiol* 1990;15:482–490.

30. USHAY HM, NOTTERMAN DA. Pharmacology of pediatric resuscitation. *Pediatr Clin North Am* 1997;44:207–233.

31. JAFFE J, MARTIN WR. Opiod analgesics and antagonists. In: Gilman AG, Rall TW, Nies AS, Taylor P, eds. *The

Pharmacologic Basis of Therapeutics. 6th ed. New York: Pergamon Press; 1990:494–525.

32. HANDAL KA, SHAUBEN JL, SALAMONE FR. Naloxone. *Ann Emerg Med* 1983;12:439–445.

33. MARTINEZ AM, PADBURY JF, THIO S. Dobutamine pharmacokinetics and cardiovascular responses in critically ill neonates. *Pediatrics* 1992;89:47–51.

34. BERG RA, PADBURY JL, DONNERSTEIN RL, et al. Dobutamine pharmacokinetics and pharmacodynamics in normal children and adolescents. *J Pharmacol Exp Ther* 1993;265:1232–1238.

35. Essentials of ACLS. In: Cummins RO, ed. *Advanced Cardiac Life Support.* Dallas, TX: American Heart Association;1997;1–33.

36. GILLETTE PC, GARSON A JR, PORTER CJ, et al. Dysrhythmias. In: Adams FH, Emmanouilides GC, Reimenschnieder TA, eds. *Moss' Heart Disease in Infants, Children, and Adolescents.* 4th ed. Baltimore, MD: Williams & Wilkins; 1989:725–741.

37. ARMSTRONG W, BOULIS N, ANTMAN E, et al. Mechanisms of cardiac arrhythmias. In: Lilly LS, ed. *Pathophysiology of Heart Disease.* Philadelphia: Lea & Febiger; 1993:180–193.

38. PERRY JC, GARSON A. Supraventricular tachycardia due to Wolff Parkinson White syndrome in children: early disappearance and late recurrence. *J Am Coll Cardiol* 1990;16:1215–1220.

39. PERRY JC. Supraventricular tachycardia. In: Garson A, Bricker JT, Fisher DJ, Neish SR, eds. *The Science and*

Practice of Pediatric Cardiology. 2nd ed. Baltimore, MD: Williams & Wilkins; 1998:2059–2101.

40. RADFORD DJ, IZUKAWA T. Atrial fibrillation in children. *Pediatrics* 1977;59:250:256.

41. JERVELL A, LANGE-NIELSEN F. Congenital deaf-mutism, functional heart disease with prolongation of the QT and sudden death. *Am Heart J* 1957;54:59–68.

42. CARBONI MP, GARSON A. Ventricular arrhythmias. In: Garson A, Bricker JT, Fisher DJ, Neish SR, eds. *The Science and Practice of Pediatric Cardiology.* 2nd ed. Baltimore, MD: Williams & Wilkins; 1998:2121–2168.

43. BERGER S, DHALA A, FRIEDBERG DZ. Sudden cardiac death in infants, children, and adolescents. *Pediatr Clin North Am* 1999;46:221–234.

44. NEUMAR RW, BROWN CG, ROBITAILLE PM, et al. Myocardial high energy phosphate metabolism during ventricular fibrillation with total circulatory arrest. *Resuscitation* 1990;19:199–226.

45. KERN KB, GAREWAL HS, SANDERS AB, et al. Depletion of myocardial adenosine triphosphate during prolonged untreated ventricular fibrillation: effect on defibrillation success. *Resuscitation* 1990;20:221–229.

46. SANDERS A, EWY G, TAFT T. Prognostic and therapeutic importance of the aortic diastolic pressure in resuscitation from cardiac arrest. *Crit Care Med* 1984;12:871–878.

47. GARSON A, et al. Atrial flutter in the young: a collaborative study of 380 cases. *J Am Coll Cardiol* 1985;6:871–878.

Index

Page numbers followed by an "*f*" indicate figures; numbers followed by a "*t*" indicate tables.

ISBN 0-8385-1542-8
90000
9 780838 515426
REITZ/CONGENTIAL CARDIAC SURG